T0188978

The complete four-volume set consists of

1   Functional Anatomy
    of Craniofacial Arteries

2   Endovascular Treatment
    of Craniofacial Lesions

3   Functional Vascular Anatomy of Brain,
    Spinal Cord and Spine

4   Endovascular Treatment of Brain,
    Spinal Cord and Spine Lesions

P. Lasjaunias   A. Berenstein

Surgical Neuroangiography

2 Endovascular Treatment of Craniofacial Lesions

With 244 Figures in 648 Separate Illustrations

Springer-Verlag
Berlin Heidelberg New York
London Paris Tokyo

PIERRE LASJAUNIAS, M.D., Ph.D.
Chef de travaux d'Anatomie, Professor of Radiology (Adj.) NYU
Service de Radiologie, Hôpital de Bicêtre,
Université Paris XI, 78 Rue du Général Leclerc,
94 275 Le Kremlin Bicêtre, France, and·

Department of Radiology, Toronto Western Hospital,
399 Bathurst Street,
M5T 2S8 Toronto, Ont., Canada

ALEJANDRO BERENSTEIN, M.D.
Professor of Radiology, Director of Surgical Neuroangiography Service
New York University and Bellevue, Medical Center, 560 First Avenue,
New York, NY 10016, USA

ISBN 978-3-642-71190-9   ISBN 978-3-642-71188-6 (eBook)
DOI 10.1007/978-3-642-71188-6

Library of Congress Cataloging-in-Publication Data. Lasjaunias, Pierre L. Surgical neuroangiography.
Includes bibliographies and indexes. Contents: v. 1. Functional anatomy of craniofacial arteries–v. 2.
Endovascular treatment of craniofacial lesions. 1. Nervous system–Blood-vessels–Radiography. 2. Nervous system–Blood-vessels–Surgery. 3. Angiography. I. Berenstein, Alejandro, 1947- II. Title. [DNLM:
1. Angiography. 2. Neuroradiography. WL 141 L344s] RD594.2.L37   1987   617'.4807572   86-26028

© Springer-Verlag Berlin Heidelberg 1987
Softcover reprint of the hardcover 1st edition 1987

Reproduction of the figures: Gustav Dreher GmbH, D-7000 Stuttgart

2127/3130-543210

To Pascale, Josée, Estelle, Erica, Vanessa, and Aude,

and to the teams of vascular technicians and nurses of both Bicêtre and New York University for their invaluable assistance.

Preface

Embolization has been performed in many European countries and in North America for over 20 years and is now beginning to gain acceptance in other countries. At first, experience with these techniques was shared in the form of individual case reports; today some centers have treated enough patients to be able to transform this anecdotal material into more concrete data. For the last 10 of these 20 years, the two of us have been deeply involved, encouraged, and stimulated by the interest created by the few pioneers in endovascular techniques.

In 1978, when we first met, our discussion on embolization could have been summarized as disagreement. It soon became obvious that these differences were primarily related to our different individual backgrounds. One of us having a strong orientation toward anatomy, and the other toward technique. We realized that these apparently opposing approaches complement each other and decided to combine them to our mutual benefit. This collaboration has matured into the search for improvements in patient care and for the safest, most reliable, and most responsible manner of treatment.

The goal of these volumes is to share what we feel useful to the performance of endovascular surgery. Vascular lesions and tumors constitute the traditional targets of embolization. Following advances in knowledge and in materials, proximal arterial endoluminal occlusion has been succeeded by the ability to produce an effect at the cellular level by means of microemboli and cytotoxic agents. The technical challenge to preserve as much as possible of the healthy tissue has led to superselectivity in the embolization of brain vessels and fourth divisions of the external carotid system. Miniaturization of devices allows us to use all our tools in newborns and infants without femoral arterial damage. The possibility of further enhancing the selectivity of delivery system placement by selective recognition of the target will create further applications of surgical neuroangiography. The development of rational protocols for specific lesions and territories, as well as guaranteed reliability and safety constitute the other objectives in the maturation of this specialty.

Embolizer, interventional neuroradiologist, surgical neuroradiologist, and neuroangiographer are the most commonly used names for the radiologists or surgeons performing embolization in lesions of the head, neck, brain, and spine. Their search for an identity may appear futile; however, it constitutes a strong psychological lever against medical bureaucracy, which often unfortunately constitutes a factor limiting innovation. The current use of "interventional" in connection with neuroradiology is too restrictive. It focuses attention on the technical aspect of our work and its imaging support. Pejorative names, such as "embolizers of pictures", enhance this feeling even more. Such a name may also convey to the public and patients the notion of an innocuous treatment. This notion is entirely untrue. As embolization techniques have become more efficacious, they have also become more aggressive and invasive. Poorly performed, they have the same potential to do harm as a poorly conceived or executed surgical maneuver. Consequently, it is imperative that operators have a sound background in functional neuroanatomy and clinical evaluation, as well as adequate technical training.

For this reason we are introducing the term "surgical neuroangiography" in the context of endovascular approaches. The adjective "surgical" refers to the use of hands and tools in treatment, and therefore better describes both our procedures and the additional clinical competence that should be acquired by the conventional neuroradiologist. The title "neuroradiologic surgery" would put a different emphasis on the link between the surgical and neuroradiological communities. Although we do not perform open surgery in a conventional sense, our treatments (therapeutic neuroradiology) or our interventions (interventional neuroradiology) require competence in certain clinical areas in addition to the actual technical skill, for example, outpatient consultation, hospital care, postoperative care and follow-up, and seminars with referring and related specialties.

Is there anything radiological in surgical neuroangiography? The angiosuite, our most expensive tool, is only a tool, and like the neurosurgical operating theaters, it can be used by others and for other purposes. Thus, concepts in surgical neuroangiography should be derived from clinical content and not from the technical surroundings. Even the angiosuite may not remain a link with radiology since ultrasound, CT, and MRI already provide much the same information as intravenous digital angiography. This type of "global angiography" will soon disappear as a diagnostic examination, leaving the angiosuite to be used almost exclusively for sophisticated invasive (surgical) measures for pretherapeutic or therapeutic purposes.

What is the persisting radiological element in surgical neuroangiography? What remains is the capability of using an image of existing conditions to make decisions and of performing therapeutic interventions without direct visual control. Stereotaxic neurosurgery uses precisely the same concept, and therefore constitutes the closest link with traditional neurosurgery.

Should we be "neurosurgeons"? We do not think so, since surgical training has to achieve specific clinical and technical goals during a difficult training program. However, there is definitely an overlap between our knowledge and that of neurosurgeons. Ideally, academic training should incorporate a common trunk, gathering all future neuroscience specialists where surgical neuroangiography and neurological surgery share certain problems. An example of such problems are the types of complications that can be encountered. Firstly, complications may be related to treatment in a general sense and correspond to the topography of the lesion and the nearness of fragile tissues (for neurological surgery) or sensitive territories (for the surgical neuroangiography). Such complications represent a real therapeutic risk which can (and should) be explained to patients in advance. Their diminution over time is due to improvements in endovascular techniques and in the selection of patients; differences in results can be attributed to the human character of surgical neuroangiographic techniques in general, and to the difference between proper and excellent patient care. Secondly, complications may be due to technical mistakes or incorrect intraoperative decisions; these represent the difference between proper and inadequate patient care. Their constant decrease in frequency is an expression of the success of modern training. Their persistence in many places emphasizes the need for individual operators to update their knowledge and skills.

We hope that these volumes will be a useful tool for those involved in surgical neuroangiography. However, one should not believe that a specifically designed instrument may compensate for insufficient training.

Surgical neuroangiography is a difficult specialty for those who choose to learn it now, and a gratifying one for those who are fortunate enough to practice it full time. The development of cytotoxic agents, techniques for the treatment of aneurysms, endovascular prostheses, and the use of lasers and angioscopes are a few of the fascinating aspects which will influence the future of the endovascular approach.

June 1987   P. Lasjaunias and A. Berenstein

Acknowledgements

We would like to acknowledge the following for their help in providing illustrative pictures: I. S. Choi, A. Roche, G. Scialfa, and K. Terbrugge.

We also wish to thank P. Burrows, J. Escridge, B. Willinsky, and J. Dion for their language editing assistance.

We are particularly grateful to C. Vachon for her help in producing the original drawings for this volume, and to D. Laclef, A. Arce, H. Helners, A. Jaladoni, and J. Scott for their photographic and secretarial assistance.

Contents

Chapter 10
**Craniofacial Hemangiomas, Vascular Malformations and
Angiomatosis: Specific Aspects**   341

CHAPTER 1

Technical Aspects of Surgical Neuroangiography

I. Introduction

Therapeutic endovascular embolization refers to the ability to occlude a pathologic territory by the introduction of embolic or chemotherapeutic agents with the goal of producing devascularization of that territory sparing normal areas.

A multitude of catheter systems, guidewires, embolic agents, and drugs have been used for a variety of indications and purposes. We believe that no single delivery system or embolic agent fulfills all needs in every case.

The purpose of this section is to express our rationale for our recommendations. This in no way means that the tools we do not use are of no value, but we believe that the ones that we have chosen best fulfill our needs in the management of our patients at present.

We would like to emphasize that the tools available cannot replace proper training nor will technical solutions replace proper knowledge of the vascular anatomy, including collateral circulation and anastomotic pathways between the various territories or between the extracerebral and intracerebral circulation. Proper understanding of functional vascular anatomy may permit the surgical neuroangiographist to compensate for any or all of the limitations of our present technology.

II. Patient Preparation

As our specialty evolves our responsibility in the management of our patients increases; a thorough discussion with the patients and their relatives is our responsibility. A patient that understands what is being done to him or her will be best prepared.

Preoperative Medications

Preoperative medications are usually not needed. Although in our early experience we used prophylactic antibiotics and corticosteroids (Berenstein, 1979), in the last six years we have stopped using these routinely aside from those needed for anesthesia or those needed for other medical conditions.

A Foley urinary catheter is placed, systematically (for one of us, AB). This permits an accurate measurement of output and will prevent patient discomfort and restlessness during the latter part of the procedure when the critical part of the embolization is being performed. In addition, narcotics for neuroleptic analgesia can cause bladder distention and retention.

III. Anesthesia of Embolization

Various types of anesthesia can be used during interventional neuro-radiological procedures in the head and neck.

1. General Anesthesia

General anesthesia is used in pediatric cases, cases requiring ethanol, an extremely painful injection, or when careful neurological assessment is not mandatory. One of us (P. L.) routinely uses general anesthesia except when carotid/vertebral occlusion will be done, or where general anesthesia is contraindicated.

The type of anesthesia used is primarily a decision of the anesthesiologist and may be modified in individual situations when specific monitoring is to be used. If using somatosensory evoked potential monitoring for spinal cord, brainstem auditory or visual cortex function (Berenstein, 1984), neuroleptic drugs are used as most of the anesthetic gases alter the evoked potentials.

Nitrous oxide (NO_2) is not used during general anesthesia in view of its risk of air expansion. If an air bubble is accidentally introduced into the circulation, nitrous oxide will expand the bubble with the risk of occluding an important vessel.

In patients with cardiac problems or very high flow fistulas (neonates and infants) where an increase in the total blood volume exists or when hypotension (primarily for brain lesions) is to be used, it may be advantageous to place an arterial line. A central venous line is not needed unless a major cerebral artery will be occluded because fluids and/or volume expanders and/or hypertensive drugs may be needed to maintain proper cerebral perfusion. If medical management of blood pressure is needed both arterial and central venous lines will be kept in the postembolization period until the patient is stable. If no medical management of blood pressure is needed the arterial line is removed at the end of the procedure but the central line is kept for 24 hours.

2. Neuroleptic Analgesia

Neuroleptic analgesia is most useful for surgical neuroangiographic procedures. It permits easy neurological monitoring throughout the procedure and at the same time gives both analgesia and sedation. It is used even in young patients, and carries less risk than general anesthesia in the older or medically compromised patient. Disadvantages of neuroleptic analgesia are: respiratory depression or airway compromise, which can usually be avoided by keeping the patient lighter, and the nausea that narcotics produce, which can be avoided by the addition of Droperidol.

The neuroleptic combination to be used is the choice of the anesthesiologist. In our experience, the best results are usually obtained with Fentanyl, an opiate derivative (0.002 mg/kg body weight) as the analgesic and Droperidol (a hypnotic 0.1 mg/kg body weight) as the sedative. The dose will vary as to the patient's weight and length of the procedure. As an alternative Demerol or morphine and Valium are used in combination.

In patients with lesions near the airway where the risks of swelling can produce obstruction, endotracheal intubation and general anesthesia are preferred. Nasogastric tube is placed in lesions that may compromise the alimentary pathway when direct ethanol embolization is used.

3. Tracheostomy

Prophylactic tracheostomy may be required where lesions at or near the airway are treated, especially if multiple procedures or surgery is foreseen.

4. Local Anesthesia

When neuroleptic anesthesia is used a long lasting local anesthetic such as Marcaine (bupivocaine hydrochloride) 0.25% is recommended to avoid the need for reinfiltration during the procedure. On occasions, the femoral nerve can be anesthetized and this will produce a motor and sensory monoplegia that will clear completely in 12–15 hours and should not be mistaken for a PNS complication.

IV. Puncture Sites

The conventional Seldinger technique is used in all of our procedures including infants and newborns. Distal pulses in the popliteal and foot area are marked prior to puncture for further reference primarily in children. If during the procedure the pulse is lost, one may inject intra-arterial vasodilators such as 40 mgr of cardiac lidocaine (without preservatives or epinephrine) through the side arm of the introducer sheath (Fig. 1.1). If every attempt to do a percutaneous puncture fails, induced hypertension with medication may be of assistance. Occasionally, one may have to resort to surgical exposure of the artery. A purse string arteriotomy with a 6–0 or smaller monofilament suture will permit repair of the arteriotomy at the end of the procedure, preserving flow through the artery.

Percutaneous Seldinger puncture may not be possible after a previous distal ligation of the external carotid artery, and surgical exposure or preferably end to side reanastomosis by an experienced vascular surgeon may be needed (Fig. 1.2). A period of 3 weeks is recommended to permit healing of the anastomosis. The advantage of reconstructive reanastomosis is that the femoral approach can be used.

Introducer Sheath

Various types of introducer sheaths are commercially available (Fig. 1.1). In general, the purposes of introducer sheaths are to

1. Permit easy exchange of catheters of the same or smaller diameters
2. Permit the use of smaller catheters without retrograde bleeding, thanks to their hemostatic valve.
3. Permit exchange of an occluded catheter without loosing access to the vascular system.

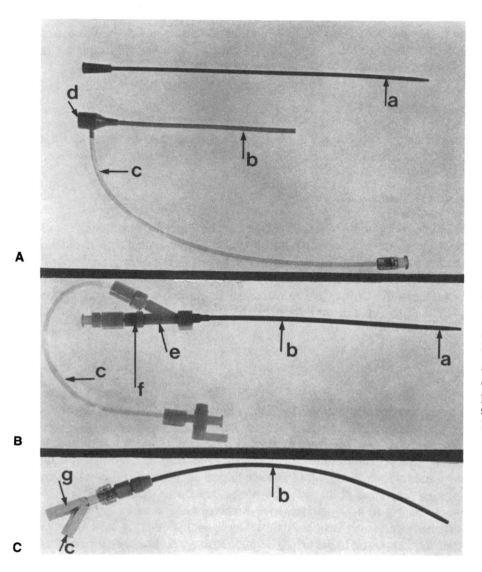

Fig. 1.1 A-C. Introducer sheaths at the arteriotomy site. **A** Cordis Model: Following percutaneous puncturing of the artery, the teflon dilator *(a)* is passed over the guidewire, followed by the thin walled teflon sheath *(b)* which has a sidearm for continuous perfusion *(c)* and a self sealing hemostatic vale *(d)*, to prevent backflow. **B** Cook Model assembled. The teflon dilator *(a)* is mounted with the teflon sheath *(b)* and has a "Y" adaptor *(e)* that has a tuohy-borst adaptor *(f)* which harbors a latex washer. This will permit to close the adaptor for catheters smaller than the sheath. Up to 1 french catheters can be used. **C** Ingenor sheath which has a transparent "Y" adapter *(g)* without a hemostatic valve or tuohy-borst adapter. It permits the easy unobstructed withdrawal of detachable balloons. (By permission from A. Berenstein, Radiology 132:619–632, 1979)

Fig. 1.2 A, B

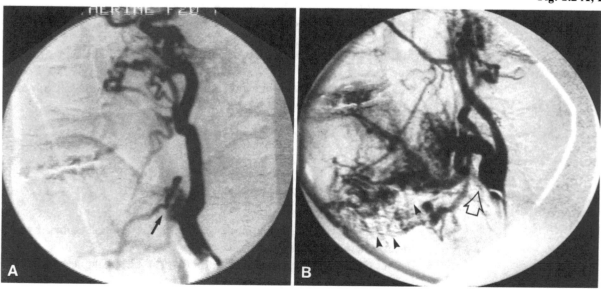

4. Significantly lessen the trauma to the artery at the puncture site while manipulating the catheter.
5. Permit finer manipulation of the catheter.

Introducer sheaths are available from 4–9 French in size (most manufacturers will make other sizes upon request). They come with a short guidewire and a leading dilator. They are usually made of thin walled teflon to maintain a large diameter (I. D.) with a relatively small outer diameter (O. D.) (Fig. 1.1 and Table 1.1). Some type of fixation of the sheath to the skin is needed to prevent accidental removal of the sheath, either with a stitch or sterile tape.

Table 1.1. Introducer sheaths

Cordis	Ingenor
Cook	UMI
USCI	BALT
Argon	

V. Catheters and Delivery Systems (Table 1.2)

1. Conventional Catheters

Two main conventional catheter sizes are used by the authors:

a) A 4 French polyethylene catheter with an I. D. of 0.032″ (0.82 mm) tapered at the tip to a 0.028″ (0.71 mm) with a 125° curve in the distal 1 cm. The curve is formed at the time of the procedure under steam and is made against the natural curve of the shaft (Fig. 1.3A) or by the manufacturer (Lasjaunias catheter Ingenor, Paris, France).

The main advantages of the 4 French catheter are the following:
1. Small O. D. that is less traumatic at the puncture site.
2. Less traumatic at the distal superselective location due to the smaller size.
3. Ability to easily catheterize arteries at the 4–6th level of branching without being wedged.
4. Sufficient I. D. to permit microparticles of various concentrations to be easily injected, or larger compressible strips such as gelfoam that can be injected into small vessels for protection (See Gelfoam, Flow Control and Protection of Normal Territories, p. 21, 48).
5. Easily can form a sidewinder curve for catheterization of difficult brachiocephalic vessels origins.
6. Injection of IBCA as a continuous column or by the "push" or "sandwich" technique without fragmentation (see IBCA Injection, p. 37).
7. Ideal for pediatric patients.

Disadvantages:
1. I. D. limit for noncompressible particles larger than 0–028″ (0.71 mm).
2. Inability to use presently available open end guidewires.
3. Less torque control.
4. Need for higher skill in manipulation.
5. Shorter curve memory.
6. Less radiopacity.

Fig. 1.2 A, B. Surgical reanastomosis. **A** Common carotid artery DSA demonstrates ligation of the external carotid artery distal to the superior thyroidal artery *(arrow)*. **B** Lateral DSA after the external carotid artery was reanastomosed to the common carotid artery *(open arrowhead)* and after the first stage microembolization of the submental region *(arrowheads)*. In general embolization should be delayed 3–4 weeks after reanastomosis, to permit proper healing of the suture lines

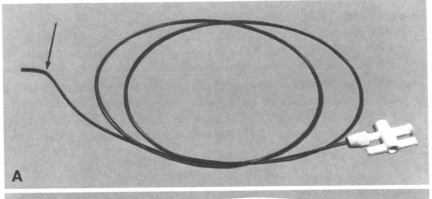

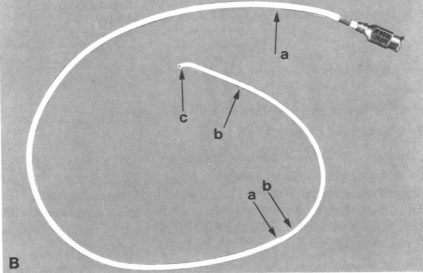

Fig. 1.3 A, B. Conventional Catheters. **A** Lasjaunias 4 French catheter with a tapered tip and a 125° distal curve *(arrow)*. **B** Berenstein catheter, 7 French, wire braided polyethylene shaft *(a)* in the proximal 100 cm. It then tapers in its outer diameter to a 5 French nonwire braided polyethylene tubing *(b)* in its distal 10 cm, maintaining a constant I.D., the last 1 cm has a 105° "hockey stick" type curve and is not tapered *(c)*

Table 1.2. Catheters[a] and delivery systems for head and neck embolizations

---

I.   *Conventional catheters*
     4 F Lasjaunias Catheter
     Berenstein 7/5 Catheter
     5.7 or 6.4 thin wall introducer (for flow guided microembolization)

II. *Balloon catheters*
     Double lumen occlusive balloon catheter (4–8 F)
     Modified (Berenstein) double lumen balloon catheter (5–7 F)
     Single (Kerber) lumen calibrated leak microballoon catheter (2.5 F)
     Single (Debrun) lumen modified leak microballoon catheter (2.5 F)
     Detachable (Debrun) latex balloon catheter
     Detachable (Hieshima) silastic balloon catheter

III. *Open end guidewires*
     USCI 0.038″ (0.97 mm), 0.035″ (0.89 mm)
     Cordis 0.035″ (0.89 mm)

IV. *Steerable microguidewires*
     ASC 0.018″ (0.46 mm) and 0.014″ (0.35 mm)
     USCI 0.018″ (0.46 mm) and 0.014″ (0.35 mm)

---

[a] Multiple catheters of a variety of diameters and configurations are available. The ones in this table represent the ones the authors use.

Fig. 1.4 A-E. Coaxial catheters and open end guidewires: **A** The Berenstein catheter *(a)* is used in the outer position. Whereas a 3 French teflon or other material catheter is used coaxially *(b)*. **B** The same catheter *(a)* is used in a coaxial manner with an open end guidewire *(c)*. The open end guidewire has a teflon cover jacket *(e)* to prevent leakage around the hollow guidewire *(f)*. The distal tip is also covered with the teflon jacket for an atraumatic insertion and has tightly woven guidewire mandrel for increased radiopacity *(g)*. **C** The open end guidewire *(c)* is used coaxially with the same catheter *(a)* and can be assisted by the use of steerable platinum tip steerable miroguidewires *(d)*.

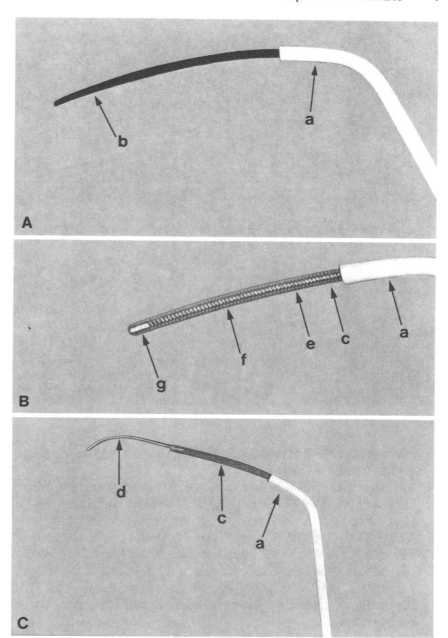

b) A 7 French wire braided polyethylene catheter in its proximal 100 cm that tapers in its outer diameter to a 5 French non wire braided polyethylene tubing in its distal 10 cm while maintaining a constant 0.041″ (1.05 mm) I.D., throughout. The tip is not tapered. A 105° "hockey stick" curve in its last 1 cm comes preshaped by the manufacturer (Berenstein Catheter, USCI, Billerica, MA) (Fig. 1.3B).

The main advantages of these catheters are:
1. Excellent torque control.
2. Larger I.D. for larger sized particles or more concentrated microparticle suspension (see Particle Embolization, p. 19), easy injection of more viscous embolic agents.

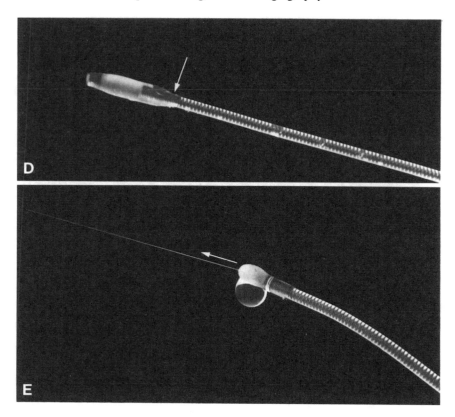

Fig. 1.4. D Open end guidewire to which a detachable Debrun latex balloon has been mounted *(arrow)*. **E** Open end guidewire to which a latex calibrated "leak" *(arrow)* microballoon has been mounted

3. May permit control of the flow by wedging the catheter into the feeding pedicle (see Flow Control).
4. The larger I. D. will allow the use of coaxial catheter assembly system or the use of 0.038″ (0.97 mm), or 0.035″ (0.29 mm) open end guidewire (Fig. 1.4, p. 21).
5. Vessels in the 3rd, 4th or even 5th level branches can be catheterized. The catheter will straighten some or most of the tortuosities which in turn will allow an open end guidewire to reach vessels at the 7th–10th level branching to be easily catheterized (vide infra). This is an important consideration when injecting liquid embolic agents or cytotoxic drugs.
6. Most useful in reaching all of the branches of the proximal or distal internal maxillary system, even when difficult turns are present in the main external carotid trunk.
7. Reliable stability of the distal catheter tip position.

Disadvantages:
1. Larger O. D. at the puncture site which may be more traumatic. We recommend progressive vessel dilatation at the puncture site prior to the introduction of a 7 French sheath for a less traumatic insertion.
2. O. D. is a limitation in the pediatric patient.
3. Need for coaxial system when attempting catheterization of small caliber arteries in the 5th, 6th, or smaller level branches.
4. The larger I. D. prevents the use of IBCA, as the column of embolic agent can easily fragment when a "push" or "sandwich" technique is used requiring a coaxial system (see IBCA Injection).

Fig. 1.5 A, B. Double lumen balloon catheters. **A** Conventional double balloon catheter. The proximal lumen is used for balloon inflation whereas the distal lumen *(arrow)* is used for distal injection of contrast material, embolic agents or infusions *(arrow)*. Bubbles of air *(×)* should be purgated prior to balloon insertion into the circulation. **B** Modified (Berenstein) double lumen occlusive balloon catheter and its assembly system. An introducer sheat *(a)* of 2 French size larger than the modified occlusive balloon catheter *(b)* is used. A smaller (2–3 French) catheter *(c)* can be used coaxially. The proximal lumen of the modified double lumen balloon catheter *(d)* is used for balloon *(e)* inflation. The tuohy-borst "Y" adapter *(f)* with a side arm *(g)* for continuous perfusion between the sheath *(a)* and the balloon catheter *(b)* is used to prevent clot formation between coaxial assembly systems. Similarly a tuohy-borst "Y" adapter is used between the proximal occlusive balloon catheter *(b)* and the small 2 French *(c)* coaxial catheter. (By permission from A. Berenstein, Neuroradiology 18: 239–241, 1979)

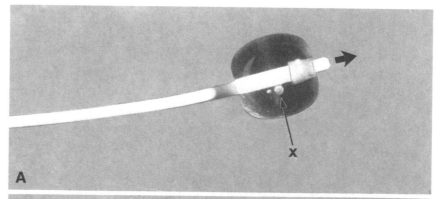

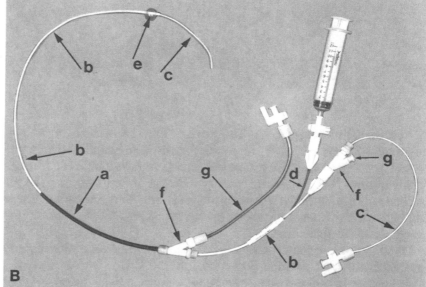

5. In tortuous origins of the brachiocephalic trunks a sidewinder curve can be formed but it may be harder to engage the origin of the vessels as the distal curve will be facing caudally. Therefore, a Simmons type catheter may be needed for engagement and a long 260 cm exchange guidewire will be needed.

We feel that each catheter offers some unique and complementary features that widen our ability to reach our goal of superselectivity.

2. Balloon Catheters

We divide balloon catheters into two main groups: Those that are used primarily for control of the blood flow or for tolerance test, and those used as the embolic agents themselves.

a) Double Lumen Balloon Catheters (DBLC)
(Meditech, Watertown, MA)

Conventional double lumen balloon catheters come in 4–8 French but may be ordered in smaller or larger sizes as special orders (Meditech, Edwards Laboratory). All balloons in these catheters are made of latex and have a

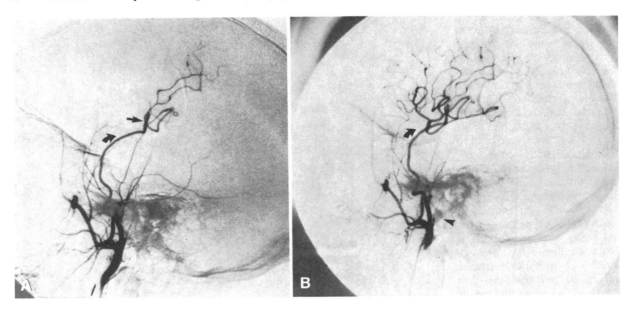

limited shelf live (Fig. 1.5A). The proximal lumen is used for balloon inflation, whereas the distal lumen is for distal injection. To free the balloons of air a low viscosity solution such as normal saline is used. A low concentration (30%) iodinated contrast material is then used to make the balloon radiopaque, while still permitting easy inflation or deflation. These catheters have a tapered distal end to prevent pericatheter leakage during percutaneous introduction.

This tapering will compromise the I. D. They are used for flow arrest and reversal during embolization (Fig. 1.19, 1.31).

At present we utilize this balloon catheter for functional investigation of tolerance to major vessel(s) occlusion (Fig. 1.6) (Berenstein, 1978) (see Tolerance test) or for flow arrest angiography for the investigation of the point of fistulization (Berenstein, 1979) (Figs. 6.25 and 6.50). *Caution:* In general, balloons inflation and deflation is easier with a small (1–2 cc) luer-lock syringe, however, if rapid deflation is needed, the larger the syringe the more negative pressure that can be applied and the faster the balloon will deflate.

In general when using conventional DLBCs, one should use an introducer sheath to prevent balloon damage during the insertion or while withdrawing the catheter.

b) Modified Double Lumen Balloon Catheters
(Berenstein, 1979)

The purpose of this modified double lumen balloon catheter is to maintain a large I. D. of the injection lumen to permit the injection of larger particles, more viscous fluids, coaxially smaller catheters (Fig. 1.5B) or open end guidewires. These catheters will increase the I. D. by approximately 30% depending of the catheter size, without changing the O. D. of the shaft. The O. D. of the nontapered tip at the site of the balloon attachment is not a problem when introducer sheaths are used. In general sheaths 2 F sizes larger than the catheter are needed.

Fig. 1.6 A, B. Double lumen balloon catheters for functional investigation. **A** Lateral subtraction angiogram of the distal left external carotid artery which demonstrates a superficial temporal artery *(curved arrow)* to middle cerebral artery bypass *(arrow)*. Note, filling of one middle cerebral artery opercular branch. **B** Lateral subtraction angiogram of the left distal external carotid artery after a double lumen occlusive balloon catheter *(arrowhead)* has been placed in the left internal carotid under systemic heparinization to test for tolerance. Note, the superficial temporal *(curved arrow)* increased perfusion to the middle cerebral artery territory (same amount of contrast material was injected). Note, the preferential flow towards the brain with poor filling of internal maxillary branches

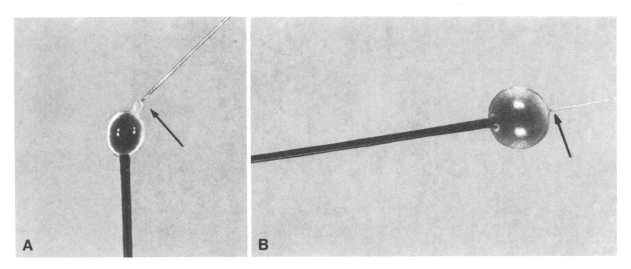

Fig. 1.7 A, B. Calibrated (leak) microballoon catheters. A Kerber model made out of a tantalum impregnated silicone shaft to which a silastic balloon has been attached. The reinforced distal tip *(arrow)* will permit perfusion through the calibrated (leak) while still inflating the balloon. **B** Latex (Debrun) calibrated leak microballoon *(arrow)* attached to a Kerber type tubing permits more reliability than the silicone model, and permits a higher rate of injection

c) Single Lumen Calibrated Leak Microballoon Catheters (Fig. 1.7)

These were introduced by Kerber (1976) and Pevsner (1977). Kerber's model (Fig. 1.6A) is made out of 2.5 french silicone tubing with an O.D. of 0.039″ (1 mm) and I.D. of 0.018″ (0.46 mm) to which a silicone balloon is attached. A silicone reinforced small orifice is made to permit the infusion of liquid agents. The Pevsner model is made out of polyethylene to which a silastic distal balloon is attached. Pevsner's catheters have an uninflated O.D. at the distal balloon portion of 0.023″ (0.6 mm) and an O.D. of the tubing at 0.015″ (0.4 mm). These types of balloon catheters are not commercially available.

The original Kerber catheter was made with a silastic balloon. The main problem was the inconsistency and unreliability of the balloon. This microballoon has been replaced with a latex microballoon (Berenstein, 1978; Debrun, 1980). One can inject through the microcatheter at a low pressure without balloon inflation or at a higher pressure that will inflate the balloons (Fig. 1.7). This is done for intravascular navigation and superselective catheterization. These catheters are used primarily for catheterization of the ophthalmic or intracranial arteries (Figs. 2.3D, 2.22C). In the head and neck there are very few indications for such a technique with the exception of very high flow lesions (fistulas or dural lesions in the pediatric group) or in the exceptional case where other techniques (4 French Lasjaunias catheter, open end guidewires, deflecting microwires) are unable to accomplish the desired superselectivity (see Vol. 4).

The silastic microcatheter is injected in a coaxial manner using a thin walled 5.7 or 6.4 French polyethylene guiding catheter.

They are too soft for torque introduction into the circulation and propelling chambers are needed for their use (Fig. 1.8) (Pevsner, 1976).

As an alternative a microballoon (Debrun #17 or #19) can be attached to a 2 F teflon tubing. A small hole can be made at its apex with a 22 to 18 gauge needle to make the leak. The shaft can then be introduced coaxially without the need for a perfusion catheter (Berenstein, 1978; Debrun, 1980).

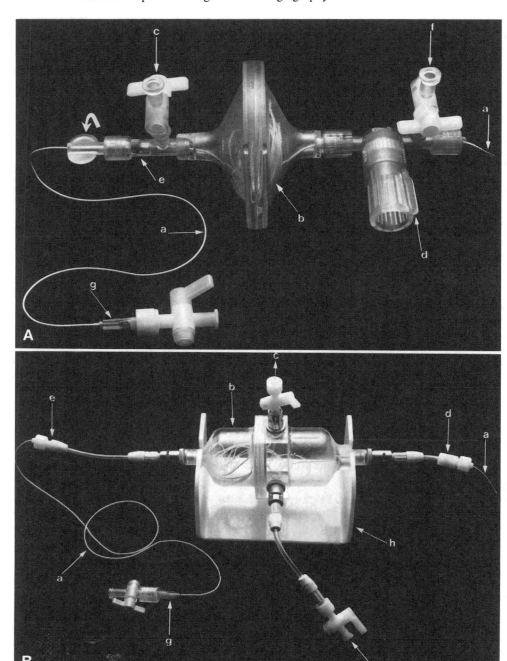

Fig. 1.8 A, B. Propelling chambers: **A** BD Pevsner model. The microcatheter *(a)* is passed through the chamber and is coiled within it *(b)*. The chamber is filled with heparinized saline through the distal stop cock *(c)*. A tuohy-borst adaptor *(d)* which is in the close position, prevents backflow towards the chamber, or if open permits propelling the microcatheter *(a)*. A second tuohy-borst adaptor *(e)* is used distally to prevent retrograde flow. To propel the microcatheter the butterfly adaptor (broken arrow) is closed when injecting through the proximal stopcock or sidearm *(f)*. This port is also used for continuous perfusion. To inject through the microcatheter the butterfly is opened until there is minimal back flow and the proximal tuohy-borst adaptor *(d)* is opened. A 23 a stub adaptor is connected to the microcatheter for injection *(g)*. **B** Ingenor model. The microcatheter *(a)* is passed through the chamber and is coiled within it *(b)* for each progression. The chamber is filled with

3. Propelling Chambers

The propelling chambers we use are of two types (Fig. 1.8): Pevsner chamber manufactured by BD (Fig. 1.8A) and the one manufactured by Ingenor (Fig. 1.8B). Both chambers work and perform similarly.

4. Detachable Balloons
(See Chapters 6 and 7; Fig. 1.9; Tables 1.2 and 1.3)

These were originally designed by Serbinenko in Russia (1974) and introduced in the western world by Debrun (1975). Detachable balloons are the embolic agent of choice for single hole fistulas of the traumatic or congenital type and are very effective when a major artery is to be occluded. The major advantages of detachable balloons when compared to other types of embolic agents (particles, coils, liquids, etc.) are the following:
1. The ability to close a vessel and/or abnormality at a precise location.
2. Flow navigation to reach distal and/or tortuous locations.
3. As they can be inflated, a vessel of larger diameter (up to 3 cm) can be occluded with a relatively small percutaneous arteriotomy).
4. They can be removed and changed if the position or size of the ballon is incorrect.
5. It can be passed into the venous side for occlusion of a pathological arteriovenous fistula with preservation of the parent artery (Figs. 6.5, 6.15 and 6.38) or into an aneurysm to exclude it from the circulation (Fig. 7.17).

Detachable balloons are made of either latex (Debrun's type) or silastic (BD or Hieshima type) (Table 1.3).

a) Latex Balloons (Fig. 1.9)

These balloons are the most frequently used by the authors. The main advantages are the following:
1. Multiplicity of sizes and shapes.
2. Reliability when hand assembled.

Table 1.3. Detachable balloons

Characteristics	Latex[a]	BD Silicone[b]	Silicone[c]
Distensibility	1:7	1:4	1:6
Hysteresis	–	+ +	+
Deflation	2–4 weeks	> 24 weeks	> 24 weeks
Shapes	Multiple	Elongated	Round
Inflation Diameter (mm)	5–30	4–8	4–35

[a] Debrun Ingenor, [b] Becton-Dickinson, [c] Hieshima

◀ **Fig. 1.8** (continued)
saline through the side arm *(f)*. To purge the air, the stopcock *(c)* is opened. To prevent back flow in this chamber model, a tuohy-borst adaptor *(d)* is closed. A second tuohy-borst adaptor *(e)* is placed on the distal part of the chamber to prevent backflow. To propel the microcatheter, the *e* adaptor is closed and the *d* adaptor is opened, while saline is injected through the side arm *(f)*. To inject through the microcatheter, a 23 g stub adaptor *(g)* is used. This chamber has a convenient plastic stand *(h)*

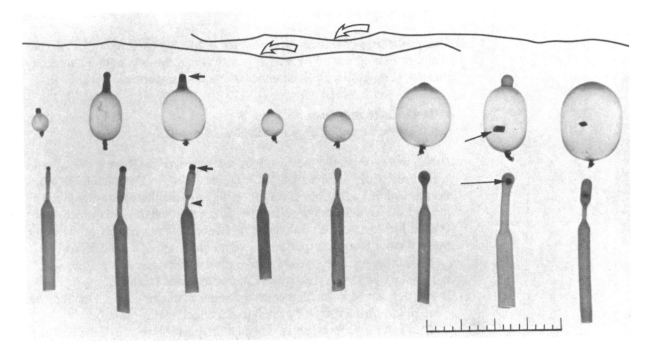

3. Latex distensibility.
4. Good memory or hysteresis even after the balloon has been inflated and deflated on multiple occasions.

The balloons come with a radiopaque marker, usually a small silver clip which permits their identification when introduced into the circulation prior to balloon inflation.

The main disadvantages are the following:
1. They must be hand mounted, therefore, experience in their assembly is mandatory for reliability.
2. Relatively short shelf life. Latex is light sensitive (Abele 1978) and should be stored with some type of cover.
3. At present regardless of the way they are attached to the catheter, they will eventually deflate. Although a theoretical disadvantage, in practice the deflation may actually be advantageous (see Chapter 6).

Debrun Latex Balloon Assembly (Fig. 1.10). The catheter assembly system consists of an introducer sheath a 6−9 French thin walled polyethylene guiding catheter that is placed into the vessel. A single curve in the outer catheter is advisable to permit catheterization of the carotid or vertebral arteries.

The balloon is attached (or transferred) to a thin walled teflon tubing with an O.D. of 0.023″ (0.6 mm) and an I.D. of 0.015″ (0.4 mm). The attachment is done with a latex thread of between 4−8 complete turns which allows a variety of balloon attachment strengths. Depending on the number of turns in the ligature and the tension placed on them, one may vary the traction and force needed to detach (Fig. 1.11). This teflon tubing is mounted coaxially with a 3 French polyethylene tubing for coaxial detachment (Figs. 1.9 and 1.11).

Fig. 1.9. Debrun latex balloons. They come in multiple sizes and shapes. Unmounted balloons have a narrow collar *(arrowhead)* where they are mounted. A radiopaque silver marker is placed in the distal part of the balloon *(arrow)* or in the balloon itself *(long arrow)*. Note, the distensibility of latex from the deflated to the inflated size. Latex threads *(open curved arrow)* are used for mounting the balloons (Fig. 1.11)

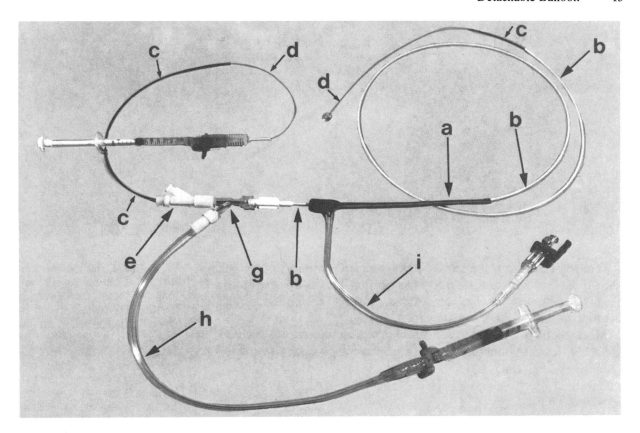

Fig. 1.10. Debrun detachable balloon coaxial system. A sheath *(a)* is placed at the arteriotomy site. A thin wall introducer (6–9 F) *(b)* is placed in the internal carotid and/or desired vessel by conventional angiographic techniques. The coaxial 3 French *(c)* and 2 French teflon balloon catheter *(d)* are introduced into the circulation via the thin wall introducer *(b)* using a tuohyborst "Y" adaptor *(e)* connected to flush solution through its second limb *(f)*. A second clear "Y" adaptor without valves *(g)* is used, through which contrast angiography can be performed via its sidearm. Prior to contrast injection *e* and *f* must be closed. Continuous perfusion through the sheath side arm *(i)* is needed to avoid clot formation

Balloon Detachment (Fig. 1.11). Once the desired position is reached, the balloon is fixed by advancing the outer 3 french polyethylene catheter by a premeasured distance. Traction is placed on the 2 french teflon catheter until detachment occurs. Careful fluoroscopic monitoring to insure no change in the balloon position is essential in preventing backward migration of the balloon. One can see the proximal neck of the balloon stretching as this maneuver is being performed with immediate return of the balloon neck to its original position once detachment occurs which is felt as a subtle "give".

Although preferable is to detach the balloon with a coaxial 3 french polyethylene catheter, in our experience this is possible in only 50–60% of cases. Therefore, while assembling the balloon a lubricant such as silicone stopcock grease or spray (Dow Corning) is put on the teflon tubing and the catheter is moved back and forth with the balloon inflated in vitro.

Many types of problems can occur during the procedure; the most frequent is related to excessive introduction of the 2 French catheter into the vessel leading to kinking; inflation of the balloon may still be possible however, deflation is impaired. When this occurs careful withdrawal of the excess 2 French tubing is done under fluoroscopic monitoring until the balloon starts moving which means the kink has been straightened. This maneuver must be done with outmost care to prevent premature balloon detachment. When advancing the 3 F catheter for balloon detachment, stretching or kinking of the 2 F tubing should be avoided; this is avoided by slight withdrawal of the 3 F catheter. Detachment at this point should be achieved by gentle traction on the 2 F tubing without the coaxial system.

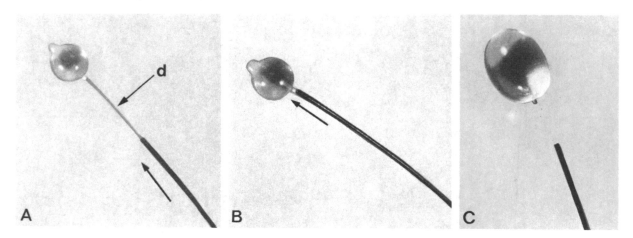

If at any time during balloon inflation one notes changes in the balloon shape, such as inflation of the distal portion (where the silver clip is) (Fig. 1.9) one *must* change the balloon. There is a high risk of balloon rupture and release of the silver clip.

More recently we have used Debrun's latex detachable balloons or calibrated leak balloons mounted on the open end guide wire (see open end guidewires, Fig. 1.4D, E).

b) Silastic Balloons

The Hieshima Balloon. This comes in two sizes and uses a miter valve for sealing. It has a 1:6 distensibility. It is attached to a 2 French polyethylene catheter and can be easily mounted, tested, and detached in vitro for inspection and reattached to the catheter shaft. It will maintain its distended size if inflated with an isosmolar contrast agent such as metrizamide, 220 mgr I/ml; when used with HEMA (Vide infra), the balloons can be used without a valve. It is easier to detach which may be a disadvantage in very high flow conditions such as AV fistulas or during manipulation. The main advantage is its ease of detachment particularly in the management of aneurysms. More recently Hieshima (unpublished data) has introduced a silastic balloon with 1:16 deflated to inflated diameter (see Vol. 4).

BD Miniballoons. Although White (1981) and Norman (1984) have used it in the management of carotid cavernous fistulas, we strongly feel that this detachable balloon catheter system offers no advantages over the Debrun or Hieshima type for surgical neuroradiology procedures and has disadvantages related to the small size (4 and 8 mm) and poor distensibility (1:4 deflated to inflated diameter).

c) Prevention of Balloon Deflation

A lot has been said and written about preventing the deflation of the various types balloons.

Silastic acts like a semipermeable membrane, whereas latex does not. Barth in 1979 demonstrated that if silastic balloons are inflated with an isosmolar solution (300 mOsm/ml) such as Metrizamide, 170 mgrI/ml, the balloons remain inflated without changes in size or radiopacity. Hieshima recommends a slightly hyperosmolar metrizamide of 220 mgrI/ml for his silicone balloons.

Debrun has advocated injecting vulcanizing silicone into the latex balloons (Fig. 6.33) using a double lumen balloon catheter to purgate the contrast filled catheter and replace the dead space of the single lumen tubing. This double lumen nylon catheter, however, is more elastic than the teflon single lumen tubing and has a larger outer diameter. Therefore, it is

Fig. 1.11 A-C. Balloon detachment. Debrun detachable balloon catheter, traction is needed for detachment. **A** Once the balloon is in the inflated and desired position, the outer 3 french catheter is advanced into the circulation *(arrow)* while monitoring the balloon position. **B** Once the 3 french tubing has reached the latex ligature and fixes the balloon gentle traction is applied to the 2 french teflon catheter *(d)*. **C** As the balloon detaches a gentle "give" is felt, this maneuver must be carefully monitored fluoroscopically

significantly harder to detach the balloon, especially if the coaxial catheter cannot be advanced. One may use a looser ligature and employ less turns to attempt to avoid this problem. In addition, if the balloon tends to move during deflation or inflation it may change its position as the contrast is being replaced by the silicone. The silicone mixture consists of equal parts of Ingenor silicone A and Ingenor silicone B made radiopaque with 1 mg/ml of black tantalum powder, 1–2 microns in size. Note that compensation for the dead space of the tubing has to be considered.

Taki (1981) suggested the use of 2-hydroxyethylmethacrylate (HEMA) which is a solidifying liquid that is soluble in water and can be made radiopaque with the addition of metrizamide powder. HEMA will mix with contrast material (metrizamide) and therefore solves the problem of dead space in the catheter shafts which prevents balloon deflation. Unfortunately, Taki's original description of this mixture is difficult to reproduce.

Hieshima (1985) has modified the use of HEMA for a more reliable application.

The modified components for polymerization are as follows:
HEMA (2-hydroxyethyl methacrylate) with 1.0 cc crosslinker to which 0.5 cc, 3% hydrogen peroxide (3% H_2O_2) is added, constitute solution no. 1.

The final component for polymerization would be the addition of the accelerator which is in the form of ferrous ion. This accelerator consists 50 mg of ferrous ion (Fe_2SO_3) per cc of solution. A total volume of this solution required to polymerize the HEMA would range between 0.05 and 0.15 cc. The 0.05 cc addition of the ferrous accelerator would have a polymerization time of approximately 60 minutes. Larger volumes of accelerator would decrease polymerization time. The addition of ferrous iron should always change the HEMA mixture to a brownish tint as the ferrous iron changes to ferric. Do not use the mixture if a precipitate of ferric oxide forms and leaves the solution clear. The working time of the polymer (time of thickening of the mixture) through the catheter is approximately 1/2 of the stated time of the polymerization.

This is for polymerization at 37° C. Polymerization at room temperature is considerably slower. In addition, polymerization with free exposure to air is also somewhat retarded. The HEMA will mix freely with metrizamide solutions. The amount of free water polymerized with HEMA should not exceed a 50% total mixture.

The obvious advantage of HEMA is that there is no need for a double lumen balloon catheter and the material is soluble with metrizamide, therefore dead space is not a problem. It can be used with either latex or silicone balloons.

The great interest that detachable balloons have created and their efficacy in embolization will result in the rapid introduction of new types of detachable balloons. All previously mentioned detachable balloons use traction detachment. However, newer types of detachable balloons that do not need traction for detachment are now being introduced. Taki (1979) and Picard (1980) have described an ingeneous detachable balloon system using high frequency electric current with thermal energy for detachment. We have had no experience with either of these types and they are not commerically available at the present time.

Romodanov and Shcheglov (1982) reported the use of their detachable balloon systems for the management of cavernous and intracranial aneurysms; however, the technology is not yet available in the west.

The use of the Prolo catheter or the Fogarty catheter for the management of cavernous fistulas or vertebral artery to paravertebral venous plexus fistulas is now only of historical interest.

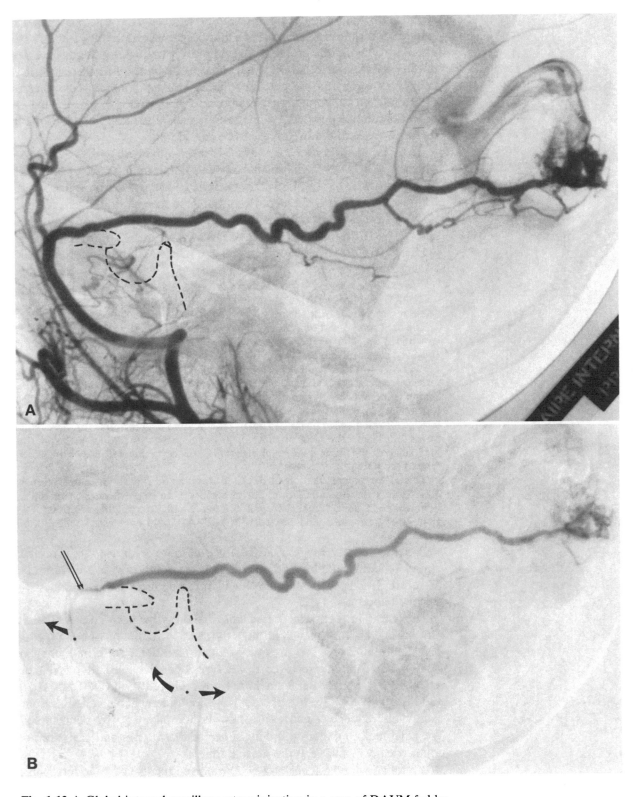

Fig. 1.12 A Global internal maxillary artery injection in a case of DAVM fed by
the temporal branch of the middle meningeal artery. **B** The tip of the open
guidewire *(double arrow)* has been advanced coaxially (femoral approach, Berenstein catheter) distal to all the dangerous branches of the middle meningeal artery
(solid arrow) namely: petrous (VIIth nerve), cavernous, ophthalmic

5. Open End Guidewires (Fig. 1.4B, C)

These have been recently introduced by industry and manufactured by USCI (Billerica, MA) for use in combination with the Berenstein superselective catheter (Fig. 1.4B). They come in 0.038″ (0.97 mm) or 0.035″ (0.98 mm). They have a removable core of either standard or softer long tapered.

To prevent leakage around the woven guidewire mandril, a teflon jacket cover is used as the outer wall. The tip consists of a tightly knitted wire for better radiopacity. They come in 145 cm lengths (although they could be made of any length), and a "J" curve can be easily molded.

Open end guidewires are assisted by the use of a small steerable deflecting guidewires (Fig. 1.4C) (ACS or USCI) that have precise control with a 1:1 torque response allowing very selective negotiation of tortuous vessels. The steerable guidewires come in 0.018″ (0.41 mm) or 0.014″ (0.35 mm) and are made with a stiff teflon coated core proximally, a flexible spring wire (30 cm), radiopaque floppy type (2 cm) and a distal welded platinum tip attached by a shaping ribbon (Young and Berenstein, 1985).

We have been using this system since 1984 and feel that it is a major technical improvement which has significantly widened our possibilities of catheterization of distal branches (Fig. 1.13).

It can be used for low concentration particulate type embolization or low viscosity liquid agents such as IBCA, chemotherapeutic drugs or 95% ethanol (Fig. 2.16). The possibility of mounting a detachable balloon or calibrated "leak" latex balloon to the open end guidewire with its obvious advantage is now possible (Fig. 1.4D).

Additional microcatheters, for more distal catheterization and specific assembly (pediatric population) will be analyzed in Vol. 4.

6. Guidewires

We employ conventional guidewires depending on the catheter I.D. In general we like the long tapered tip (10 cm) and use various curves either premade by the manufacturer or formed by us at the time of the procedure. The Bentson floppy guide is also very useful (Bentson, 1975).

VI. Embolic Agents (Table 1.4)

The choice of embolic agents will depend on the goal of the procedure, selectivity accomplished and vascular anatomy of the pathological territory. They are divided into solid particles or liquid agents by their physical characteristics and into absorbable, nonabsorbable, or cytotoxic types by their biological behavior.

1. Particle Embolization

Particle embolization refers to a mechanical blockage of a vascular territory utilizing precut particles that may be of uniform or variable sizes and shapes. Their ability to occlude is related to their size, shape, and

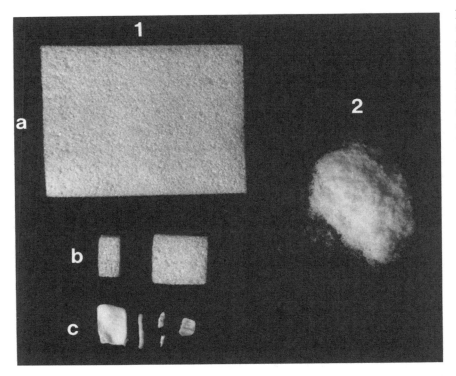

Fig. 1.13. Gelfoam emboli. *(1)* Gelfoam particles of different sizes *(a, b)* which can be compressed then soaked in contrast material and cut in various size particles *(c)* swelling will occur following contrast moistening of the gelatin sponge; or it may come as a powder *(2)* with particles 40–60 microns in size

Table 1.4. Embolic agents presently used by authors for head and neck embolizations

I.   Absorbable (biodegradable)
  a. Gelfoam powder (40–60 μ)
  b. Gelfoam particles (any size)

II. Nonabsorbable (particulated)
  a. Polyvinyl alcohol foam (PVA):
     Microemboli 40–1000 μ in suspension of iodinated contrast material
  b. Detachable balloons

III. Nonabsorbable (liquids)
  a. Isobutyl-2-cyanoacrylate (IBCA) (Adhesive)
  b. N. butyl cyanoacrylate (NBCA (Adhesive)

IV. Cytotoxics
  a. 95% ethanol
  b. Chemotherapeutic agents

coefficient of friction. Particulate emboli used during surgical neuroangiographic procedures are of two main types: 1. absorbable and 2. nonabsorbable materials. More recently there is interest in a 3rd particulate agent for chemotherapy – Time releasable microparticles (Vide infra, cytotoxics).

a) Absorbable Materials

Emboli such as autologous clot, avatine, or gelfoam can be used (Djindjian, 1973). We have found gelfoam to be the best one for our purpose and do not use any of the others.

Gelatin Sponge (Gelfoam; Upjohn, Fort Lee, NJ) was first used to control hemorrhage during surgical procedures by White in 1945. The first report of the intravascular use of gelfoam was by Speakman in 1964. He tried it for occlusion of a traumatic carotid cavernous fistula via the internal carotid artery. Djindjian in 1973 reported 60 cases treated with the aid of percutaneous catheter embolization using gelfoam as the occluding agent. Since that time it has been noted that although gelfoam is readily available and easy to use, the vascular occlusion accomplished by it is temporary and recanalization occurs from 7–21 days after embolization (Gold, 1975; Barth, 1977). It is available as powder (40–60 microns in size), as a sheet or as cubes from which pieces of varying sizes can easily be cut, placed in contrast material and injected through small lumen catheters (Fig. 1.13).

α) **Gelfoam Powders** (Berenstein, 1981). We use gelfoam powder for occlusion of vascular neoplasms prior to surgical removal (Figs. 1.29C, 1.30, 1.31). In these cases the embolic occlusion occurs at the capillary or precapillary level. The tumor bed is deeply penetrated, allowing no possibility of subsequent collateralization. Perivascular tumor necrosis may be observed pathologically (Fig. 1.14). The particles are injected after mixing the powder in 60% iodinated contrast material until a homogeneous suspension is obtained. Injection is accomplished under fluoroscopic monitoring using a 1–3 cc luer-lock syringe held in a horizontal position. Depending on the size of the lesion, small amounts (0.3–0.5 ml) of the suspension are injected during systole (see external carotid physiology, p. 20) and the contrast material washout is fluoroscopically monitored to follow the progressive obliteration of the tumor microcirculation. If changes in vascular resistance are noted, the catheter is purged backwards and rinsed thoroughly. A low pressure injection of contrast material is done under fluoroscopic monitoring to evaluate the distal territory remaining after the embolization. In general, gelfoam powder should be carefully used in the external carotid due to the multiple anastomosis between the external carotid system and the intracerebral circulation. As the embolized territory is progressively occluded, one may opt for a slower rate of injection and if necessary, larger particles to prevent passage of the microemboli through the anastomotic pathways.

In the middle meningeal territory, in addition to the collateral circulation to the carotid and ophthalmic systems, one should spare the proximal segment of the middle meningeal artery when using powder to a point 15 mm beyond the foramen spinosum where the petrosal branch of the middle meningeal artery arises and supplies the peripheral VIIth nerve. The proximal middle meningeal artery can then be closed with a gelfoam strip to maximize preoperative thrombosis. Horton (1984) used gelfoam powder as a "lubricant" to facilitate the flow of PVA particles. We, however, use one or the other as we feel that one can have better control and safety if there is more uniformity of particles. One of us (A.B.) has been using a combination of gelfoam powder, 95% ethanol, and metrizamide in the management of malignant lesions at the base of the skull (Figs. 2.2, 2.20).

β) **Gelfoam Particles.** These larger particles have been used for preoperative hemostasis, however, they do not enter the tumor and necrosis is not observed pathologically. At present, we do not use gelfoam in particles for

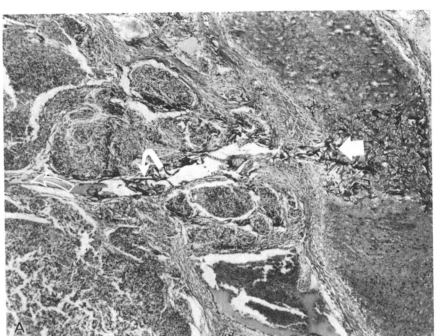

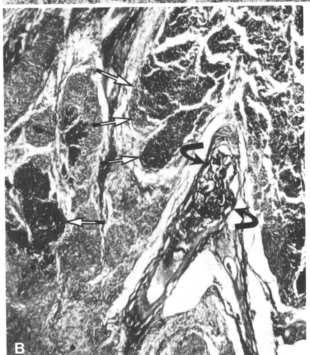

Fig. 1.14. A Pathological specimen after gelfoam powder embolization of a meningioma. HE stains at low magnification powder, demonstrates aggregated gelfoam particles *(solid arrow)* as they enter a small capillary distally occluded *(broken arrow)*. Note thrombosis of the vessel distal to the microparticle *(open curved arrow)*. **B** Azocarmin stain at larger magnification demonstrates the foreign body gelfoam *(broken arrows)* as well as darker areas of perivascular early necrosis *(white arrows)*. (By permission from Berenstein, AJNR 2:261–267, 1981)

occlusion of abnormal vessels even as a preoperative measure. We use a permanent particulate agent such as polyvinyl alcohol foam or liquid agents, primarily isobutyl-2-cyanoacrylate (Berenstein, 1980).

The use of gelfoam particles to devascularize a vascular lesion prior to surgical removal carries an immediate risk similar to that encountered with any permanent agent. If an intracranial vessel is occluded with any agent (absorbable or not) this complication is the same.

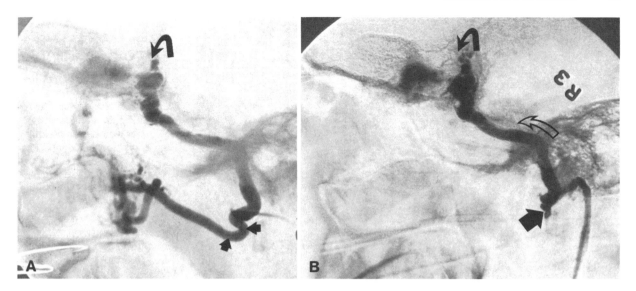

Fig. 1.15 A, B. Gelfoam particles for vessel protection. AV fistual in fibrous dysplasia of the sphenoid bone. **A** Lateral substraction angiogram at the origin of the middle meningeal and internal maxillary arteries. The middle meningeal artery is markedly hypertrophied and supplies an arteriovenous fistula of fibrous dysplasia of the sphenoid bone *(broken arrow)*. The middle meningeal artery could not be superselectively catheterized without continuous filling of the internal maxillary artery *(arrows)*. **B** A gelfoam strip was placed in the internal maxillary artery for protection *(solid arrow)*. Now there is direct flow towards the fistula *(broken arrow)* through the middle meningeal artery *(open curved arrow)*. (By permission from Berenstein, 1982)

When superselectivity cannot be accomplished and a permanent agent must be used, a gelfoam particle, 1×2 or 1×3 mm or even larger in size may be injected to occlude and protect normal vessels (Fig. 1.15) partially or completely. The occlusion needs to be sufficient to change the hemodynamics of the involved territory so that at the time of injection of the permanent agent, only pathological vessels will be filled (Figs. 1.15, 3.5). Theoretically, gelfoam absorption when used in this manner is an added advantage as late recanalization should result in restoration of flow to the normal vessels that were temporarily occluded.

In cases of traumatic arterial hemorrhage or traumatic aneurysms (Fig. 7.20), gelfoam particles are probably still the best choice as they are easy to inject and produce the desired hemostasis in the majority of cases. A possible exception is when the vessel is larger in diameter than the particles. In these instances, expansile polyvinyl alcohol foam, detachable balloons or IBCA will easily occlude a large vessel (vide infra). A point of caution when using gelfoam particles to protect a distal territory is related to the tendency for gelfoam to fragment as suggested by Picard (1976) with isotopically labelled gelfoam particles. These fragments may theoretically penetrate small collaterals between the extracranial and intracerebral vessels with unwanted complications. Although we have used gelfoam particles for more than 10 years and have not observed this phenomena in clinical practice, if in doubt, an alternative is the use of a small coil (see Flow Control, Fig. 1.29).

Gelfoam comes in sterile, single use packages.

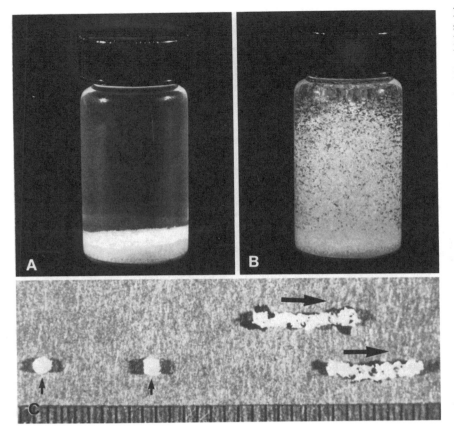

Fig. 1.16 A-C. PVA suspension. **A** PVA microparticles layered in the bottom of the bottle after blending, filtration, resuspension and sterilization. **B** After decanting the sterile water the microparticles are resuspending in contrast material. After a moments shaking a relatively homogeneous suspension is obtained. (By permission from Berenstein, Radiology 145:846–850, 1982). **C** Dry compressed PVA discs *(arrows)* can be seen to expand after rewetting *(large arrows)*. (By permission from Berenstein, Radiology 132:631–639, 1979)

Fig. 1.17 A

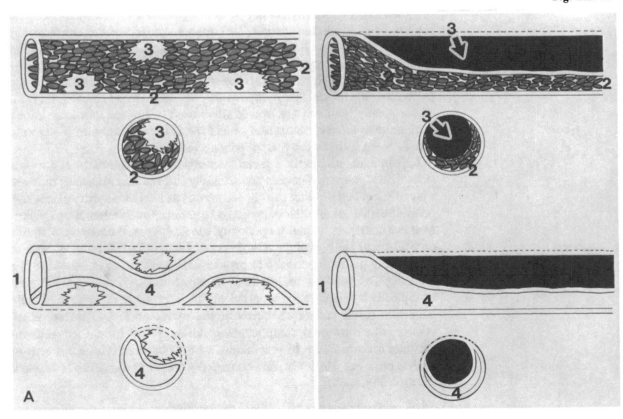

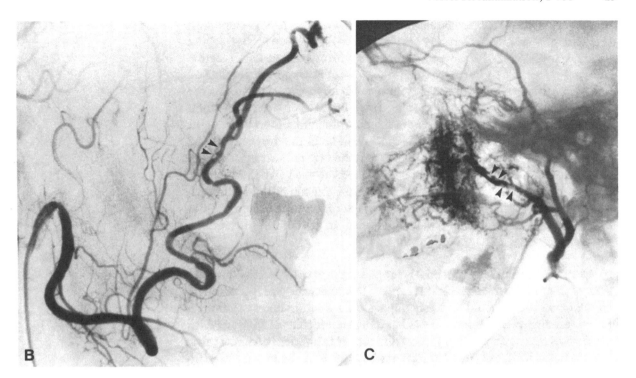

Fig. 1.17 A-C. Recanalization of nonbiodegradable embolic agents. **A** Diagramatic representation of the various embolic agents *(3)* and the recanalization *(4)* of the autologous clot *(2)* with re-endothelial lining of the embolic agents. Although the material is not biodegradable, the vessel (and territory) is revascularized *(1)* vessel wall. **B** Lateral substraction angiogram of the facial artery which has recanalized after PVA embolization. Note, the filling defects of the endothelial covered PVA particles *(arrowheads)*. **C** Lateral substraction angiogram in a 24 year old patient with a capillary vascular malformation which was previously embolized with silicone spheres in the internal maxillary and transverse facial arteries. Note, the contrast material is surrounding the substracted radiopaque spheres *(arrowhead)*. See Fig. 1.18

b) Nonabsorbable Particulate Materials

Multiple materials of the nonabsorbable particulate type have been introduced. The oldest one being silastic spheres originally introduced by Luessenhop (1964). This agent has been primarily used for embolization of cerebrovascular malformations. Although they have been used in head and neck embolizations we feel that this agent offers no advantages over other available agents and may produce recanalization which may make management of vascular lesions more difficult (Fig. 1.17). For head and neck embolization, both authors feel that the nonabsorbable particles of polyvinyl alcohol foam are probably best suited. Dura mater appears to be a good agent although no animal studies or human studies as to their toxicity and tissue tolerance are available (Djindjian, 1975) when used intravascularly.

α) Polyvinyl Alcohol Foam (PVA) unproperly called Ivalon (Fig. 1.16). Chemical Properties: The sponge is a water insoluble material made by the reaction of polyvinyl alcohol foam with formaldehyde. It is resilient when wet but semirigid when dry. The wet volume is about 20% greater than the dry volume. It is a nonabsorbable, biocompatible sponge. It has been used in the repair of patent ductus arteriosos (Bentson, 1972), skin graft (Hogeman, 1961), colon surgery (Boutsis, 1974) and as an embolic agent (Tadavarthy, 1979). In the dry compressed form only gas sterilization should be used. The sponge expands 10–15 times in length (depending on its original thickness) approximately 30 seconds after contact with moisture (Fig. 1.16). PVA is useful for occluding a medium to large sized vessel for it expands to occlude an artery larger in diameter than the internal diameter of the catheter. This material is difficult to handle in the dry, compressed state. However, if small discs are made from the original sheet by catheter hand punchers, or the NYU introducer catheter is used (Kricheff, 1979), the injection of compressed PVA is facilitated. PVA can be made radiopaque with 60% barium sulfate, however, the addition of tantalum powder may add further radiopacity to small particles. In general, at present, the dry compressed PVA is seldom used.

β) **PVA Suspension.** The material is supplied in dry particles of either 140–250 or 590–1000 microns in diameter. The particles are prepared in formalin and they should be washed in a sterile solution before embolization to eliminate any residue. PVA has a high coefficient of friction which sometimes makes a smooth injection difficult. Heat sterilization may cause the particles to aggragate. Various maneuvers have been suggested to overcome this problem, including the back and forth passage of the precut particles between two syringes (Kerber, 1978) or the addition of gelfoam particles or powder to the PVA microparticles (Horton, 1983). The back and forth maneuver takes time to separate the aggregated particles. The mixture of PVA and gelfoam particles of various sizes may produce proximal occlusion with the large particles or unwanted embolization through extracerebral to intracerebral anastomosis with the powder.

Our ready to use PVA particle preparation (Berenstein, 1982) is made by taking the desired quantity of the dry PVA particles of either size and adding it to a sterile water in a blender. The blender is operated at low speed for 15 minutes followed by high speed for 5 minutes or until the particles are suspended uniformly. The suspension is then filtered through paper filter. The separated particles of washed PVA are deposited into small glass jars with heat resistant plastic cups (Fig. 1.16A, B). The jars are then filled with sterile water to resuspend the particles. Sterilization is done at 270° for 20 minutes with the caps loosely fastened, later tightened under sterile conditions. Bacteriological testing has shown that the suspension remains sterile for at least three months. Prior to placing the material in bottles for sterilization, the agent is passed through progressively decreasing sized vibrating sieves to separate the various sizes (Herrera, 1982). In microscopic examination of the blended particles of PVA, particles as small as 40 microns in size can be detected. To insure a uniform size, we divide blended PVA into three sizes: below 150 microns, between 150 and 250 microns, and between 250 and 500 microns in size.

Immediately prior to use the sterile water is decanted and the particles are resuspended in 60% iodinated contrast material (even with digital subtraction angiography). This results in homogeneous uniform suspension which can easily be injected.

As an additional measure for smoother injection, the PVA contrast material suspension is mixed with 10–15 ccs of human albumin (Herrera,

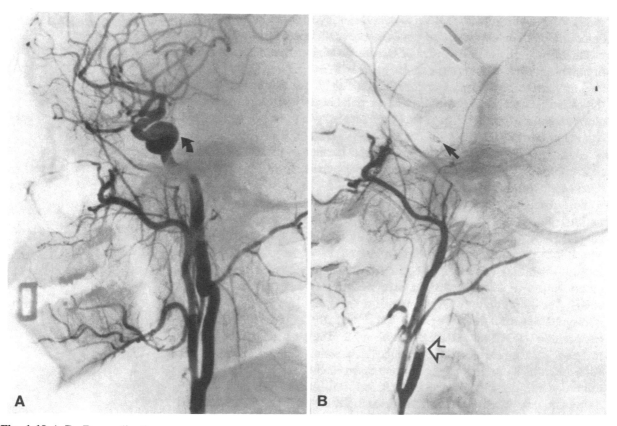

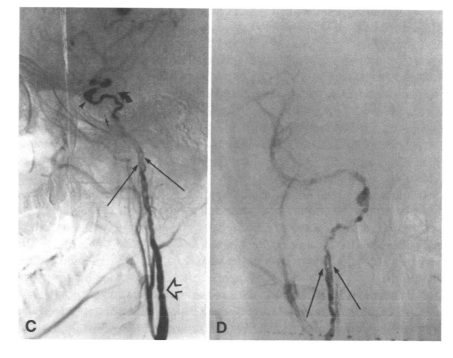

Fig. 1.18 A-D. Recanalization from a prematurely deflated balloon. **A** Lateral subtraction angiogram of the common carotid artery demonstrates an ICA cavernous sinus aneurysm *(curved arrow).* **B** Immediate postembolization common carotid artery study demonstrates a detached balloon approximately 2 cm distal to the origin of the internal carotid artery *(open arrowhead),* a second balloon is in the cavernous segment of the internal carotid artery *(arrow).* **C** lateral and **D** frontal subtraction angiogram three month later demonstrate an area of narrowing where the previous proximal balloon was placed *(open arrowhead).* Two separate channels had recanalized *(arrows).* In the cavernous ICA the recanalized lumen corresponds to the angiographic dome of the aneurysm *(curved arrow).* The internal carotid artery then acquires its normal caliber at the level of the ophthalmic artery *(arrowhead)*

1982). This will further assist to smoothness of injection permitting detection of change in washout or resistance at the time of injection.

The microparticles of PVA can be injected in various manners depending on the objectives. These particles (as other with irregular margins) may or may not enter the abnormal angioarchitecture of a vascular lesion. Factors that will affect the final position include superselectivity, force of injection, concentration of particles per cc of contrast and the presence or size of a capillary "barrier".

Quisling (1984) showed that the irregular surface of precut PVA has a high coefficient of friction which permit the particles to stop against the vessel wall without completely occluding it.

This irregular partial occlusion may stagnate blood, producing a combination of PVA and autologous clot that will eventually recanalize (Fig. 1.17A), producing re-endothelialization of the nonabsorbed PVA. The dilute concentrations of PVA microparticles are useful with small internal diameter catheters or open end guidewires and are best in the embolization of lesions with an arteriocapillary "barrier" (Berenstein, 1980). We start the embolization with a relatively low concentration of microparticles for a deeper penetration (Fig. 1.20). As the smaller vessels are occluded, we change to a more concentrated suspension or a larger size to "pack" the larger vessels with embolic material. One must be familiar with the capacity of the delivery system to avoid clogging the system. If the lumen of the delivery device is occluded, one uses a 1 cc syringe with nonopaque material (normal saline) and gently pushes the aggregated particles producing the plug. As a general rule, if one is unable to easily and smoothly unplug the delivery system, it is best to change it. The guidewire should *not* be used to attempt to unplug the lumen as it usually worsens the problem by impacting the emboli even further.

Although PVA particles are not reabsorbed (Tadavarthy, 1977; Latchaw, 1979) follow-up in our patients, where an apparently excellent embolization was achieved, later may result in complete irregular recanalization (Fig. 1.17 and Vol. 1, Fig. 13.3). Therefore, we feel that the best indication for PVA is for preoperative devascularization (tumor, some vascular malformations, flow rerouting in preparation for IBCA or ethanol injection), especially in those situations where IBCA or ethanol are not indicated (epistaxis).

In our experience, even after dense packing PVA has recanalized. We infer from these observations that a similar recanalization can occur with any other particles: dura, or silicone sphere. Interestingly spheres are of uniform size with smooth borders and are not adhesive or reactive. The recanalization that we have observed suggests a similar phenomena where the endothelial lining covering the spheres and the vessel are being opened above and below (Fig. 1.17C). Recanalization has been seen with detachable balloon, deflated prematurely (Fig. 1.18). Similar occurence has been observed by us and others in IBCA embolization of brain AVMs and will be discussed in Vol. 4.

c) Flow Directed Particle Embolization (See also PVA Particles)

When particles are used for devascularization, a careful analysis of the angioarchitecture to be embolized is done to evaluate vessel size and the presence or absence of "dangerous" anastomosis, to select the best particle size. The smallest possible size is best to result in a more distal occlusion. As the embolization is progressing one must be aware that previously not visualized "dangerous" anastomosis may now fill. In these situations the catheter should not be wedged so that one can follow the distal wash out and its behavior as the flow is slowing.

We must emphasize that particulate emboli should not be injected through stopcock adapters as they may get trapped in them.

A catheter through which emboli have been injected should NOT be used for angiograms of important (internal carotid, vertebral) arteries.

If very small particles are used and after multiple injections no gross change is seen in the abnormality, one can increase the particle concentration accordingly. A high concentration usually results in faster devascularization but probably less penetration.

Important considerations are to continuously rotate or change the syringe position to prevent sedimentation and/or aggregation of the particles at any one part of the syringe which will result in catheter occlusion. A meniscous at the catheter hub should always be made with normal saline or clean contrast material to prevent accidental introduction of air bubbles which will change the flow hemodynamics as the air emboli exits the catheter. Catheters full of emboli should be thoroughly backflushed and rinsed with nonopaque agents to know that the catheter is free of embolic material.

2. Gianturco Coils

These are small pieces of guidewire to which the inner core has been removed and a foreign body such as cotton or dacron is added to promote thrombosis. They have very little use in head and neck embolization and may even be contraindicated if used as the main agent to obtain devascularization. In our experience coils frequently do not produce thrombosis and become an obstacle to reach the pathological territory with other agents. Their main uses are to protect a normal vessel or anastomosis (see Flow Control, Fig. 1.29). They are easily introduced with the assistance of a conventional guidewire and can be made of various gauges and lengths. In our experience in the head and neck very small coils, no more than 1 cm in length with a 0.038″ (0.90 mm) diameter or smaller, are usually best (see Vol. 4).

3. Nonabsorbable Liquids

Liquid embolic agents are nonabsorbable. They must be liquid at the time of injection and should solidify when they have reached the pathological angioarchitecture producing an endovascular cast of the area without passing to the venous circulation. The ideal liquid embolic agent would be the one that if injected into an undesirable location, could be dissolved (with nontoxic byproducts) and be nonabsorbable. As these agents are as yet not available we have used 3 main types of liquid agents: a) liquid silicone, b) IBCA, c) cytotoxics. Each has specific physical, chemical and biological characteristics. These characteristics can modify the selection of one over the other depending on the goals of treatment.

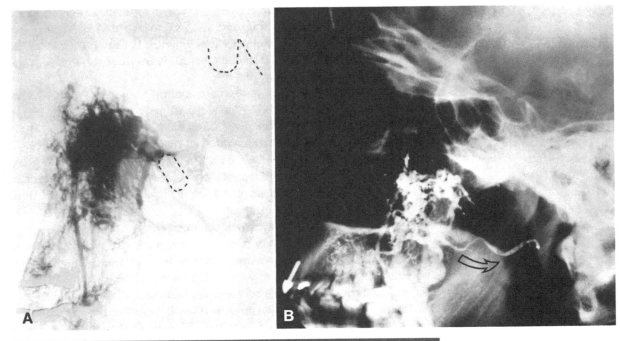

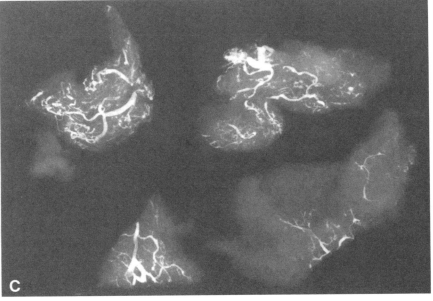

Fig. 1.19 A-C. Silicone fluid embolization under flow arrest: **A** Lateral subtraction angiogram of the distal internal maxillary artery under flow arrest using a double lumen occlusive balloon catheter (in *dotted lines*). **B** Lateral plain radiogram demonstrates the excellent radiopaque cast obtained with the liquid silicone and tantalum mixture. Note, some silicone in the draining vein *(open curved arrow)*. **C** Radiogram of the fragmented specimen demonstrating the deep penetration of the liquid radiopaque silicone mixture. Same patient as Fig. 10.14

a) Silicone Fluid Mixture

Silicone fluid is a permanent biocompatible agent made radiopaque with tantalum powder. Superselectivity is mandatory prior to injection.

The mixture consists of Dow Corning silastic elastomer 382, a silicone of relative high viscosity (50,000 centistokes C.P.) that contains a filler necessary for vulcanization, and medical grade Dow Corning silicone fluid 360, a clear fluid with a lower viscosity (20 C.P.) that acts as the dilutant to the more viscous silastic elastomer.

These two silicones are thoroughly mixed in a 1:2 to 1:5 proportion depending on the viscosity desired. 1 mg of tantalum powder is added per cc of mixture for radiopacity. Two catalysts are required for vulcanization: Dow Corning Catalyst M (stannous octate) as reported by Doppman (1972) and a co-linker, tetraethyl-silicate introduced by Hilal in 1976. The co-linker permits a prompt, reproducible

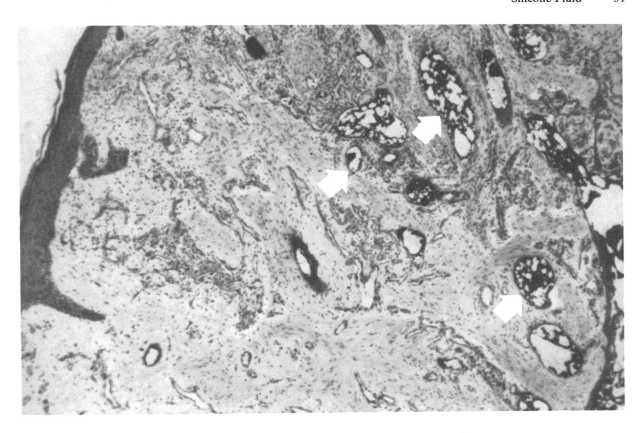

Fig. 1.20. Photomicrograph of a biopsy specimen in a patient with a high flow vascular malformation. Note the ability of the low viscosity silicone to penetrate into very small vessels in the range of 40–60 microns. Black material in all the blood vessels represents the silicone *(open arrowheads)*. No inflammatory reaction is noted

vulcanization of the low viscosity fluid silicone mixture; and has made silastic embolization a practical technique. We have also used tetra-N-propoxysilane as the co-linker. There appears to be no practical difference in the performance of these two co-linkers. However, less stannous octate is needed if the silane is used. Typically one 21 gauge needle drop of catalyst and one drop of colinker per cc of mixture will produce vulcanization in 3–4 min. In order to accurately assess vulcanization time a sample of the mixture to be used is tested in vitro just prior to injection by continuously stirring the liquid to compensate for body temperature.

Complete stasis will considerably facilitate the injection of silicone fluid. A double lumen balloon catheter may be used alone (Fig. 1.19) or coaxially for a more distal catheterization and still maintain some degree of flow control with the more proximal balloon (Berenstein, 1979). The small inner coaxial catheter is advanced to the main arteries feeding the lesion. Flow stasis is monitored fluoroscopically and the amount of fluid necessary to obtain the desired embolization is measured by contrast material injection. Liquid silicone may be injected in the less viscous form and can fill vessels as small as 40 microns in diameter (Fig. 1.20). The balloon is deflated and the catheter assembly removed after the predetermined vulcanization time has elapsed as judged by prior and concurrent in vitro testing of the mixture. There is no risk of catheter "gluing" with this agent and a true cast of the lesion can be obtained (Fig. 1.19).

Doppman et. al. have reported distal migration of a silicone cast in a parathyroid adenoma. To prevent distal migration, the cast should be anchored in vessels of progressive diminishing diameter.

If the silicone is not well mixed, air bubbles may be trapped in the fluid. Such air will reabsorb and the cast will retract and possibly migrate distally (Berenstein, 1978).

Silastic may be used in a more viscous mixture in the form of flow guided radiopaque globules (Sano, 1976). We have modified Sano's original techniques by using our modified double lumen balloon catheter to control the flow. A drop of fluid is injected with the balloon deflated, the silicone globule is carried out by the blood flow until the progressively decreasing vessel diameter stops its flow, due to its relative high viscosity. If the silicone does not stop, slow controlled inflation of the balloon causes the drop to flow distally until it reaches the desired position: the balloon is then further reinflated and the material is allowed to vulcanize. The balloon should not be deflated again until full vulcanization has occured.

The short and long term results of patients treated with liquid silicone has been excellent, including patients treated exclusively by silicone emboliza-tion, with no recurrence and good clinical outcome (Figs. 1.21, 1.23, 3.8) the main advantage of silicone is its liquid form that permits a good cast without the associated clot (as seen in the discussion of a recanalization in particles, Fig. 1.19), therefore, recanalization is less likely. More recently in vascular malformations, we have been using IBCA with similar result as with silicone.

Silicone produces no inflammatory response (Doppman, 1976; Hilal, 1978; Berenstein, 1979). In histological specimens only minimal foreign body giant cell reaction (Fig. 1.20) is seen. Some of the reaction seen histologically is related to the ischemic insult and not histocytoxity (as will be discussed in IBCA). The main disadvantage of silicone fluid emboliza-tion is related primarily to the difficulty in mastering injection, and the frequency of pulmonary embolization.

When using this agent (and other liquids) in or near skin surfaces, its excellent penetration can produce significant tissue damage which will manifest itself as marked swelling (Fig. 1.21A) which will then progress to necrosis (Fig. 1.21B). Therefore, when using liquid agents of this type, proper planning is important. To be considered are the following:

1. Is the lesion going to be removed after embolization?
2. What tissue (skin) can be sacrificed?
3. What tissue (skin) has to be preserved?

In deep lesions not involving the skin or mucous membranes, necrosis is usually not a problem as it will be incorporated by fibrous tissue (Fig. 3.8). However in skin or mucous membranes necrosis (mostly if of significant size) can be a problem unless it will be part of the planned resection (Fig. 1.21C). When using aggressive agents and swelling occurs, surgery should be delayed until full demarcation occurs. The necrotic area is not painful and proper local care is advisable to prevent infection. A prophylac-tic antibiotic may be warranted.

b) IBCA

Isobutyl-2-cyanoacrylate (IBCA) is a vinyl monomer of the alkyl-2-cyanoacrylates. These compounds range from the methyl to the ethyl monomer. Several methods are available for preparing alkyl cyanoacry-lates, eg. by reacting formaldehyde with alkyl cyanoacrylate to obtain a polymeric material and the depolymerizing of the material by heating and distill of the liquid monomer. A crucial problem during preparation is that of removal which causes the monomer to polymerize; several liquid and

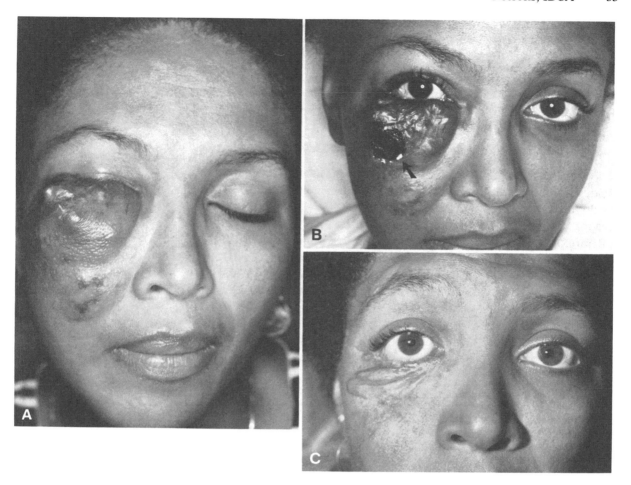

Fig. 1.21 A-C. Postembolization swelling and necrosis following embolization near skin surfaces. **A** Five days after silicone embolization of the infraorbital and facial systems with radiopaque silicone. **B** Three weeks later there is a significant shrinkage of the lesion with an area of well circumscribed necrosis, note the white silicone rubber *(arrow).* **C** After resection of the lesion with removal of the excess skin. The patient has had further reconstruction of the lower eyelid with excellent results (same patient as Fig. 9.8)

vapor phase polymerization inhibitors are used, phosphorous peroxide, O-sulfobenzoic anhydride, nitric oxide or sulfur dioxide.

An exothermic reaction occurs with alkyl cyanoacrylate polymerization which can be initiated by free radicals or anions, IBCA polymerizes upon contact with an ionic solution such as contrast material, saline, blood or endothelium. The polymerization may be retarded by a low ph. The speed of polymerization is a function of the alkyl side chain monomers those with smaller chains (4–6 carbon atoms) such as IBCA will polymerize within seconds. In addition, the larger the chain the less flexible the material. In general, cyanoacrylates generate heat as they are transformed from monomeric to polymeric form, a fact that may be relevant in considering hystotoxicity.

The compound has a low viscosity of 1.6 centipoises at 25° C and a low exothermic polymerization, approximately 10 kcal mol produces less than 0.5° C of temperature elevation at the site of deposition in humans (at volume of 0.5 ccs of IBCA or less). Polymerization may occur by free radical in the presence of Lewis acid or hydrogen peroxide by an anionic initation with very weak bases, e.g., water or alcohol. The bounding characteristics of IBCA are the result of nonionic polymerization occuring between two adherents. The catalytic effect of water or weak bases are maximized by spreading the adhesive in a thin film. Solvents for the polymer includes N-dimethylformamide and nitromethane. Preliminary work with these agents have suggested little biotoxicity in small diluted solutions (1–5%) still maintaining effective solvent characteristics. Storage of IBCA at 4–7° prolongs its shelf life, but is not an absolute requirement (Pevsner, 1980).

Polymer Retardants (Table 1.5). These retardants include polyphosphoric acid, octanoic acid, monoalkyl phosphoric acid ester, ethyl-10-(iodophenyl), undecanoate (pantopaque) (Lafayette, Indiana), nitric acid (vapor phase), and sulfur dioxide (vapor phase) (Pevsner, 1982). The mixture of ethyl-10-(iodophenyl) undecanoate or pantopaque with IBCA has proven to be a good choice on theoretical and practical grounds (Cromwell, 1979). The compound remains in solution with IBCA and has a pH of 6, preventing an ionic polymerization. The rate can be controlled based on stoichiometric mixtures. Thus, polymerization can be achieved in 1–30 seconds. The main disadvantage of pantopaque is its high viscosity of more than 20 C.P. although it has not been a problem with microballoon catheter injection.

Table 1.5. Opacifying agents/retardants

Tantalum powder (1–2 μ) black powder
Tantalum oxide (1–2 μ) white powder
Pantopaque (used with IBCA primarily to retard polymerization time)
Meterizamide powder
Acetic acid retards IBCA polymerization time

Cromwell's work shows a close relationship between the amount of pantopaque and polymerization time in laboratory setting, in practice 0.2 to 0.5 ccs of pantopaque per 1 cc of IBCA will retard polymerization 4–8 seconds. Additional factors must be considered in the ability of the agent to penetrate into the abnormal territory, such as vessel caliber, blood flow, flow control, and injection rate.

The pantopaque can be mixed with IBCA without tantalum and can be seen with good fluoroscopy or with digital subtraction; however, we usually mix it first with tantalum powder (1 gram per 1 cc of IBCA) for best radiopacity. In very high flow conditions where vessels occlusion is the goal and there is no "nidus" to be permeated, IBCA and tantalum may be injected without pantopaque.

More recently Vinuela (1985) has used acetic acid (0.01–0.05 cc) to keep the IBCA pantopaque tantalum mixture in an acid media which will further retard the polymerization time and may be more applicable to brain embolization (Vol. 4). The viscosity problem of the IBCA pantopaque tantalum mixture may be solved (Pevsner, 1982) by using octa- or decaionic acid, mild alkyl acids, or a monoalkyl phosphoric acid ester (Testwet 1143: Intex products, Greenwall, SC). All of these have little biological effect and are low viscosity agents (3 CP). They can be sterilized with liquid chloroform which is easily evacuated by vacuum. The addition of 0.1 to

1.0% by volume of a 1% solution of any of these compounds will give a polymerization time of 1–30 seconds. Control's can be established in citrate blood. The addition of one of these agents further reduces the problem of intraluminal polymerization and intravascular fixation of the microballoon catheter. For opacification of the IBCA mixture one uses tantalum powder or titanium oxide to decrease the CT artifacts produced by radiopaque markers (Pevsner, 1982). The viscosity of IBCA and tantalum powder is around 4 C.P. and adding pantopaque it increases to 8–12 C.P. depending on the mixture. This viscosity is not a problem in head and neck embolization.

Histotoxicity. In the various toxicity studies performed by Lehman (1966, 1967) and Gottlieb (1967) the isobutyl-2-cyanoacrylate and the N-butyl-cyanoacrylate (NBCA) appear to be the most suitable agents for endovascular applications. This opinion is shared by Vinters (1985) in his review of the histotoxicity of cyanoacrylates. Lehman demonstrated that the shorter alkyl substitute compounds are less toxic. Cultures performed on this agent demonstrates that this material fails to produce any bacterical growth when tested in dogs cerebral cortex and monkeys chiasm. There was no evidence of neurological deficit when applied in the cortex.

In Lehman's (1967) experience the isobutyl-2-cyanoacrylate was present nine months in the dog and 14 months in the chimpanzee. In none of the animals had it disappeared. In his long term studies of isobutyl-2-cyanoacrylate in chimpanzees, there was no suggestion of tumor formation. Zanetti (1972) was the first one to use this material for endovascular occlusion of aneurysms and renal arteries in dogs. He noted that when injected, IBCA rapidly polymerized to form a sponge like mass that increased in size. The dose of the adhesive required was approximately 75% of the original measured aneurysm volume with the apparent discrepancy being explained by the tendency of the adhesive to trap fluids within its clefts.

Manelfe (unpublished data, 1979) confirmed the increased volume obtained by and IBCA-blood mixture.

The entrapped red blood cells would not hemolyze after 24 hours, but a faint fibrillar structures suggesting fibrin can be seen at pathology (Zanetti, 1972). White cells composed of about equal number of neutrophilic granulocytes and mononuclear cells tended to concentrate adjacent to the polymer at 3 hours. By 24 hours these cells had not increased in number and many were degenerating. At one week, very few erythrocytes remained in the entrapped blood which had taken on a uniform dark eosinophilic stain. A few fibroblasts were disseminated in it while focal groups of macrophages and granulocytes were scattered in the periphery. By 2 months the IBCA itself showed little change. However, the interstices were densely fibrotic and a few scattered foreign body giant cells lay adjacent to the polymer (Fig. 1.22) most surfaces of the matrix were found to be covered directly by fibrous tissue. The reaction of the internal surface and endovascular wall was of particular interest to the authors because of its relationship to the problem of adhesion and toxicity. The polymer was in direct contact with only about 15% of the endothelial surface and entrapped blood occupied the remainder. After 3 hours at points of contact with the wall of the artery, the polymer seems to be touching the internal elastic lamina rarely with a degenerating endothelial cell interposed. Often the internal elastic lamina

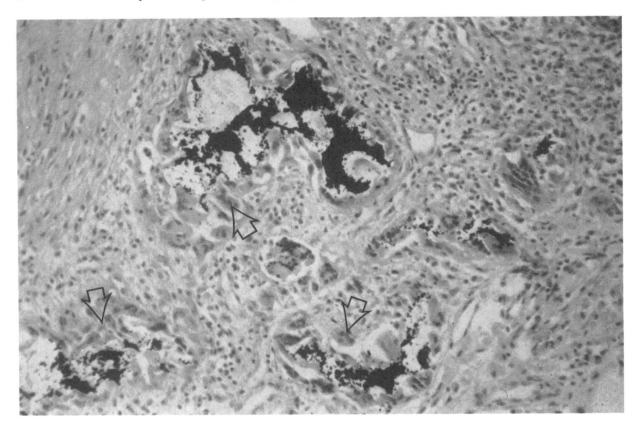

seems to be dented slightly outwards. The media was altered only by shrinkage and hyperchromatism of a few nuclei adjacent to the internal elastic lamina with no changes in the adventitia. There was no progression of degeneration at 24 hours or at 3 month. White, et al. (1977) in their pathological studies noted that the IBCA found in arteries and arterioles manifested as a nonstaining, slightly retractile network surrounded by a large number of foreign body giant cells and organized thrombosis. There were varying degrees of chronic inflammation manifested by lymphocytes and plasma cells in the thrombosed and surrounding vascular tissue. The vascular outlines were retained although the internal elastic lamina were often focally disrupted as noted by Zanetti (1972). In many cases the arteries appear to be dilated by their contents. IBCA and associated giant cells were found in very small arterioles within the submucosa in a gastric ulcer and within fibrous areas of splenic and hepatic infarcts. Zanetti injected IBCA into surgically constructed aneurysms and one week after injection the thrombi did not intrude into the lumen. Fibrous tissue had replaced the blood entrapped in the spongy matrix near the wall of the aneurysm and had not yet reached the central portion. The smooth muscle wall of the aneurysm had degenerated and fibrous tissue running through it. A fibrous capsule about 1 mm thick surrounded the aneurysm. Specimens at 1, 2, 3 months had endothelial lined fibrous walls at the mouth of the aneurysm. The interstices of the IBCA mass were sealed with fibrous tissue containing a few scattered foreign body giant cells. The walls of the aneurysms were fibrous but did not extend beyond the original venous graft. Vinters in 1981 reviewed the pathology of two arteriovenous

Fig. 1.22. Photomicrogram after IBCA embolization, the IBCA and tantalum mixture is seen in black. Note, the inflammatory reaction with foreign body giant cell infiltration *(open arrow)*

malformations previously embolized with isobutyl-2-cyanoacrylate, one 42 days after embolization and the other 1 year after embolization. His findings were consistent of those reported by Lehman (1966), Zanetti (1972), and White (1977).

Interestingly enough, they found that many, although not all, vascular channels were thrombosed and contained a particular black substance representing the IBCA tantalum mixture. The lack of filling of some of the branches is probably related to the form of IBCA injection in vivo. In some sections, IBCA was seen within the walls of the embolized vascular malformation channels and in some it was seen extending into the surrounding gliotic brain parenchyma. Vinters (1981, 1985) did not consider the possibility that the extravascular IBCA seen may be artifactual. In the parenchyma no foreign body giant cell or particulated material was observed. Vinters in 1985 review, an additional 7 patients that were studied pathologically after IBCA embolization with similar pathological findings; one patient had the IBCA for 16 month. The IBCA persisted and could be demonstrated by the black tantalum powder or using a modified oil red O stain. In this publication, Vinters and coworkers did a more detailed histological analysis of the IBCA embolized AVMs. In addition to the previously mentioned histological findings, they found patchy transmural necrosis of portions of some vessels within days or weeks of IBCA embolotherapy. Some vessels containing IBCA thrombus had undergone recanalization; in other the IBCA thrombus was lined by endothelium and with time there was actually smooth muscle cell hyperplasia between the endothelial lining and the IBCA. These findings correlate with Quisling's histological findings with PVA; supporting our theory that it is the autologous clot mixed with any type of nonbiodegradable embolic agent the one that recanalizes, covering any truly nonabsorbable embolic agent by endothelium and virtually making it "extravascular" (Fig. 1.17).

As to the question of potential carcinogenesis of the alkyl cyanoacrylates in general and the isobutyl monomer in particular, the preponderance of hystotoxicity studies seem to point to a purely inflammatory reaction rather than a neoplastic tissue reaction. No reports of neoplasms in man exists in over 18 years that the agent has been used in humans.

An absolute statement denying carcinogenicity however cannot be made. Marck (1982) who studied the mutagenicity of N-butyl-2-cyanoacrylate and that of isobutyl-2-cyanoacrylate using the Ames test in bacteria where a positive result implies that that the product under study is mutagenic for man, found a weak mutagenicity of the isobutyl-2-cyanoacrylate. Although the extrapolation of this study to human neoplasms is not absolute mainly with the small doses used during embolotherapy, the material should be used with care and discrimination and it is our duty to keep good long term follow-up in our patients. At present this agent is the most practical in clinical practice.

IBCA Injection. Thanks to its low viscosity, even when mixed with pantopaque and tantalum powder, IBCA can be easily injected through microcatheters or open end guidewires. As we have discussed, polymerization will occur when the material gets in contact with any ionic solution such as contrast material, blood vessel intima or a basic pH solution. Therefore prior to any injection of IBCA through any delivery system, the catheter must be rinsed with a nonionic solution such as 5% dextrose solution to prevent the plastic from hardening within the catheter.

The material can be injected as a continuous column or pushed in between a nonionic solution as a "sandwich".

1. Continuous Column. If superselectivity is accomplished and no normal or "dangerous" vessels are present, one can inject IBCA as a continuous column to produce an intravascular cast. In general, the amount of IBCA needed to reproduce the same filling as the contrast material estimated is 50–75% of the original test (see above).

Fluoroscopic monitoring of the IBCA progression is done by observing the first material that enters the circulation as it will be the first to polymerize and is usually a good guidance of how much IBCA can be injected prior to backward flow of the acrylic toward the catheter which can result in reflux, filling of previously nonvisualized arteries or adherence the catheter to the cast.

In very high flow situations one may need some form of flow control: double lumen balloon catheters, calibrated leak microballoon, or less no retardant (pantopaque or acetic acid). In general, IBCA should be injected through small lumen delivery systems (less than 0.028″ (0.71 mm) to prevent fragmentation of the acrylic which will produce an IBCA clot mixture that can result in clot recanalization. IBCA injection is best performed with a coaxial delivery system; if IBCA refluxes or a small amount of acrylic remains at the tip of the delivery system, the outer catheter will prevent undesirable reflux and can separate the excess acrylic at the tip of the delivery system. Polyethylene and teflon usually do not adhere but they may. Therefore, the most distal delivery system should be withdrawn immediately after IBCA deposition when using a continuous column technique unless the tip can be detached (such as balloons).

When performing IBCA embolization certain precautions should be considered prior to injection.

Position of the catheter tip: 1. If the catheter tip is at a sharp vessel curve or loop, the IBCA may hit the vessel wall first preventing proper antigrade flow which will result in a proximal occlusion (even if sufficient retardant is used) or even reflux. To avoid this, the catheter is advanced, if it is not possible, it will be slightly withdrawn. 2. If the catheter tip is at a bifurcation attention should be paid to the preferential flow; if it is towards the main target, the injection will usually result in a good deposition. If the preferential flow is towards the less important feeder or towards normal territory (and if better selectivity cannot be accomplished on the main pedicle), one may try to protect or block that territory first (see Flow Control). Alternatively the IBCA column may be injected in two movements: first a small amount is injected; it will flow towards the less desirable path, as this small amount slows or stops, the vessel is occluded proximally and the second injection is then started which fills the main trunk.

2. "Sandwich" Technique: In situations where the arterial feeder to the target is not reached by the delivery systems, one may protect normal territories with particulate agents (see Protection of "Dangerous" Vessels, p. 48) or by use of the continuous column technique. If the proximal vessel is to be spared, the delivery system is rinsed with a 5% dextrose solution. A small predetermined amount of IBCA is then loaded in the delivery system (preceded by the 5% dextrose solution), and the IBCA is injected in a "sandwich" fashion.

To assess the amount of IBCA needed and the rate of injection, tests are done with 60% contrast medium "sandwiched" between nonopaque saline. This technique, as all others, must be mastered in an experimental setting.

This technique gives additional flexibility for embolization. Example, in vascular lesions with multiple small channels (like DAVMs) or in situations where previous interventions (surgical ligations, proximal embolization) have taken away a direct access one must use small collaterals to reach the lesions (Fig. 6.49). In these situations, small amounts of acrylic (0.05–0.2 ccs) are used. The delivery system will remain patent and additional depositions are possible (see Figs. 2.14C, 6.49, 10.19). If a second liquid deposition is to be performed, the stopcock valv must be changed, and back flow established.

3. In situ injection. IBCA may be injected directly into the nidus of a vascular lesions in selected instances, if flow control can be achieved (Figs. 9.13, 10.6).

VII. Opacifying Agents (Table 1.5)

1. Tantalum Powder

Tantalum powder is an inert biocompatible metal first reported by Burke in 1940. He placed it into the fractured and unfractured tibia and femur of dogs and rabbits. Burke could find no detectable microscopic or roentgenologic evidence of bone or soft tissue irritation. In 1942, Pudense and Ottman showed that strips of tantalum implanted over the surface of the brain caused little reaction. Additional uses of tantalum in man have included tantalum plates for cranioplasty (Echols, 1945) without adverse tissue reaction even when the tantalum is in contact with nervous tissue. The use of tantalum in nervous tissue was reported by Whitcomb as a method for marking the plane of section in the open lobotomy operation on postoperative skull roentgenograms. Bailey, et al, studied the reaction to powdered tantalum introduced into various areas of the nervous systm of cats and monkeys. The response to tantalum was minimal in all areas except the basilar system.

The tantalum dust (Kenna Metal, Latrobe, PA) comes in two preparations; tantalum powder, a black powder and tantalum oxide, a white powder (Kerber, 1980). The powder comes in various sizes, the 1–2 micron particles are best for embolization.

It does not alter the chemical characteristics of the embolic agents, but will increase the viscosity of the mixture. It is important to remember that the black tantalum powder may produce skin discoloration in white patients (Fig. 1.23) whereas the white powder will not even in black patients (Fig. 1.21). The main disadvantage of tantalum oxide is that it is of lesser weight, therefore more material is needed for similar radiopacity, increasing further the viscosity of the mixture.

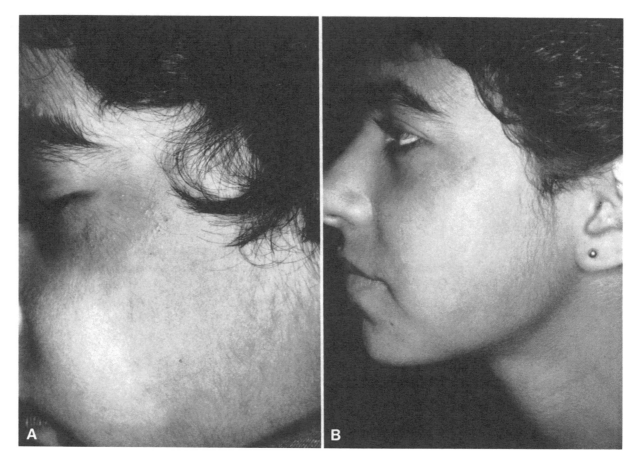

2. Metrizamide Powder

The metrizamide powder may be used to make ethanol or other embolic agents radiopaque. The ideal concentration is one that will give an equivalent of 190 mg of iodine %. In situations where the metrizamide is used for radiopacity, the metrizamide powder is diluted in the ethanol instead of the conventional dilutant. It does not change the characteristics of the ethanol or it may be used with water soluble vulcanizing substances such as HEMA for detachable balloons (See Detachable Balloons).

VIII. Ethyl Alcohol (95% Ethanol)

Ethyl alcohol is gaining popularity as an effective and aggressive embolic and cytotoxic agent (Ellman, 1979; Buchta, 1982). It is available in any hospital in a 95% concentration. It can be easily injected through any delivery system presently available. It produces no immediate mechanical blockage, only secondarily, due to its cytotoxicity on blood cellular elements and endothelium as well as adjacent tissues. It then produces an ischemic or anoxic insult and cytotoxic damage. The local effects of ethanol are related to its potent denaturant and hydrophopic property in high concentrations. In our measurements of systemic concentrations of ethanol in blood using Widmark's factor during endovascular treatment and using up to 60 cc of ethanol (in venous vascular malformations of an adult) at any one treatment, blood levels of alcohol have been well below systemic toxic

Fig. 1.23 A, B. Skin discoloration due to black tantalum powder. **A** 7 year old female treated with liquid silicone and tantalum powder for the management of an extensive vascular malformation of the maxillofacial area. Embolization was the only treatment. Note, the ash discoloration of the cheek. **B** 10 years later skin discoloration has fainted but remains. The patient is free of disease and has been well controlled over 10 years with liquid silicone exclusively. She has had menstrual cycles without changes on her clinical condition. White tantalum oxide will avoid this problem

levels. When the ethanol reaches collateral circulation or the venous outflow, it becomes diluted and nontoxic.

Ellman (1981, 1984) and Buchta (1982) in various experiments and in pathological specimens demonstrated the effects of ethanol. However, no head or neck or cerebral vasculature was studied.

In the renal vasculature Buchta showed vascular pruning and spasm in the distal circulation with stasis in the segmental and main renal arteries and an absence nephrogram in the immediate arteriogram following slow infusion of 95% ethanol.

Pathologically changes were noted as early as 2 minutes and consisted of protein precipitation and fibrinoid necrosis at the tissue level; the blood vessels were congested but not thrombosed. E. M. studies demonstrated severe cellular changes at various levels with necrosis of endothelial, epithelial, and mesenchymal cells with distortions of all intracellular elements. In the intravascular space erythrocytes were congested, lysed or agglutinated. Ellman in 1984 showed the difference in damage produced by rapid (2 ml/sec) versus slow (less than 0.5 ml/sec) injection of intra-arterial ethanol. Rapid infusion produced more tissue damage and less blood cellular element aggregation, whereas slow infusions permitted a higher contact of blood cellular elements with the alcohol producing damage to the cells, aggregation and thrombosis.

He demonstrated no gross differences between the rapid intra-arterial injection and those produced following balloon occlusion to permit evaluation of the cytotoxic damage in the absence of blood cellular elements in the renal circulation.

The conclusions of Ellman's (1984) and Buchta's (1982) studies suggest that a better way to produce tissue damage may be to produce flow arrest to permit a long contact between the ethanol and the endothelium, in the absence of blood cellular elements.

1. Ethanol Injection in the Arterial System

In view of its cytotoxic effect ethanol seems to be a suitable agent when necrosis and not only devascularization is the main objective, such as in malignant or aggressive tumors (Fig. 5.6) (Choi, 1985). Alcohol is not indicated in very high flow conditions where the objective is a mechanical blockage where detachable balloons or IBCA may be best.

In very hypervascular (but not high flow) lesions, one may use a combination of ethanol and particulate agents such as PVA (Wallace, 1984), gelfoam powder or collagen. This has the advantage of producing alcohol stagnation.

When using ethanol the final result will not be apparent immediately (Figs. 2.2, 2.20, Meningioma Chapter). One may opt for injecting a strip of gelfoam at the end of the infusion to maximize its effects. The end point of alcohol infusion is difficult to judge as vessel spasm may give a false picture. Furthermore, spasm may occur proximally at the tip of the catheter where the highest concentration of the ethanol is in contact with the vessel wall; caution must be taken to prevent reflux. If spasm occurs it may be advisable to work on another pedicle and return to the first one at a later time. When ethanol is injected in the arterial system, it must be done with outmost selectivity, particularly in skin and mucous membrane areas.

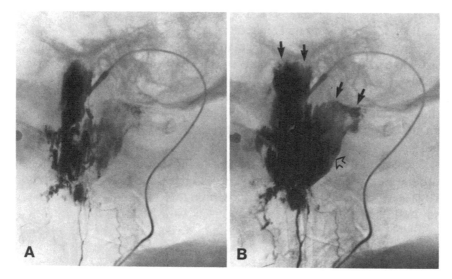

Fig. 1.24 A, B. Venous vascular malformation of the parotid area. **A** Following injection of 5 cc of radiopaque ethanol. **B** After 25 cc. Note the upper body limits of the pouch *(arrows)* and the convex aspect of its posterior margins on the styloid muscles *(open arrow)*. Note the very poor venous outflow

2. Ethanol Injection in Venous Malformations (Fig. 1.24)

Patient preparation: the procedures are performed under general anesthesia with endotracheal intubation. Tracheostomy and nasogastric intubation are indicated if the clinical evaluation and preliminary CT scan already demonstrate the lesion near the airway or alimentary passages. The puncture site is chosen at a normal area near the lesions in most instances. The skin is prepared in the usual antiseptic manner. We employ an 18–21 gauge angiocatheter connected to a venotube. In general, the angiocatheter is placed in a dependent orientation to facilitate backbleeding and prevent air embolism. Blood samples are obtained from the lesion and examined for $P_a O_2$, CBC, PT, PTT and fibronolytic splitting product. Following needle placement and venous sampling under fluoroscopic monitoring, 5–10 ccs of contrast material are injected. Stagnation or very slow flow of the contrast agent is usually observed. Gentle manual compression is then applied in an attempt to empty the lesion or clear the contrast material from the tip of the angiocatheter, therefore, insuring its intravascular position.

Depending on the lesion size or compartment, progressive injection of 5–10 ccs of contrast are performed and monitored to determine the volume of the lesion or a specific compartment of the lesion. Multiple septations can be seen as contrast material enters the pouches and starts unfolding the venous spaces. As the lesional compartments are filled, the walls will bulge outwards or will follow anatomical landmarks such as bone (Fig. 1.24). The venous drainage demonstrated is usually very poor in this type of malformation. On occasion, the transition from abnormal looking vein to a more normal appearing one can be seen. When considering management with sclerosing agents such as alcohol, special attention should be paid to the venous drainage which may involve the ophthalmic vein, cavernous sinus or the vertebral epidural plexus (Figs. 10.42, 10.43).

Ethanol injection: depending on the preestimated volume of a lesion or compartment, 95% ethanol made radiopaque with metrizamide powder is injected. Five ccs are slowly injected every 3–5 minutes. We do not inject contrast following alcohol infusion to prevent displacing the alcohol beyond

Fig. 1.25. Capillary venous and venous vascular malformations. 7 year old female with a venous vascular malformation of the right upper lip. Note, two areas of ulceration secondary to ethanol. These ulcerations were preceded by a blister and healed completely without scarring

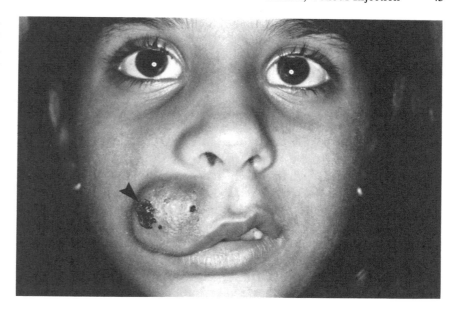

the lesion. One must check backbleeding each time or if no blood returns, antigrade flow is checked under gravity by elevating the venotube above the heart level.

If there is no spontaneous backflow or antigrade flow is not obtained, no alcohol is injected and a new puncture is done. Usually, we inject up to 1/3 the estimated contrast volume at any one lesion or compartment and the maximum alcohol we have injected in any one sitting is 60 ccs.

In tongue localization, one must establish the venous outflow and ethanol should be injected from a more distal to a more proximal position to prevent thrombosis of the already compromised venous outflow.

At the end of the alcohol injection, hemostasis is easily achieved using a suspension of hemostatic agents such as Avatine and Gelfoam powder mixed with normal saline or a large strip of gelfoam. Injected as the angiocatheter is withdrawn to seal off the tract.

Following ethanol infusion, the area becomes swollen, indurated, noncompressible, but it is not tender. This process starts within the first minutes and reaches maximum in approximately 3–7 days. Resolution occurs in 1–5 weeks. One can then evaluate refilling of portions of the lesion and additional treatment can then be planned, limited necrosis can be observed (Fig. 1.25), it usually heals spontaneously.

IX. Infusion Chemotherapy

In head and neck tumors, however, available intravenous chemotherapy and radiation therapy appears as effective as simple intra-arterial infusions but no sufficient interest has been apparent as yet. Part of it may be due to the need for long repeated infusions as exemplified in intra-arterial chemotherapy in the rest of the body and the still prevailing fear of cerebral embolization with long and repeated implanted devices in the carotid artery. We have used chemotherapy drugs in few occasions with promising results (Figs. 2.1, 2.21). Functional vascular embolization should maximize the effectivity of this approach, permit higher concentrations and decrease toxicity and should be encouraged.

Time Released Microcapsules (Chemoembolization)

Time released microcapsules have created a significant amount of interest outside the interventional field for many years. And only recently has attention been paid to the synergic application of these two modalities. It is quite attractive to use the arterial route to deposit microcapsules that can release in a very selective manner high concentrations of cytotoxic agents and add to the insult the effects of ischemia. It would avoid the need for long, tedious, and repeated catheterization and infusions. Unfortunately, there has been slow progress in developing reliable easy to manufacture and use time released microparticles. The principle of microencapsulated agents have been applied to ethyl cellulose (Kato, 1978) or carnauba wax (Madoule, 1981). Although still not in general use, this has a very promising role in our pursuit of an endovascular approach to various pathological entities and this includes not only presently treated hypervascular conditions but also hypovascular problems that may be even more sensitive to ischemic insults.

X. Other Potential Agents

A new development is boiling contrast material to produce a thermal injury in the vascular tree (Amplatz, 1984). To our knowledge this has only been done in human veins and in animal models. Radiation therapy of brain AVMs as done by stereotactic radiation (Steiner, Kjellberg) produces a thermal injury of the endothelium and it is the repair of that thermal injury that produces the permanent occlusion.

Other possibilities include the use of laser technology which at present is inpractical, but is a promising technology of the future.

1. Ethibloc

A promaline corn zen protein mixed with 60% ethanol which will solidify in 10–15 minutes has been used for obliteration of kidneys by Kauffman (1981) and Ellman (1984) and by Riche (1983) in venous vascular malformations. At present limited biocompatibility studies are available.

2. Collagen

This is used in dermal inplants and recently was used experimentally for endovascular occlusions by Strother (1983). It has the potential of a recanalization, probably related to collagen blood mixture (see Ethyl Alcohol section).

3. Estrogen

The efficiency and pathophysiology of exogenous estrogen are discussed in chapter 3. The most promising use is in conjunction with microcapsules primarily in patients with Rendu Osler Weber, possibly some AVMs or some tumors with hormonal dependence (see Chapters 2, 8 and 10). It has already been infused in situ for meningioma, DAVM (Suzuki 1980).

XI. Miscellaneous

1. Syringes

We believe that all syringes should be of the luer-lock type. As a matter of precaution syringes used for flushing or contrast injection should be of different size and/or marked differently than those used to inject embolic materials. When learning or testing the flow characteristics in an individual situation, the same type of syringe used to do the testing should be used to inject the embolic material or provocative drugs (Xylocaine, Amytal).

2. Stopcocks and "Y" Adaptors

One way luer-lock stopcocks are recommended for best fitting transparent plastic stopcocks are best to detect any air bubbles prior to injection. However, in superselective works back flow may not be present in these instances a fluid meniscus is needed to avoid air emboli.

When using a coaxial system, "Y" adaptors that have a side arm for continuous perfusion between two catheters, or that can permit control angiography are very useful, in addition a tuohy-borst fitting will permit the use of catheters or guidewires of a variety of sizes without backleakage (Fig. 1.26). When using detachable balloons no proximal washers or tuohy borst adaptors are used, to prevent accidental balloon detachment when withdrawing or changing the balloon catheters (Fig. 1.10).

Fig. 1.26. "Y" adaptors for coaxial catheterization. *a* ACS transparent "Y" adaptor with a sidearm for perfusion *(curved open arrow)* and a tuohy-borst adaptor with a silicone washer *(arrow)* to prevent leakage arround variable sized catheters and guidewires is closed by rotation of the screw *(broken arrow)*. This adaptor is ideal to prevent accidental introduction of air bubbles into the system. *b* Ingenor "Y" adaptor without hemostatic valve or washer. It is used in the manipulation of detachable balloons to prevent accidental balloon detachment if the balloon catheter has to be withdrawn. *c* Cook "Y" adaptor with a latex washer in the tuohy-borst end *(broken arrowhead)* that permits variable sized catheters or guidewires to be introduced

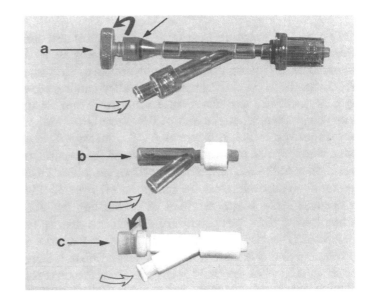

3. Tray Containers

As with the syringes different containers can be used for contrast or emboli to prevent accidentally mixing one for the other.

4. Flushing Solutions

Flushing solutions may or may not contain heparin.

One of us (PL) uses normal saline without the addition of heparin. Whereas the other (AB) uses 4000 units of heparin sulfate for each 1000 ccs of flushing solution. In adults 0.9% normal saline is used, whereas in children a solution of 0.35 normal saline and 2.5% dextrose to which 2000 units of heparin are added per 1000 cc of solution is used.

The results and experience are similar with both regimens.

5. Systemic Heparinization

During routine head and neck embolizations heparinization is not used by either author. Only when performing a tolerance test occlusion or when multiple catheters are used to obtain flow control will systemic heparinization be used (Fig. 1.6, and Chapters 3 and 8). When needed, systemic heparinization is done for the tolerance test using 10000 units of heparin sulfate in a 70 kg adult and is given as an IV push. Prior to balloon occlusion of the parent vessel an activated coagulation time (ACT) test is obtained to confirm proper heparinization. At the end of the tolerance test and/or the procedure, reversal is done based on the information of the ACT sample (Scott, 1985). When heparinization is used for multiple catheter work, 3000 units are used, supplemented by 1000 units per hour (usually given through the flush solution).

When using calibrated leak catheters in intracerebral catheterization, systemic heparinization is also recommended (Vol. 4).

6. Activated Coagulation Time (ACT) Monitoring

One of us (AB) routinely uses an ACT measurement during our intreventional procedures (Scott, 1985). The monitoring is done by using a hemochrome (International Technidyne Corp, Edison, NJ). A baseline ACT sample is obtained immediately after gaining access to the arterial system usually a 2 cc blood sample is drawn via the side arm of the catheter introducer sheath. At the end of the procedure, prior to removal of the sheath and/or catheter, a repeat ACT is measured. Protamine sulfate is then administered intravenously to reverse the heparin and normalize the ACT prior to the removal of the sheath or catheter. We give 20–35 mgr of protamine (depending on the patients age) over 10 minutes if the postprocedure ACT is greater than twice the baseline ACT. 10–20 mg is administered if the postprocedure ACT is less than twice the baseline. A repeat ACT is then measured 5–10 minutes after the administration of protamine and it is determined if a second dose is necessary. Once the normal ACT value is obtained the sheath of the catheter is removed and manual compression is applied to the arteriotomy site for 15–20 minutes.

7. Corticosteroids

The use of prophylactic steroids may be of benefit to reduce postembolization pain and swelling. One of us (PL) uses it routinely, administering 4 mg of Decadron TID 3 days after the procedure and tapered over the next 3 days. The other (AB) will only use it if some normal territory has to be occluded during the embolization. If needed, IV Solumedrol in doses from 16–125 mgr IV of 4–6 hours is used, depending on the patients age, weight and the indications.

8. Normal Physiology of the External Carotid Arteries

To best understand flow control as it relates to embolization a brief analysis of normal physiology of the external carotid artery is necessary.

The normal hemodynamic characteristics of the external carotid artery is the absence of diastolic flow as demonstrated by Doppler ultrasonography (Fig. 1.27). Therefore, emboli injection during diastole carries a higher risk of reflux. As a general principle, particulate emboli are injected in small intermittent injections during systole.

Du Boulay (1975) demonstrated in the baboon, the arterial autoregulation response down to a blood pressure of 60 mmHg.

This autoregulatory mechanism is noted to be more effective in the internal maxillary and pharyngo-occipital system, whereas in the facial artery no real autoregulatory mechanisms were noted. Vasoconstriction in response to hypertension is a function of large and medium sized arteries, while true autoregulation is seen in more distal branches.

Fig. 1.27. Doppler ultrasound of a normal external carotid artery. Note, the elevation during systole whereas there is no flow during diastole. See below for comparison of the normal internal Doppler with its diastolic flow

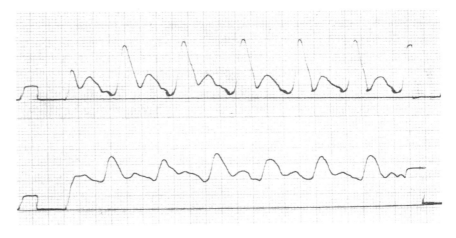

XII. Flow Control

Flow control refers to our ability of altering the flow characteristics in abnormal or normal territories. It may represent a deliberate augmentation, dimunition or arrest of flow, using the collateral circulation, with the aim of reaching a target, sparing normal noninvolved territories.

In our analysis of the functional anatomy of the head and neck we have illustrated the various anastomosis between the neighboring territories. Some have more dangers than others, as the anastomosis supply more vital territories: visual system, brain, peripheral nervous system, mucosal or musculocutaneous territories (Fig. 1.28). Anastomoses must be respected, their presence however does not represent a contraindication to embolization, but some type of control in the direction of their flow is mandatory for safe and proper embolization (Fig. 1.30).

1. Protection of a "Dangerous" Anastomosis

a) Mechanical Blockage

The simplest and most obvious way to protect a "dangerous" anastomosis is to mechanically block them. This can be done with a coil or a large particle such as gelfoam. After this anastomosis is blocked, embolization can be done with microparticles or other embolic agents (Figs. 1.15, 1.29).

b) Reversal of Flow in a "Dangerous" Anastomosis

Reversal of flow can be done with an occlusive balloon catheter proximal to the anastomosis or with a wedged catheter. The aim is to impose the flow through the dangerous anastomososis away form the dangerous territory (vertebral artery for example) and redirect the flow towards the "non-dangerous" distal target or lesion (Fig. 1.30A). This reversed flow will assist or "push" the emboli towards the abnormality. Prior to emboli injection various test hand injections are done to determine the tolerance and/or pressure needed not to fill the anastomosis. When one sees contrast material flowing towards the anastomosis, one stops or decreases the rate of injection; it can be observed under fluoroscopy that the contrast material is reversed and is washed out by nonopacified blood toward the abnormal territory (Fig. 1.30B). As the embolization begins, the contrast and emboli mixture is gently injected and monitored as the nonopacified reversed blood flow (away from) the vertebral washes the emboli distally toward the desired territory. As the embolization is progressing one starts noting that the washout is slowing and more careful injections are required. When the flow is significantly slowed, the embolization is stopped (Fig. 1.30C).

c) Protection of a "Dangerous" Anastomosis by Distal Catheterization

An obvious safety feature would be catheterization beyond the "dangerous" point. This is not always possible, but the introduction of coaxial open end guidewire and steerable microwires are improving our ability to accomplish this (Fig. 1.12) (see section on open end guidewires).

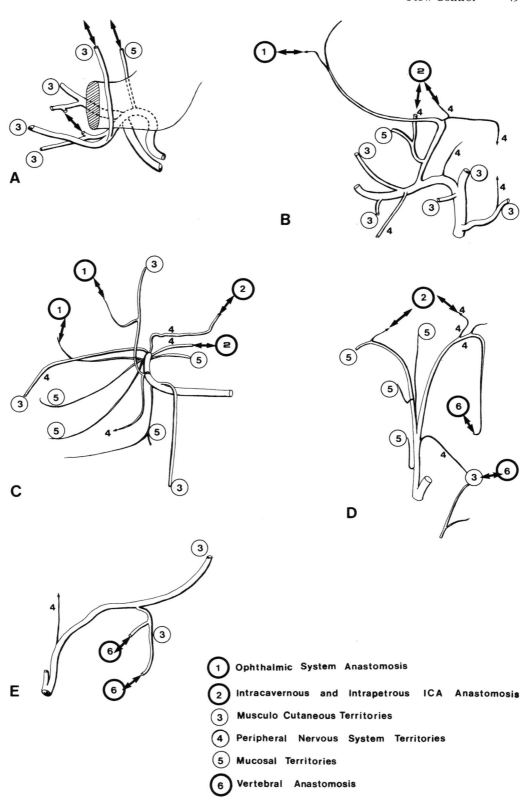

Fig. 1.28 A-E. Diagramatic representation of the various territories and the bidirectional flow through the collateral circulation. **A** Lingual and facial arteries. **B** Proximal internal maxillary artery. **C** Distal internal maxillary artery. **D** Ascending pharyngeal and cervical arteries. **E** Occipital artery

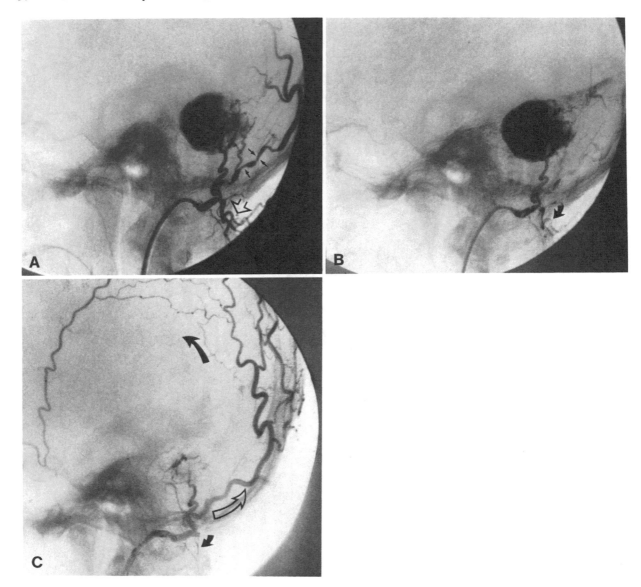

Fig. 1.29 A-C. Mechanical protection of a "dangerous" anastomosis with Gianturco coil. Hemangiopericytoma (also see Fig. 2.4). **A** Subtracted angiogram of the left occipital artery. Catheterization distal to the C 2 anastomosis *(open arrow)* could not be accomplished. While attempting distal catheterization, spasm in the occipital artery at and distal to the transmastoid branches was produced *(small arrows)*. **B** A minicoil (0.038–1–3) was used to block the "dangerous" anastomosis *(curved arrow)*. Note, the preferential flow towards the tumor with no filling of the normal distal occipital artery. Complete flow control exists and is dependent on the rate of injection. **C** Towards the end of the embolization, the "dangerous" anastomosis is still protected *(curved arrow)*, the tumor has been embolized with 40 microns gelfoam powder. At this pressure of injection, flow is antigrade to the distal occipital artery *(open curved arrow)*. Although powder has been used, thanks to the reversal of flow all the distal microanatomosis between the occipital and superficial temporal arteries *(curved arrow)* have been preserved

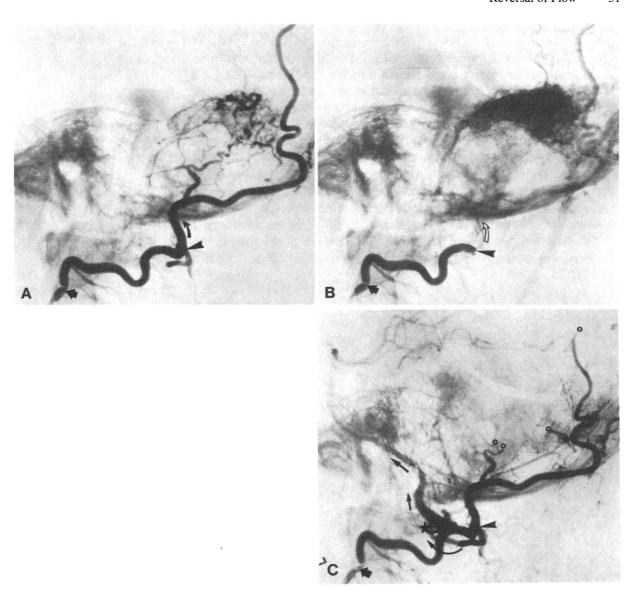

Fig. 1.30 A-C. Reversal of flow in a "dangerous" anastomosis. **A** Lateral subtraction angiogram of the left occipital artery supplying a meningiosarcoma invading the sigmoid sinus. The catheter is wedged in the occipital artery *(arrowhead)* obtaining flow control of the proximal segment of the occipital artery from the tip of the catheter to the C 2 anastomosis *(arrowhead)*. The increased pressure of injection forces contrast material towards the distal occipital artery *(curved arrow)*. **B** The injection is stopped, arrested contrast material is seen from the wedged catheter *(solid arrow)* until the C 2 anastomosis *(arrowhead)*. The nonopacified flow from the vertebral artery is reversed at C 2 and washes of the distal occipital artery *(open curved arrow)*. The resversed flow on C 2 can therefore be used to push the emboli into the tumor. **C** Post embolization control of the occipital artery, the tumor has been embolized with 40 microns gelfoam powder (○) while the anastomosis has been preserved. Note that at this rate of injection, the C 2 collateral has reserved its flow and fills now the vertebral artery *(star)* and basilary system *(arrows)*

2. Intralesional Flow Control

Monocompartmental vascular lesions such as some vascular malformations, some paragangliomas and some intratumoral AV fistula (Figs. 2.2;
5.12) may permit us to reach the nidus within the lesion through one,
feeding pedicle. This will permit us to use the less critical or "dangerous"
pedicle sparing the more vital one. To determine if this is possible prior to
embolization, a relatively high pressure, high volume injection is done with
the aim of overcoming the intralesional pressure to reflux into the other(s).

Multiple test injections with contrast material are done to determine the
rate of injection and to estimate the volume of embolic agent needed to
accomplish occlusion of the nidus without reflux into the "dangerous
vessels." This technique is only accomplished with liquid emboli such as
IBCA. We must emphasize that a good understanding of all the factors
involved is mandatory to accomplish this result safely (Figs. 3.5; 5.12;
10.19).

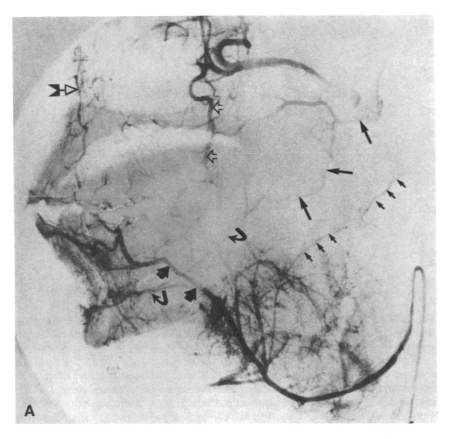

Fig. 1.31 A-C. Balloon flow reversal in a capillary-venous vascular malformation.
A Selective right facial injection demonstrates filling of the collateral circulation
with filling of the inferior to superior masseteric arteries *(small arrows)* transverse
facial *(arrows)* and distal facial arteries *(broad arrows)*, mid mental to inferior
dental *(broken arrows)* buccal to internal maxillary artery *(open arrowheads)* and
the infraorbital point *(flagged arrow)* with only modest opacification of a capillary
venous vascular malformation of the submental area. **B** Using a double lumen
occlusive balloon catheter in the proximal facial artery *(flagged arrows)*, one can fill
the capillary venous vascular malformation to best advantage. Note, the superior
ascending palatine circumferential artery *(open curved arrow)* and only very modest

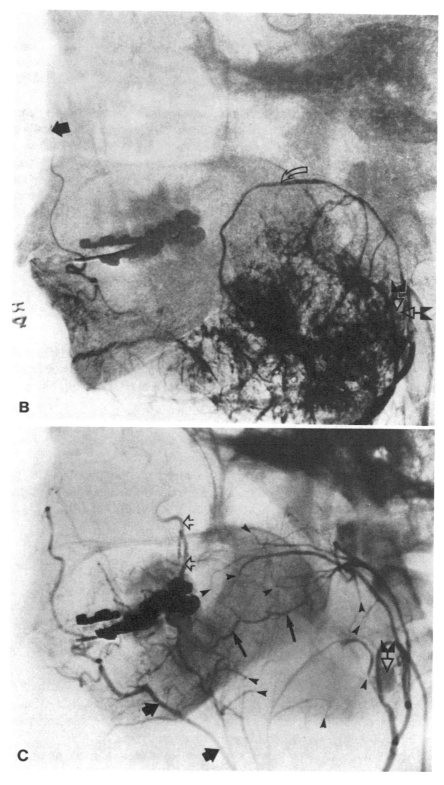

Fig. 1.31 (continued)
opacification of the distal facial artery. Under fluoroscopic monitoring, the reversal
of the flow through the collateral anastomotic pathways towards the lesion could be
seen. **C** This permitted an excellent microembolization with 40 microns gelfoam
powder *(arrowheads)* preserving the collateral circulation

3. Occlusive Balloon Flow Reversal

In hypervascular lesions that do not have a "sump" effect or when preferential flow does not exist, injection of emboli into a feeding pedicle may not reach the lesion and/or only partially occlude it. Many of the emboli will therefore enter normal territories.

Thanks to the ability of the collateral anastomosis to carry flow in either direction one can use a double lumen balloon catheter placed proximally at the origin of an artery such as the facial artery (Fig. 1.31). This will then force the collaterals from the maxillary, transverse facial, or opposite side to supply the facial territory (and therefore a lesion in its territory). One must have absolute control in the proximal facial trunk. If contrast materal is progressively injected, one can observe nonopacified blood "pushing" the contrast material into the lesion. If the right pressure of injection is used all of the contrast will then enter the abnormality, sparing the normal territory (Fig. 1.31B). The same maneuver is then repeated with the appropriate size of microparticles until the lesion is devascularized.

4. Functional Rearrangement of the Supply to a Territory

This is primarily used for rearrangement in malignant lesions prior to infusion chemotherapy with the need to infuse an entire territory through one single pedicle (see Chapter 5) or to disconnect a lesion with bilateral supply and to convert it to a unilateral one.

5. Surgical Flow Control

Surgical ligation of the anterior ethmoidal arteries or nasal branches of the ophthalmic artery is a very useful adjunct to lesion with dual supply; this will convert the lesion to a purely external carotid artery one (Fig. 8.13). It is also used for control in some cases of epistaxis.

XIII. Provocative Test

Primarily designed to test the safety of endovascular obliteration in a specific distribution; 3 territories are of importance:

a) Central nervous system, can be tested with 50 mg of sodium amytal and it is primarily used in brain and spinal cord work (see Vol. 4).

b) Peripheral nervous system: cranial nerve dysfunction in the distribution of external carotid branches can be tested with superselective infusion of 50 mg of cardiac xylocaine (Horton, 1985). It is also useful for pain control during the procedure and to prevent spasm.

c) Mucocutaneous territories: are primarily determined by anatomy. Discoloration of skin follows the superselective injection of a 60% concentration contrast agent, or the superselective injection of low concentration methylene blue (Djindjian, 1978), represent alternative solutions.

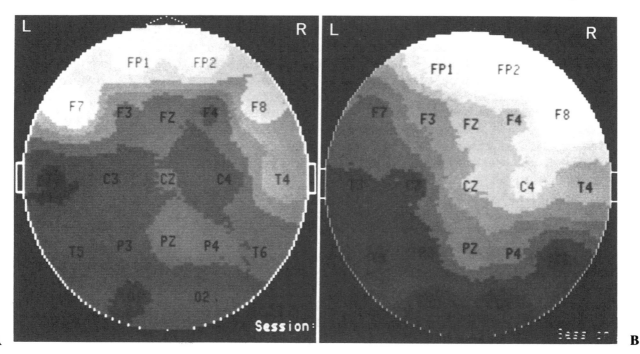

Fig. 1.32 A, B. EEG monitoring during carotid occlusion. **A** Axial view of the EEG wave activity at baseline. The lighter areas represent increased % in delta activity. **B** EEG monitoring 5 minutes after the left internal carotid artery was temporarily occluded with a double lumen balloon catheter under systemic heparinization. Note, the increase in the delta activity on the right (contralateral) middle cerebral and anterior cerebral territories. The patient had left sided weakness during ipsilateral carotid occlusion. The increased delta activity on the right (nonoccluded) side was interpreted as a hemodynamic steal towards the occluded side

XIV. Electrophysiological Monitoring (EPhM)

The use of EPhM is primarily used in spinal (Berenstein, 1982) or cerebral (Berenstein, 1985) embolizations (Vol. 4). In the craniofacial area the only present assistance is during the tolerance test of a carotid or vertebral artery, and the EEG can be of assistance by the increase in delta activity, as one of the earliest signs of poor cerebral perfusion (Sundt, 1984) (Fig. 1.32).

XV. Angiographic Equipment

For the most part, head and neck embolization can be performed with almost any conventional fluoroscopic unit; however, with available technology, the minimum equipment necessary for proper, safe and accurate surgical neuroangiography, is the use of optimal fluoroscopy with the largest possible field size, a C arm or biplane type fluoroscopic capabilities. Digital subtraction angiography with immediate life subtraction and road map capabilities, is a major advancement. All the optimal tube, small focal spot, film screen combination are all of importance but their description is beyond the scope of this text. However, the angiographic suite should be serviced as a conventional operating room.

XVI. Postembolization Care

In routine head and neck embolizations the usual precautions following a percutaneous femoral stick are followed namely by bed rest for 5 hours. In situations where detachable balloons are used or major cerebral arteries are occluded, bed rest for 24–48 hours is warranted as well as standing orders for antihemetics, as severe vomiting had dislodged a balloon on two occasions (Fig. 6.27). Analgesics for the most part are given on a PRN basis, as pain is usually not a problem. In the management of some patients with giant aneurysms or some patients with CCF (Fig. 6.4) severe headache will occur as the lesion is thrombosing.

These types of headaches will require heavier analgesia, including narcotics. In general, it lasts 3–5 weeks before subsiding. Following VAF repair, a soft neck collar is advisable for better stabilization.

XVII. Special Care

1. Neurological Deficit

In head and neck embolization, cerebral and/or ophthalmic complication may occur in 0.5–1% of cases. When it occurs close cooperation with clinicians familiar with the management of stroke is advisable. Although in general there is little that can be done, the use of volume expanders, hypertensive medications, or the need for EC-IC bypass (Fig. 1.6) should be considered in the individual situations.

The use of a recovery room and/or ICU with strict bed rest is advisable with patients undergoing occlusion of a major cerebral vessel (internal carotid, vertebral artery) (see Chapter 7).

2. Post-Op Swelling

In most arterial embolizations, swelling starts within 24 hours. Usually it represents embolization of normal territory (similar to trismus) und usually resolves spontaneoulsy in a few days; and respond to corticosteroids when needed. On the other hand, painless swelling after direct alcohol injections for venous lesions (see Vascular Malformations) is the rule. No treatment is generally needed, however, if there is a problem with closure of an eye or airway impairment, IV diurectics and postural drainage is indicated.

3. Skin Necrosis

If skin necrosis occurs in skin that is going to be part of the resection, no special care, except hygiene is needed (Figs. 1.21, 1.25). If in normal skin, it will heal spontaneously by granulation (Fig. 1.25). Only when a previously compromised territory is embolized, or if too large, grafting will be needed. In the authors experience, only on one occasion was grafting needed (see Fig. 10.12).

XVIII. Follow-Up

It is the responsibility of the surgical neuroangiographer to monitor the benefits or lack of benefits in his or her patients. Therefore periodic monitoring is advisable. The use of follow up angiography will depend on the primary problem (such as aneurysms or fistulas), individual and cultural environments. Particular cases and individual problems are discussed in each chapter.

CHAPTER 2

Dural and Bony Tumors

I. Introduction

Because of the rich blood supply of the dura and bone, tumors involving these structures are frequently hypervascular. The unique dual function of the dura as the periostium of the inner table of the skull, and as a protective covering for the central nervous system, makes tumors affecting the dura and/or bone of particular interest. Presenting complaints may involve central nervous system manifestations, or, if the lesion grows outward local changes in the bone, muscle or skin.

II. Meningiomas

1. Epidemiology

a) Origin

The term "meningioma" was introduced by Harvey Cushing in his 1922 Cavendish Lecture on tumors arising from the meninges. Although known to exist for many decades they had previously been called by a variety of names.

Meningiomas originate from cell elements that form the meninges, usually the arachnoid cells, packing the arachnoid villi, which protrude as finger like projections into the walls of the dural veins and sinuses. They may also arise from dural fibroblasts and pial cells (Rubinstein, 1972).

The most frequent sites of origin of these tumors are, therefore, those where the arachnoid villi are normally the most numerous i.e., the major dural sinuses and along the root sleeves of the existing spinal nerves.

Meningiomas may, however, originate anywhere along the arachnoid membrane. Rarely they may arise from stromal cells in the spaces that surround the perforating blood vessels or the intracerebral infoldings of the leptomeninges as they form the villi interposita and the stroma of the choroid plexus giving rise to intraventricular meningiomas. These rare extracalvareal or "ectopic" meningiomas are believed to arise from ectopic arachnoid cell inclusions.

b) Incidence

Meningiomas account for 13–18% of all primary intracranial tumors and 20–25% of intraspinal tumors (Rubinstein, 1982). They occur at any age, but typically affect adults between 20–60 years of age with a peak incidence at age 45. In adults, intracranial meningiomas are more frequent in females, with a female to male ratio of 2.5:1 (Kepes, 1982). It is interesting to note that this female predominance applies primarily to symptomatic middle age adults. At the extremes of life one does not find these features.

Wood (1957), in his study of meningiomas encountered incidentally at autopsy, found a female to male ratio of 1:1. Sano (1981) and Deen (1982), in their review of meningiomas in patients under 20 years of age, found a female to male ratio of 1:1. The rapid growth of meningiomas during pregnancy was noted as early as 1929 by Cushing and Eisenhart and in 1958, by Bickerstaff; tumors in these women are most frequent near the sella turcica, and their clinical behavior is probably related to their proximity to the optic nerve and chiasm; the changes in visual acuity produced by tumor growth are quickly noticed by the patients.

As with other tumors the relationship of sex hormones to tumor growth is a very interesting and puzzling phenomena. One may argue that the changes which occur are secondary to direct hormonal activity of the tumor, such as occurs with breast or endometrial cancers, or that they are due to hydropic swelling with vacualization, suggesting tissue edema (Weyand 1951). It is difficult to estimate the relative importance of tumor enlargement by hormonal factors versus the role of cerebral edema during the hyperemia of pregnancy. Michelson and New (1969) demonstrated a decrease in mass effect of a frontal meningioma after pregnancy was terminated. Unfortunately this was reported prior to the era of CT, and the reduced mass effect documented by serial angiography may have been due to a decrease in white matter edema and not tumor size. Even in carcinoma of the breast or endometrium, where estrogens are thought to play a role in the formation or growth rate of the tumor, these effects are believed to be slow and cummulative. Probably some combination of hormonal stimulation and hydropic swelling contribute to the growth of meningiomas and the edema which is frequently associated.

c) Association of Meningiomas with Other Tumors

Breast Carcinoma: There are numerous reports of patients suffering from both of these tumors. Schoenberg (1975), in his analysis of a possible relationship between nervous system tumors and primary cancers in other sites found a statistically significant correlation only between meningiomas and breast carcinoma. Fenyes (1956) reported a patient with carcinoma of the breast and a cerebellar metastasis who at autopsy was found to have multiple meningiomas; one of these harbored a tumor embolus from the carcinoma. This association between meningioma and breast cancer is of clinical importance, patients with known breast cancer who develop symptoms and signs of an intracranial mass must be evaluated very carefully, as the cerebral lesion may be a curable lesion rather than a metastasis (Haar, 1972).

Multiple meningiomas occur incidentally in 1–2% of cases (Kepes, 1982) but are typically associated with the central form of von Recklinghausen's neurofibromatosis, which also has a hight incidence of neurinomas and gliomas. The occurrence of gliomas or other central nervous system tumors in association with meningiomas in other patients is felt to be coincidental (Russel and Rubinstein, 1977).

d) Sex Hormone Receptors in Meningiomas

Donnell (1979) demonstrated estrogen receptors in four out of six meningiomas, at a high level in two. Interestingly, one of the four patients with a positive tumor was a male. Poisson (1980) studied 22 meningiomas; he found estrogen receptors in 59% and receptors for progesterone in all 22 cases. This may explain why meningiomas appear to grow more rapidly during pregnancy. Schnegg (1981) found androgen receptors in two of ten patients with meningiomas; both were postmenopausal females.

These sex hormone receptors may be important in cases of nonresectable, partially resected, or in malignant meningiomas, as some form of hormonal therapy may play a role in the management of these patients in the future.

e) Chromosomal Patterns in Meningiomas

The relationship between chromosomal abnormalities and meningiomas has interested many investigators. Robbins (1979) states that most human cancers are aneuploid. Zang (1967) reported 8 meningiomas cultured for 4–9 days. The karyotypes showed loss of a chromosome from the 22nd pair in the G group (monosomy G) suggesting a tendency for meningiomas to lose chromosomes during their karyotypic evolution. Benedict (1970), in studying recurrent meningiomas and their incidence of malignancy, suggests that this karyotypic aberration may prove useful in the future prediction of malignancy (See discussion on Malignant Meningiomas).

f) Meningiomas in Children (Fig. 2.1)

Meningiomas occur in frequently in children; they represent from 1.1% (Taptas, 1961) to 2.3% (Crous, 1972) of all meningiomas and less than 2% of all intracranial tumors in children (Kepes, 1982).

Congenital meningiomas are even more rare, but a few cases have been reported (Kepes, 1982).

Childhood meningiomas have some special characteristics:
1. Higher incidence of malignancy: a 33%–38% incidence of meningiosarcomas has been reported by Crause (1972), Russel and Rubinstein (1977), Sano (1981) (Fig. 2.1).
2. Relatively high incidence of intraventricular tumors: 27.2% in Kandel's (1966) and 11.1% in Sano's (1982) series.
3. High incidence of cyst formation within the tumor (Sano, 1982).
4. No sex predilection.
5. High incidence of association with the central form of neurofibromatosis (Deen, 1982).
6. High incidence (39%) of tumor recurrence (Fig. 2.1E) (Deen, 1982).
7. Decreased 15 year survival (68%) (Deen, 1982).
8. Relatively poor surgical results reported even in the presence of benign tumors (Kepes, 1982).

g) Familial Occurrence

It has long been recognized that patients with neurofibromatosis, a hereditary autosomal dominant condition, are suspectible to meningiomas which are often multiple.

However, there have been reports of multiple occurrence of meningiomas in families without stigmata of von Recklinghausen disease (Kepes, 1982). In most cases, however, it is probably justified to assume the presence of neurofibromatosis with incomplete expression in these families.

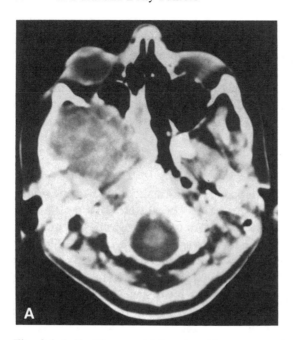

Fig. 2.1 A-E. 16 year old female with a recurrent malignant meningioma with extracranial extension into the subtemporal fossa and face. **A** Axial CT after intravenous administration of contrast material. Note, the extension to the right subtemporal and pterygoid region of a homogenously enhancing lesion. **B** Lateral subtraction angiogram in late arterial phase demonstrates the marked tumor hypervascularity, its intracranial, epidural extension into the middle cranial fossa, parasellar and cavernous area *(small arrows)*, as well as its downward and anterior extension to the face. **C** Lateral subtraction angiogram of the distal internal maxillary artery *(arrow)* shows the tumor hypervascularity to best advantage. Note, the inhomogeneous stain with some puddling but no arteriovenous shunting. Note, flow reversal in the collateral circulation via the ascending palatine, buccal and infra-orbital arteries *(curved arrows)*. **D** Control postembolization (PVA preoperative) angiogram of the ascending palatine artery *(arrow)* demonstrating filling of the ascending palatine and buccal arteries *(curved arrows)* in an antegrade fashion. There is no opacification of the tumor. **E** Eight months later the significant recurrence of the tumor. (Same patient as Fig. 2.21)

h) Incidence, Prevalence and Mortality of Meningiomas

Benign meningiomas are not infrequently found incidentally at autopsy. The larger symptomatic tumors are usually removed during life and will therefore fail to show up in post mortem statistics.

Choi (1970) in his epidemiological study of central nervous system neoplasms found that only 6.8% of patients dying from brain tumors had meningiomas.

i) Etiology of Human Meningiomas

It is probably accurate to say that the etiology of most naturally occurring meningiomas is yet unknown. Nevertheless, there are some factors that may play a role in their occurrence:

1. *Genetic Factors:* As we have seen in the central form of neurofibromatosis there is a definite genetic factor.
2. *Trauma:* Cushing (1938) introduced a theory linking head trauma and meningiomas, but this association has not since been substantiated and is not felt to be valid.

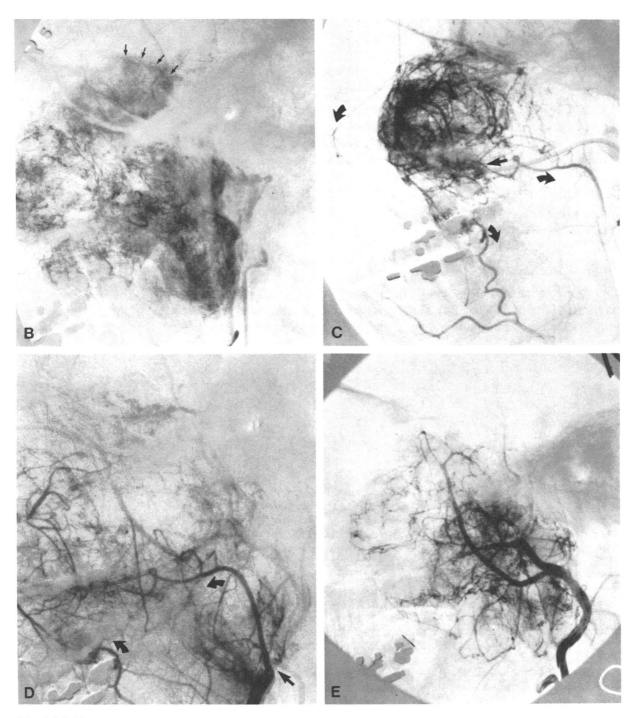

Fig. 2.1 B-E

3. *Radiation:* There is definitely an increased incidence of meningiomas in patients who have received either high dose irradiation for other neoplasms (Kepes 1982) or low dose radiation to the scalp for the treatment of tinnea capitis (Modan 1974). Furthermore, Soffer in 1983 demonstrated that post irradiation meningiomas have distinctive characteristics. They typically occur at the site of maximal irradiation and demonstrate the following differences from spontaneous meningiomas:

1. More rapid growth and aggressive biological behavior.
2. Higher incidence of calvareal locations.
3. Higher proportion of multiplicity.
4. Higher recurrence rate.
5. Higher proportion of histological malignancy.

The time interval between radiation therapy and the clinical manifestation of meningiomas has been reported to be from 5–25 years (Kepes, 1982, p. 13). We have seen a mesenchymal chondrosarcoma of the petrous cavernous area in a young female 4 years after radiation therapy, which rapidly increased its rate of growth (Fig. 2.2). This tumor was considered a nonresectable meningioma and was radiated without a tissue diagnosis, but the possibility of malignant transformation of a benign lesion must also be considered.

j) Oncogenic Viruses

Oncogenic viruses have been used with success to induce meningeal tumors in animals (Kepes, 1982, p. 10). However, there is no conclusive evidences that oncogenic viruses play a role in the induction of these tumors in humans (Kepes 1982, p. 14).

Fig. 2.2 A-H. 23 year old female who in 1980 presented with a vascular tumor in the cavernous-petrous area and was treated with radiation therapy at that time. Proven mesenchymal chondrosarcoma (1984) (see also Fig. 5.12, same patient). **A** Lateral carotid angiogram of 1980 demonstrates narrowing of the internal carotid artery starting in its precavernous segment *(arrowhead)* with some hypervascularity. **B** Lateral subtraction angiogram of the distal external carotid artery in 1980 demonstrates only ᠌minimal hypervascularity from the petrosal branch of the middle meningeal artery *(arrowhead)*. **C** 4 years later the patient was referred to us because of rapid increase in the size of the tumor. Lateral digital subtraction angiogram (DSA) of the middle meningeal artery *(arrow)*. Note, the marked change in the tumor hypervascularity. **D** Lateral DSA of the left internal carotid artery after a balloon *(open arrowhead)* has been detached distal to the cavernous branches to protect the brain. Note, the development of a malignant fistula between the petrous segment of the internal carotid artery and the tumor *(arrowheads)*. This tumor-fistula eroded both the petrous carotid and middle meningeal arteries producing an unusual anastomosis. **E** Lateral film of the skull following 95% ethanol infusion of the tumor bed after the distal internal carotid artery was protected by a detachable balloon *(open arrow)*. A second balloon was placed more proximally to trap the carotid artery *(arrow)*. Note, the stagnant alcohol metrizamide mixture in the tumor bed *(small arrows)*. The middle meningeal (Fig. 2.2C) accessory meningeal and ascending pharyngeal were also treated with ethanol (not shown). **F** Contrast enhanced CT prior to ethanol infusion shows tumor filling the temporal fossa, and suprasellar cistern and invading the petrous bone. **G** CT 1 week after the ethanol treatment. Note the significant reduction in size of the infused area. **H** CT follow up 16 months later (contrast could not be given for technical factors). The patient underwent partial resection of tumor which was mostly necrotic and remained stable. There has been subsequent calcification in most of the remaining tumor

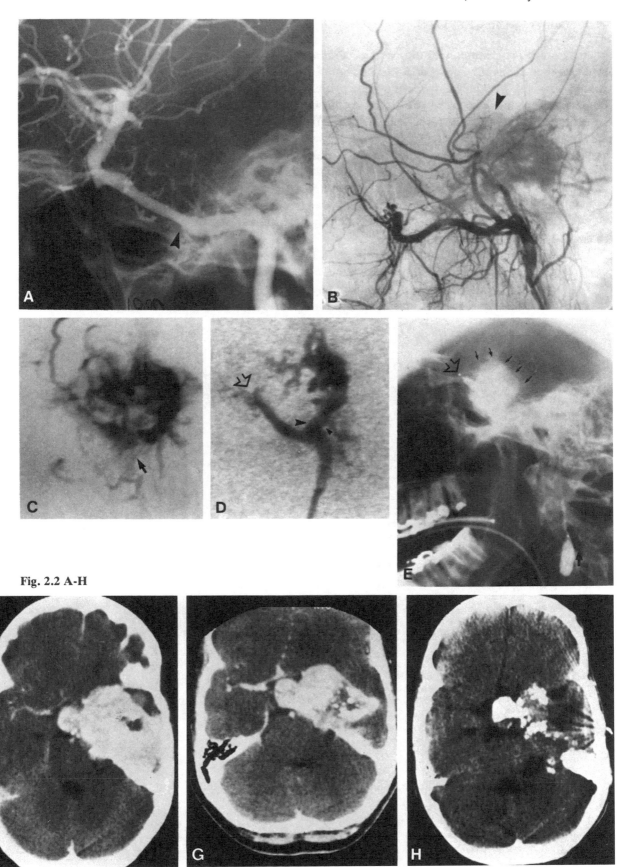

Fig. 2.2 A-H

2. Pathology (Rubinstein, 1972)

Meningiomas are characteristically well circumscribed globular or lobu-lated tumors which are clearly demarcated from the brain. They are firm, tough, grayish, or pinkish gray and rather homogeneous. They may compress adjacent structures, but do not infiltrate neural tissue with exception of the very rare sarcomatous type. Calcium, bone, or rarely cartilage can be found in them. In general, necrosis is not present in meningiomas, except in the rare malignant type, and spontaneous hemorr-hage and cyst formation within the tumor are also unusual. Arachnoidal entrapments may occur at the periphery of the tumor. Hyperostosis of the adjacent skull may be the presenting features; it represents extensive new bone formation which may or may not be associated with invasion of the marrow spaces by meningioma cells.

The microscopic appearance is highly variable. The fundamental cell of origin, however, is the meningothelial arachnoid cell.

The histological variants have been designated by the different structural patterns. Two major classifications exist: That adapted by Russell and

Table 2.1. Classification of meningiomas (Russel and Rubinstein 1977)

Syncytial
Transitional
Fibroblastic
Angioblastic
Malignant

Table 2.2. WHO classification of tumors of meningeal and related tissues (Kepes 1982)

A. Meningioma
  1. Meningiothelioma (endotheliomatous, syncytial arachnotheliomatous)
  2. Fibrous (Fibroblastic)
  3. Transitional (mixed)
  4. Psammomatous
  5. Angiomatous
  6. Hemangioblastic
  7. Hemangiopericytic
  8. Papillary
  9. Anaplastic (malignant) meningioma

B. Meningeal sarcomas
  1. Fibrosarcoma
  2. Polymorphic cell sarcoma
  3. Primary meningeal sarcomatosis

C. Xanthomatous tumors
  1. Fibroxamthoma
  2. Xanthosarcoma (malignant fibroxanthoma)

D. Primary melanotic tumors
  1. Melanoma
  2. Meningeal melanomatosis

E. Others

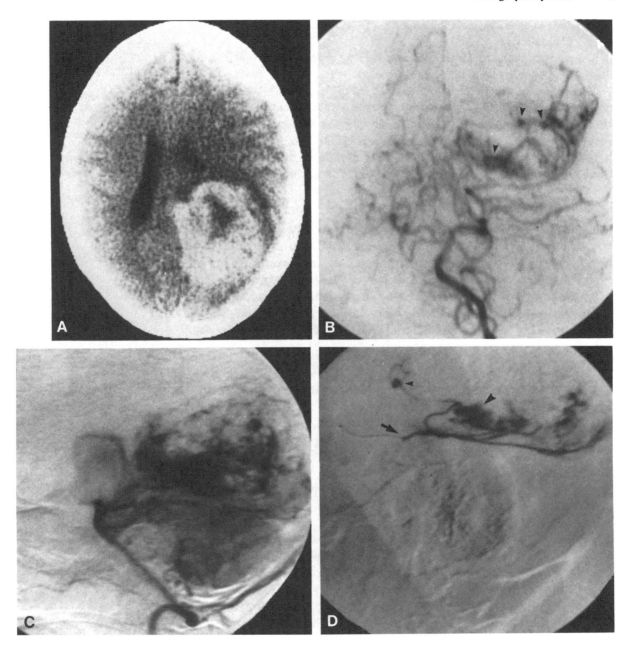

Fig. 2.3 A-D. 42 year old female with relatively rapid onset of severe headaches, papilledema and a homonymous hemianopsia. Histologically proven hemangiopericytoma. **A** Axial CT after intravenous administration of contrast material. Note the lobulated irregular tumor with a central area of decreased absorption coefficient suggesting necrosis, and the peritumoral edema. **B** DSA of the left vertebral artery in frontal view, mid-arterial phase. Note the two branches of the posterior cerebral artery supplying a hypervascular tumor which demonstrates some puddling *(arrowheads)*. **C** Late arterial phase of the left vertebral artery injection in lateral projection showing the inhomogeneous tumor blush. **D** Lateral DSA of the superselective catheterization of one of the two posterior cerebral branches supplying the tumor with a calibrated leak microballoon catheter *(arrow)*. The feeding vessels are not markedly hypertrophied and show the tumor puddling to best advantage *(arrowheads)*. For management (see Fig. 2.23) additional dural supply from the left occipital artery was present (not shown)

Rubinstein (Table 2.1) and a more comprehensive one proposed by the WHO (Table 2.2).

The various histological variants exemplify the multipotentiality of the arachnoid cell from which these are derived.

Except for the rare atypical examples [the papillary type (vide infra)] and possibly the angioblastic type, no prognostic significance can be attached to these histological variants. A description of these variants is beyond the scope of this text. With the possible exception of the angioblastic or hemangiopericytoma type (Fig. 2.3), the different histologic patterns do not have distinguishing radiologic or angiographic features.

a) Growth and Spread

Meningiomas are characteristically benign; they are slow growing, circumscribed, and do not invade the compressed brain, but may infiltrate or invade other supportive mesodermal tissues. They may invade the dura on both sides, dural sinuses and their tributaries, the bone marrow, or when they extend outside of the cranial cavity, the pericranial musculature and other tissues including the skin may be involved. Inferior frontal meningiomas invade the optic nerve sheath and infiltrate the extra-ocular muscles.

b) Malignant Meningioma

The rare highly invasive meningioma may be considered to be sarcomatous (Fig. 2.1) and cannot always be differentiated from the primary meningeal sarcoma (Fig. 1.30). This unusual tumor although circumscribed and grossly similar to other meningiomas, may have atypical cytologic features and in some patients gives rise to extracranial metastasis. In many cases. however, the future behavior of an individual tumor cannot be predicted by its histological appearance. As stated previously, cytogenetic studies may prove useful in the future to distinguish those tumors that will behave aggressively (Thomas, 1981). At present, however, one must still rely on clinical and pathologic criteria; malignancy is diagnosed in the presence of a history of rapid recurrence over histological anaplasia and metastases. Mitotic figures are exceptional in typical meningiomas and if present in large number indicate aggressive growth. Although any histological variant may behave aggressively, the angioblastic and/or hemangiopericytoma type is particularly likely to do so (Fig. 2.3). Papillary formation or transformation to a papillary form of meningioma has been recognized as a reliable sign of malignancy or malignant transformation (Kepes, 1982) and carries a poor prognosis with a high incidence of local recurrence and distal metastasis (Kepes, 1981).

In general, features suggestive but not specific for malignancy include: necrosis, mitosis, increased cellularity, invasion of small blood vessels within the tumor, anaplasia, and cerebral invasion (Kepes, 1982).

The presence of distant metastasis is incontrovertible proof of malignancy, although patients with distal metastasis may live for years.

Strang (1964) estimated the incidence of distant metastasis to be about 0.1% and metastasis within the neural axis to be even less common. Most metastatic tumors have histological hallmarks of malignancy, although a few of them appear histologically benign both in the primary tumor and its metastasis.

Three possible mechanisms of spread have been postulated:

1. Seeding through CSF: This is very rare and only 12 cases of such spread have been reported (Kepes, 1982); nine had histological features of malignancy, whereas three did not. Conceivably, surgical intervention could mobilize clusters of tumor cells and cause subarachnoid seeding. Eight of these 12 reported patients had previous surgery, but 4 did not. Six (50%) had additional extraneural implants. If one considers the thousands of surgical interventions for these tumors, the role of surgical mobilization of tumor cells cannot be considered significant. Exfoliative meningioma cells are generally not found in the cytological analysis of CSF of patients with meningiomas (Kepes 1982).

2. Extraneural metastasis: There is a slight male predominance of 1.2:1, and although as a whole metastases are more frequently seen in adults; they proportionally are more common in children. The site of the primary tumor is of limited significance, as it is the history of previous surgery. However, invasion of the scalp by the primary tumor may facilitate metastasis to cervical lymph nodes. Invasion of major dural sinuses has a questionable role, as this phenomena is so frequent in benign meningiomas. The most common sites for distal metastasis are the lungs, liver, lymph nodes, bone, pleura, kidney, pancreas, thyroid, mediastinum, breast, urinary bladder, thymus, superior vena cava, heart, stomach, colon, skin, vulva, thigh, finger, ocular fundus, and adrenal gland.

   Most, although not all, reported patients with metastatic meningiomas also had local recurrence.

3. Local recurrence: Although not properly classified as metastasis, local recurrence is the most common presentation of malignant meningiomas and occurs far more frequently than distal metastasis.

c) Angioblastic Meningioma and/or Hemangiopericytoma (Figs. 2.3, 2.4)

Some controversy exists regarding the inclusion of the meningeal hemangiopericytoma in the meningioma group (Kepes 1982, Rubinstein 1972).

Electron microscopic studies by Houten (1977) showed some features to be common to both meningothelial and hemangiopericytic tumors.

All authors, however, concur that this group of meningeal tumors exhibits the most malignant behavior of the meningiomalike tumors. Jaaskelainen (1985) reviewed their experience in 21 patients with hemangiopericytomas. He found an incidence of 1.9% among his 936 meningiomas; a comparable figure of 1.6% was reported in Jellinger's series with a higher incidence in males (1.4:1) and a younger mean age of 38 years. 86% were supratentorial, and there was a higher incidence of occipital lesions. They were frequently attached to the sinus (Fig. 2.4) and bled profusely at operation. All 21 primary tumors were solitary, but 2 patients hat multiple recurrences. The recurrence rate was 19% after the first operation and 43% after the second operation in Jaaskelainen's series; an 80% recurrence rate was reported in 1975 by Jellinger. Operative mortality was as high as 24% due to uncontrollable bleeding. Distant metastases occurred in 14% of Jaaskelainen's series and in up to 23% in Jellinger's series. Radiotherapy although not proven, is thought to be of some value (Fukui, 1977; Cerella, 1982; and Jaaskelainen in 1985). None of the 3 hemangiopericytomas

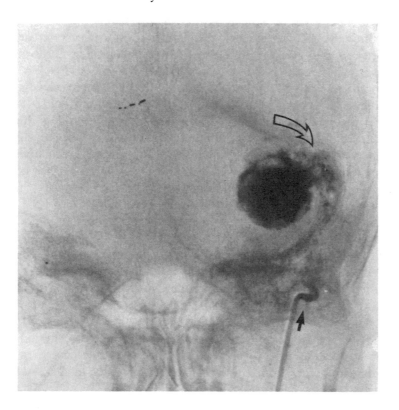

Fig. 2.4. Angioblastic meningioma, sometimes called hemangiopericytoma; in the posterior fossa with extension into the sigmoid sinus. Frontal selective subtraction angiogramm of the occipital artery *(arrow)*. Late arterial phase. A well circumscribed highly vascular tumor is seen attached to the inferior border of the sigmoid sinus with some tumor blush extending into the sinus *(open curved arrow)*, confirmed at surgery. The patient was embolized with gelfoam powder and the tumor was surgically removed (same patient as Fig. 1.29)

Fig. 2.5 A, B

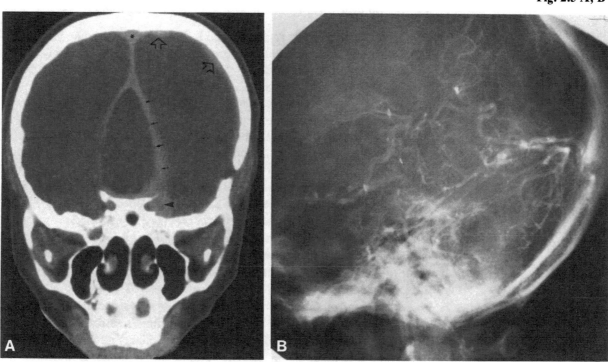

Fig. 2.5 A-D. Meningiomatosis. **A** Representative CT scan in coronal view after intravenous administration of contrast material demonstrates marked thickening of the free margin of the tentorium *(arrows)*, left cavernous area *(arrowhead)* as well as multiple areas of thickening and lobulation of the dural surfaces *(open arrowhead)*. There was involvement of the sinuses by tumor *(asterisk)*. Biopsy of dural and tentorial surfaces demonstrated meningeal infiltration. **B** Lateral angiogram of the left vertebral artery in late venous phase which demonstrates multiple collateral venous pathways with complete obliteration of the occipital portion of the superior sagittal sinus and confluent sinus by tumor invasion. **C** Lateral subtraction of the left internal carotid artery of the posterior portion of the superior sagittal sinus with collateral venous drainage towards cavernous sinus. **D** Lateral subtraction angiogramm of the middle meningeal artery which demonstrated tumor blush in the region of the torcular and the sigmoid sinuses *(small arrowheads)*

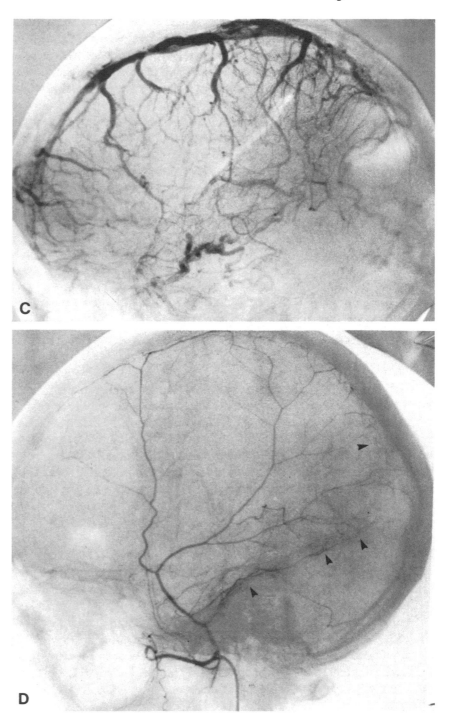

reported by Hayword (1983) had progesterone receptors; this contrasts the almost invariable presence of these receptors in all other histological types of meningiomas.

Marc (1975) and Jaaskelainen (1985) reviewed the angiographic features of hemangiopericytomas and found a high incidence of dual supply from the meningeal and cortical arteries, a hypervascular network of small corkscrew tumor vessels, an intense persistent blush and absence of early venous drainage (Fig. 2.3). This angiographic pattern is best appreciated by superselective angiography of both dural and pial vessels (Fig. 2.3 and Fig. 1.29). It correlates with Angervall's (1978) pictures of the microangioarchitecture of hemangiopericytomas which demonstrated that numerous capillaries are responsible for the intense tumor stain and thin walled channels which show up as corkscrew vessels.

Preoperative irradiation, as suggested by Fukui to reduce vascularity, is felt to be indicated primarily because the vascular supply from cortical vessels makes these tumors unfavorable for embolization. Berenstein and Ransohoff (1985) have proven that it is possible and safe to superselectively catheterize and embolize some of these cortical branches (Fig. 2.3D). Embolization of hemangiopericytomas would provide a major benefit, as the effects of radiation therapy are on these tumors controversial. Yamakama (1980) reported positive tumor response to radiation therapy: however, Enzinger (1976) and Mira (1977) felt that a significant number of these tumors do not respond. Jaaskelainen in 1985 reported that only one of 3 tumors responded to radiation therapy. Major disadvantages of preoperative radiation therapy include the risk of skin atrophy which impairs wound healing, risk of secondary induced neoplasia and the length of time necessary before the effect on the local blood vessels occurs (Steiner 1984).

d) Meningioangiomatosis

This is a rare condition in which a portion of the cerebral cortex is diffusely involved with an ingrowth of both meningothelial cells and blood vessels, with a variable ratio of the two. These lesions do not behave in a malignant fashion. Indeed, they are probably more of a hamartomatous than a true neoplastic lesion (Kepes, 1982) and are frequently but not always associated with the central form of neurofibromatosis (Rubinstein). It presents in the second or third decade of life, frequently with focal epilepsy, and may show cortical calcification on CT. The frontal and temporal gyri are most frequently involved.

e) Meningeal Meningiomatosis

Rubinstein describes another variant which he calls meningeal meningiomatosis or primary sarcomatosis. This is a multifocal neoplastic disease that involves the leptomeninges diffusely without the presence of a definitive mass (Fig. 2.5); it presents mainly in infants and children and clinically resembles the course of meningo encephalitis. It is frequently accompanied by small nodules of subarachnoid tumor at various sites along the cerebral spinal axis. Microscopically they may be indistinguishable from the polymorphic type of intracranial sarcoma.

3. Clinical Presentation

Meningiomas, for the most part, are slow growing neoplasms. Earle's (1969) review of the Frazier-Grant collection in 1969 showed the average length of time between the onset of symptoms and the diagnosis of tumor to be 2 1/2 years.

Headaches, visual impairment, and focal seizures are the most common complaints, in that order; seizures are usually the first symptom of meningiomas involving the convexity.

Most of the clinical symptoms and signs in patients with meningiomas are caused by local effects of the tumor mass, except perhaps with "en plaque" meningiomas. There is always some pressure on the underlying tissues with resulting damage to cortex or other parts of the brain.

The tumor may be large enough or may grow rapidly enough to produce increased intracranial pressure. Other effects include vascular occlusion, either venous or arterial, and hemorrhage or cyst formation in adjacent tissue. Meningiomas may also affect more distant portions of the brain, e. g. incisural obstruction with resultant hydrocephalus.

Some "indirect" effects may be due to local pressure on the pituitary gland or hypothalamus, with endocrine dysfunction (Korsgaard, 1976) or diencephalic syndromes of emaciation in children (Campiche, 1972).

"Distant" effects that are derived from the mere presence of the tumor or its chemical constituents may be seen. Mahaley (1971) found some degree of immunologic anergy in 17 patients with meningiomas which did not improve after removal of the tumor. In the same group of patients lymphopenia and a decrease in humoral antibodies was also present. Mazzei (1976) found tetany and hypocalcemia in one patient which disappeared after removal of the tumor. The significance of these distant manifestations (Kepes, 1982) are beyond the scope of this text.

Significant symptoms related to the specific locations of these tumors will also be present. We will therefore review the sites of presentation without reviewing the obvious symptoms that they will produce however, in specific sites important diagnostic features will be pointed out.

a) Sites

The most frequent site of intracranial meningiomas is the parasagittal region (Figs. 2.6, 2.7, 2.16), followed by the lateral cerebral convexity (Fig. 2.8). A significant number of tumors arise from the falx cerebri and these may extend laterally on both sides of the dura, or anteriorly into the

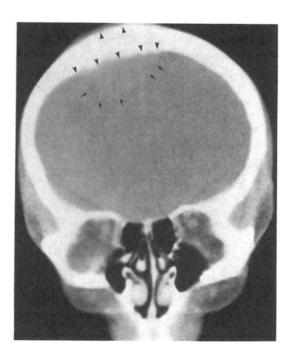

Fig. 2.6. Parasagittal meningioma. Axial CT with bony window demonstrates a parasagittal tumor (arrows) with bony hyperostosis that crosses the midline and extends into the extracranial soft tissues (arrowheads)

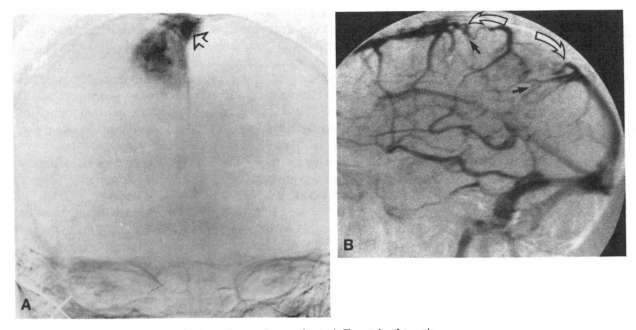

Fig. 2.7 A, B. Parasagittal meningioma in another patient. **A** Frontal subtraction angiogram of the left middle meningeal artery in late phase showing a right parasagittal tumor. Note, the tumor blush on the right side as well as a dense tumor blush in the superior sagittal sinus *(open arrowhead)*. **B** Lateral DSA demonstrating occlusion of the parietal portion of the superior sagittal sinus *(open curved arrows)* with collateral venous bridges *(arrows)*. To properly document sinus occlusion filling of both carotid arteries is necessary either by high volume angiography or manual compression. In addition, collateral bridging veins to explain cerebral venous drainage have to be documented

Fig. 2.8 A, B

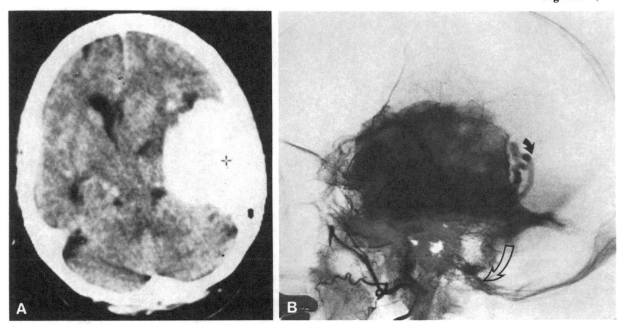

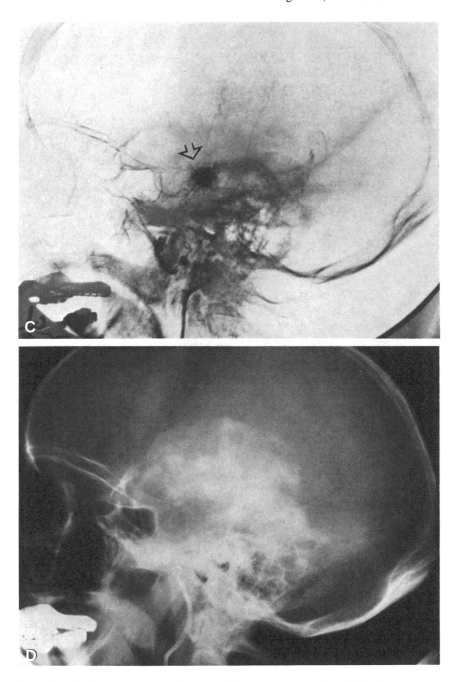

Fig. 2.8 A-E. Convexity meningioma. **A** Contrast enhanced axial CT demonstrates a relatively well circumscribed homogeneously enhancing hyperdense lesion (+) associated with minimal irregularity in its most anterior medial portion and a moderate amount of surrounding edema. Note, the significant shift of midline structures. **B** Lateral subtraction angiogram of the middle meningeal injection, late phase. The tumor was exclusively supplied by the middle meningeal artery. Note, the homogeneous tumor blush compatible with the CT appearance. Note, a dural venous structure draining the tumor *(curved arrow)* and filling the sigmoid sinus *(open curved arrow)*. **C** Lateral subtraction angiogram after microembolization with gelfoam powder. 95% of the tumor blush has disappeared. Note, a small area of stasis *(open arrowhead)*. **D** Plain film of the skull in lateral view showing the stagnant gelfoam powder and contrast material mixture showing a cast of the embolized tumor (compare to **B**).

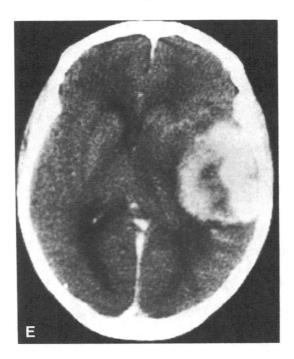

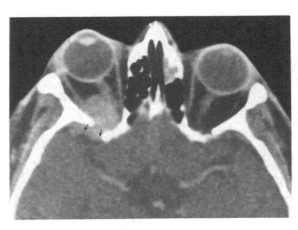

Fig. 2.8. E CT scan 12 hours after embolization. Note the intratumoral lucencies and decrease in midline shift. At surgery a completely avascular necrotic well circumscribed tumor was found (see Fig 1.14)

Fig. 2.9. "Dumbell" orbital tumor. Axial CT at the level of the orbits demonstrates a well circumscribed homogenously enhancing mass which is primarily in the orbit with extension into the middle cranial fossa in a "Dumbell" manner *(small arrows)*. Supply to this tumor location is usually ophthalmic in its intraorbital part, but the middle meningeal artery may reach part of the intracranial extension

orbit (see Intraorbital Meningiomas) to form the so called "dumbell" tumor (Fig. 2.9). Another frequent location is the sphenoid ridge (Fig. 2.10) and tuberculum sellae. Other sites include the olfactory groove (Fig. 14.8, Vol. 1., p 327), cerebellopontine angle, petrous ridge (Fig. 2.11) (this may be at the cavum of Meckel, which presents clinically with a Vth nerve dysfunction) or the peritorcular area. Less frequently seen are those on the lower surface of the tentorium cerebelli, the cerebellar convexity in the posterior fossa, and the foramen magnum (Fig. 2.12) and clivus (Fig. 2.13).

With exception of the malignant form and hemangiopericytoma, meningiomas more often involve the anterior half of the cranial cavity than the posterior half.

In all locations the tumor tends to be related to a major dural venous sinus (Figs. 2.4–2.7). Those arising in the convexity abut the sagittal sinus in about 50% of cases (Figs. 2.6, 2.7, 2.16).

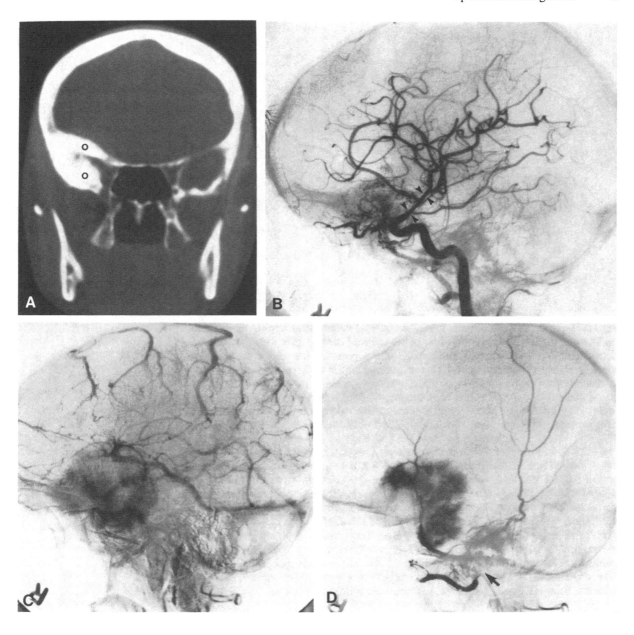

Fig. 2.10 A-D. Sphenoid Region Meningioma presenting with marked hyperostosis and narrowing of the superior orbital fissure with exophthalmus and ophthalmoplegia. **A** Axial CT with bony windows demonstrates the encroachment of the fissure by marked hyperostosis of bone (○). Significant intracranial extension was seen in the conventional axial CT with soft tissue window (not shown). **B** Lateral subtraction angiogram of the internal carotid artery in mid arterial phase. Note, the significant narrowing of the supraclinoid carotid artery *(arrowheads)*. Tumor blush could be seen anterior, posterior, medial, and lateral to the carotid artery. An important consideration is to differentiate compression from encasement. **C** Late phase of the common carotid injection demonstrating the homogeneous tumor stain lasting far into the venous phase without AV shunting. **D** Lateral subtraction angiogram of the middle meningeal artery *(arrow)*. Note, the different compartment opacified by the middle meningeal artery. The most anterior medial portion was supplied by the ILT and ethmoidal arteries as shown in **B**

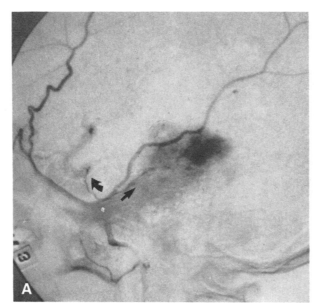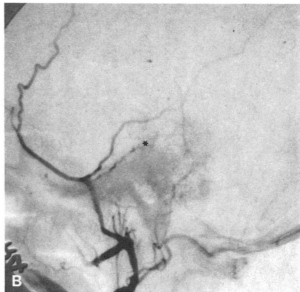

Fig. 2.11 A, B. Petrous meningioma. **A** Lateral subtraction angiogram of the middle meningeal artery. Note, filing of the internal carotid artery via the inferior lateral trunk *(curved arrow)* and filling of the petrosal branch of the middle meningeal artery supplying the tumor *(arrow)*. This represents a danger for microembolization unless flow control to permit reversal of flow in the ILT can be accomplished. **B** Lateral subtraction angiogram after microparticle embolization under flow control by gentle hand injection with microparticles larger than the anastomosis. Note, complete devascularization of the tumor *(asterisk)*

Fig. 2.12 A-C. Foramen magnum meningioma, MRI scan. **A** T1 image demonstrating a well circumscribed extra-axial mass with a broad basal attachment on the anterior dural surface. Note, in the T1 image the multiple areas of void signal (black) which represent hypervascularity. **B** Frontal subtraction angiogram of the right ascending pharyngeal artery *(arrow)* which demonstrates the main supply to the tumor. **C** Control left ascending pharyngeal injection *(arrow)* in frontal view, demonstrates tumor supply from the left ascending pharngeal artery. Refilling of the contralateral ascending pharyngeal artery via the clival arcade demonstrates the point of occlusion following embolization of the right ascending pharyngeal artery *(arrowheads)*. The left ascending pharyngeal artery was also embolized with microparticles. (PVA 250 microns, low concentration)

"En plaque" meningiomas are a special group with some specific characteristics. They have a marked predilection for females, even more so than other meningiomas. They usually provoke hyperostosis of neighboring bony structures. For the most part they do not compress the adjacent brain or produce increased intracranial pressure (Fig. 2.14). When present in the pterional region, or when the sphenoid bone is involved (Fig. 2.10) they often present with exophthalmus. The cranial hyperostosis is caused by a diffuse process which does not spare the midline structures (Fig. 2.6) if develops near the sagittal plane. This is an important sign in the differential diagnosis with hyperostosis frontalis interna that does not cross the midline.

Meningiomas may also occur without dural attachment (pial forms) in the depth of major fissures (such as the sylvian fissure). Intraventricular meningiomas arise either from the tela choroidea or from the stroma of the choroid plexus. Although they may occur in any ventricle there is a distinct

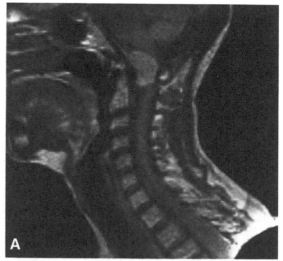

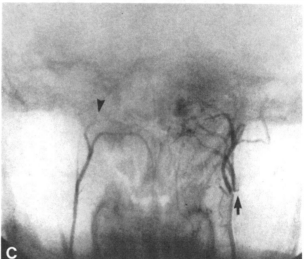

Fig. 2.12 A-C

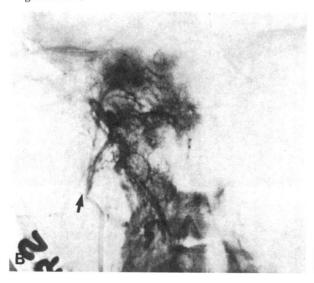

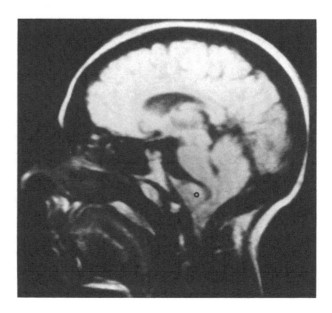

Fig. 2.13. Clival meningioma, ▶ MRI scan on T2 weighted image demonstrates posterior displacement of the brain stem by extra-axial mass effect, produced by a clival meningioma. Note, the similar signal given in the T1 weighted image by meningioma and normal brain. This may make tumors in the convexity more difficult to detect

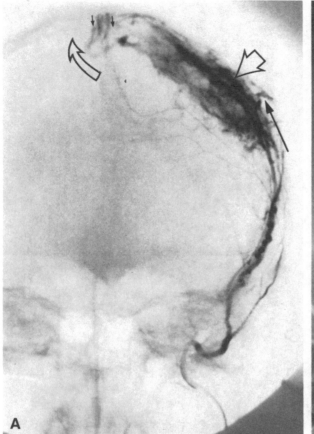

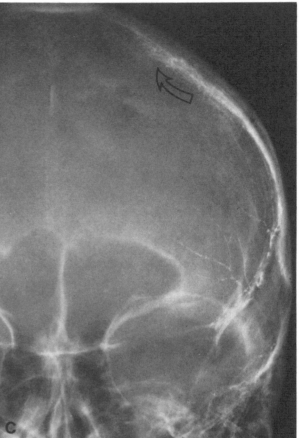

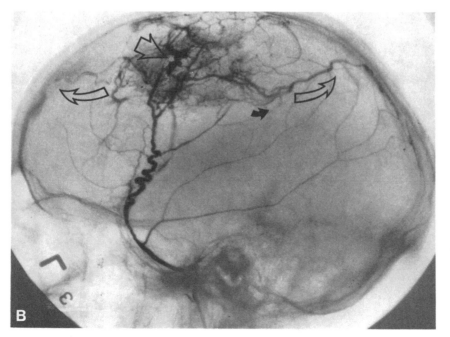

Fig. 2.14 A-C. "En Plaque" Meningioma of the left parietal region presenting in a 36 year old male (these tumors are more frequent in females) presenting with seizures. **A** Frontal subtraction angiogram in late arterial phase of the left middle meningeal artery injection. The en plaque meningioma is seen following the convexity of the brain but without compression. There are transbony emmissary veins *(arrow)*, diploic *(open arrowhead)*, dural *(small arrows)* and cortical *(open curved arrowhead)* venous drainage. **B** Lateral subtraction angiogram of the same patient. Note, the dural to cortical venous anastomosis *(small curved arrow)* draining into a cortical vein *(curved open arrows)*. The diploic venous lake *(open arrowhead)* is well visualized. Embolization will not be successful in stopping the venous bleeding from this diploic drainage. **C** Frontal skull radiogram of the same patient following IBCA "sandwich" embolization. Note, the excellent cast of the en plaque tumor *(white open curved arrow)*. And the associated hyperostosis. The outer table is not involved (compare with **A**). A facial nerve palsy occurred following embolization, and resolved in 3 months

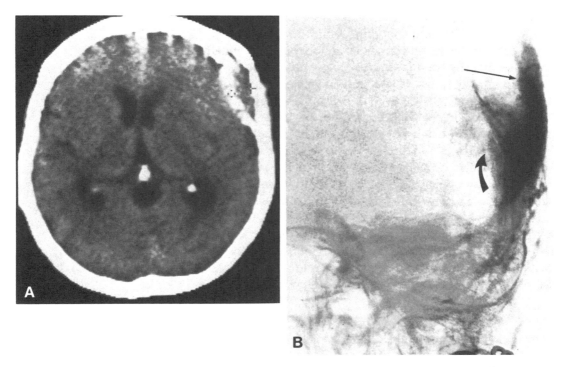

Fig. 2.15 A, B. Epidural meningioma. **A** CT scan with bony windows demonstrates splaying of the outer and inner table. **B** Frontal subtraction angiogram in late phase of the left middle meningeal artery demonstrates the diploic *(long arrow)* and epidural *(curved arrow)* tumor

preference for the lateral ventricle in general, and the left lateral ventricle in particular. Intraventricular meningiomas are more frequent in children.

b) Epidural Meningiomas (Fig. 2.15)

By far, most cranial meningiomas develop deep to the dura mater, with or without attachment to the membrane. Some can grow right through it. Much less frequently the main bulk of the tumor is in the epidural space, and therefore, in the bone itself (Fig. 2.15). These may grow through the bone into the soft tissues of the scalp. These epidural tumors are frequently associated with hyperostosis and may be palpable on examination. In some cases a "purely" intraosseous tumor may be found without involvement of the dura, the so-called "primary intraosseous meningioma". These may or may not involve the diploic space (Kepes, 1982).

c) Meningiomas of the Orbit (Fig. 2.9)

Reese (1976) found meningiomas to account for 3% of expanding lesions of the orbit. There is a higher incidence in younger people, especially young white females below 20 years of age (25%, Karp, 1974); 16% of these patients have the central form of neurofibromatosis.

Meningiomas present in the orbit by three mechanisms. The most frequent type invades the orbit as an extension from an intracranial tumor, usually but not exclusively, from the middle cranial fossa through the optic foramen and superior orbital fissure.

Meningiomas also originate from the anterior portion of the optic nerve sheath. They may develop in the optic foramen region and form a "dumbell" tumor with intracranial extension (Fig. 2.9). Finally, a rare type of tumor may arise from ectopic arachnoid nests in other orbital tissues.

Ocular signs may be related to impingement on the optic canal and obstruction of the superior orbital fissure. "En plaque" meningiomas (or tumor invasion, Fig. 2.10) of the pterion can cause exophthalmus secondary to tumor growth or hyperostosis and may endanger vision. Optic nerve sheath meningiomas usually lead to severe optic atrophy (Karp, 1974). Additional ocular circulatory problems may be caused by the shunting effect of ectatic opticocilliary veins that develop in patients with orbital meningiomas (Zakaka, 1979). Rarely the tumor will penetrate the globe and invade the choroid and the retina (Henderson, 1977). Tumors near the optic canal cause prechiasmal optic nerve compression with slowly progressive loss of vision characterized by near normal acuity, but poor color perception, and Marcus Gunn pupils but with a normal appearance of the disc. This is important in the differential diagnosis with optic nerve gliomas.

d) Meningiomas Involving the Cavernous Sinus

These tumors, in view of their difficult location for surgical removal, have a relatively high incidence of oculomotor palsies and recurrences. On occasions a good embolization may provide relief of cranial nerve dysfunction.

e) Meningiomas in Other Unusual Sites

This group of tumors is considered separately in view of its relative infrequency, and its clinical importance to surgeons, and radiologists that may be involved in the diagnosis and treatment.

α) Meningiomas can originate from extracranial and extraspinal arachnoid cells in or near the foramena that serve as exit points for cranial nerves.

β) Most of those arising in the parapharyngeal region are related to cranial nerves, particularly the VIth nerve. Additionally the IX, X, XI, XII cranial nerves may be the site of origin. Those arising from the base of the skull usually occur in association with spinal nerves (Hawkins, 1979) or sympathetic nerve roots (Wilson, 1979).

γ) Truly ectopic meningiomas with no obvious connection to foramena or nerves can occur at remote sites. These originate from embryonic rests of arachnoid. They may arise from the outer table of the skull, particularly the frontal or temporal bone. In the orbit they are seen without involvement of the optic nerve (Lloyd, 1982).

The most frequent location for ectopic meningiomas is the paranasal sinus and naso-oral cavity (Geoffrey, 1983) (see Nasopharyngeal Tumors).

δ) Distal metastasis from intracranial meningiomas (see Malignant Meningiomas).

Ectopic meningiomas have been reported at multiple sites (Farr 1973), including those reviewed and also in the parathyroid glands, ear, mediastinum, and skin (Kepes, 1982).

Lopez in 1974 reported 25 cases of cutaneous meningiomas; he divided them into three types.

1. Those in the scalp, face, and paravertebral skin. These are most frequently seen in children and are usually benign.
2. Those in the skin near the sensory organs.
3. Meningiomas originating intracranially or intraspinally may reach the skin by growing through the bone or through a bony defect; these have the poorest prognosis (Figs. 2.1, 2.2).

f) Intracranial Vascular Involvement

Infarcts or hemorrhage may be included in the differential diagnosis of meningiomas, and may actually be the presenting symptom of these tumors (Moore, 1954). Massive hemorrhage as a complication of a meningioma has been reported by Skultety (1968) but this is rare. When meningiomas do cause hemorrhage it may be intracerebral, subdural, subarachnoid or intratumoral (Modesti, 1976). The majority of reported hemorrhagic complications in meningiomas have been found in tumors which are highly vascular at histology.

The subdural hematomas seen with meningiomas may be caused by growth of tumor into the subdural space producing rupture of bridging veins or by direct hemorrhage from the tumor into the subdural space.

Askenazy (1960) reported two patients with subarachnoid hemorrhage as the presenting symptom. In both, the meningioma involved the choroid plexus of the lateral ventricle. It may also be seen with tumors outside the ventricular system (Kepes, 1982).

Intratumoral hemorrhage may be present as an acute and even fatal episode due to rapid enlargement of the tumor mass (Helle, 1980). Venous occlusions occur more frequently, usually in the presence of meningiomas which arise near a major sinus which is occluded either by extrinsic pressure (Fig. 2.16) or actual tumor invasion (Fig. 2.7). If this ocurs slowly (as is usually the case) it will be tolerated, due to the development of bridging or collateral pathways of drainage (Fig. 2.7C) (see Pretherapeutic Evaluation). Rapid occlusion of a major sinus may cause a venous infarction.

Another complication of venous occlusion is increased intracranial pressure and papilledema.

Arterial occlusion is less frequent, but may occur secondary to tumor "encasement" of an artery (Fig. 2.10).

g) Peritumoral Edema in Meningiomas

The presence of cerebral edema in association with meningiomas is well known, and its cause has been a topic of great interest to many investigators. Multiple theories have been proposed however, none has been definitive. Therefore, we will only describe some pertinent and practical aspects of this phenomenon. The edema of meningiomas is of vasogenic origin (Klatzo, 1967). Stevens in 1983, analyzed the literature and his own experience of peritumoral edema in meningiomas, based on CT scans in 160 patients. Edema was present in 46%; it occurred most frequently in the centrum semiovale and the deep white matter around the ventricular trigone and frontal horns reflecting the size of the interstitial spaces adjacent to the tumor. Cyst like spaces of various types were observed in 20%. Edema usually resolved within 3 months after surgery, except in very large lesions. Atrophy in the underlying cortex was related to tumor size

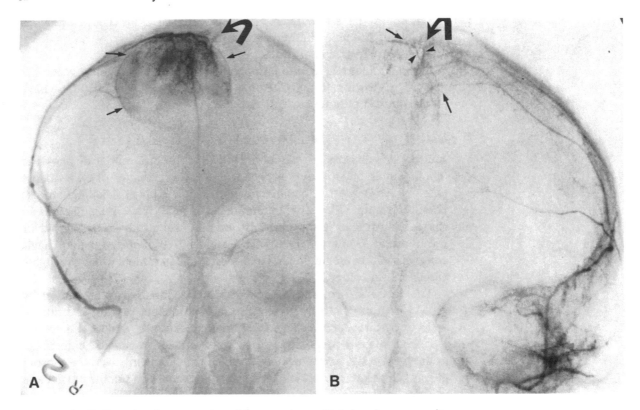

Fig. 2.16 A, B. Functional compression of the superior sagittal sinus in a parasagittal meningioma. **A** Frontal subtraction angiogram of the right middle meningeal artery. The catheter is at the level of the foramen spinosum. Note, the well circumscribed tumor *(arrows)*. The superior sagittal sinus is pushed medially *(curved arrow)* but is not invaded (compare with Fig. 2.7). **B** Frontal subtraction angiogram of the left middle meningeal artery after embolization of the right side. The meningeal artery demonstrates the wall of the sinus, with a characteristic triangle configuration and is shown compressed, but free of tumor *(arrowheads)*. Note the filling of the same capsular artery as in **A** *(arrows)*, but no tumor visualization, confirming the ability of gelfoam powder mircroparticles to enter the tumor angioarchitecture. Furthermore, proximal larger particle embolization of the right middle meningeal artery would have not devascularized the tumor. Closure of this left middle meningeal artery is also advisable in preparation for surgery. To avoid the need of opening the left side and maximize the effect of devascularization

and not the edema. Increased edema after surgery could nearly always be ascribed to a definable complication. He found a statistically significant positive correlation between edema production and tumors of large surface area, tumors that were flat and lobulated, tumors that spread across the midline, those located in the anterior parasagittal region, those involving the sinus, and those with a short clinical history. Significant negative correlations were found with small tumors, presence of Ca++, and relatively low vascularity. Although the exact cause of the edema is still unclear, he points to hydromechanical factors as predominant.

4. Pretherapeutic Evaluation

At the present time, CT scanning has proven to be the best diagnostic test for the proper localization of a suspected meningioma.

It has replaced plain skull films, complex motion tomography, soft tissue radiography, or radioisotopic brain scanning. The impact of MRI on the diagnosis of meningioma in still being assessed.

a) CT Scanning in Meningiomas

This topic has been well reviewed by various authors. A brief review of the CT findings is pertinent.

On the noncontrast scans the lesions are hyperdense compared to brain in over 55% of cases, isodense in 20%, hypodense in about 10% and calcified in about 14%. Surrounding edema is noted in 46% and associated cyst-like spaces are seen in about 20% of cases (Stevens, 1983).

Following intravenous contrast material the lesions usually show well circumscribed borders and marked enhancement as compared to normal brain; this enhancement measures in the range of 25 to 40 HU. The tumor enhancement is homogeneous in over 85% of cases (Figs. 2.8A, 2.9). Russell found that 14% of lesions had "atypical" features such as areas of lucency, which seemed to correlate with more aggressive behavior (Fig. 2.3A). Tumor necrosis is also unusual and is suggestive of aggressive behavior.

Meningiomas are found near dural surfaces, usually with their broadest margins abutting it (Figs. 2.3A, 2.6). Signs of an extra-axial origin can usually be detected, including buckling of the white matter (George, 1982) which is very useful in evaluating large lesions.

Bony window imaging is necessary to detect hyperostosis (Figs. 2.6, 2.10A) and/or bone expansion which is suggestive of marrow involvement or frank destruction (Fig. 2.15). Soft tissue windows are useful to detect extracranial or extraorbital (Fig. 2.9) extension of the tumor, including subtemporal and zygomatic fossa involvement. "En plaque" meningiomas or epidural tumors are best seen with the higher windows.

Although CT is excellent in determining the site of origin and/or attachment of most tumors, this may be impossible to determine for very large lesions. In these cases superselective angiographic studies may provide this information. Sinus invasions and/or thrombosis can often be predicted from CT, although it is best documented by vascular studies (Figs. 2.7 and 2.16).

Additional pertinent information such as mass effect, ventricular size, presence of additional tumors, areas of intratumoral hemorrhage, or the presence of associated lesions such as extra-axial or intra-axial collections (subdural, intracerebral or subarachnoid hemorrhage) can be assessed.

Although CT findings in meningiomas are usually characteristic, in some rare exophytic intra-axial tumors the diagnosis is not obvious, and for these, superselective vascular studies usually resolve the diagnostic dilemma.

b) MRI Scanning (Figs. 2.2A, 2.13)

This new imaging modality is still in its early stages and not readily available in all centers; however, reports of MRI in meningiomas are starting to appear in the literature (Zimmerman, 1985). At present CT scanning seems

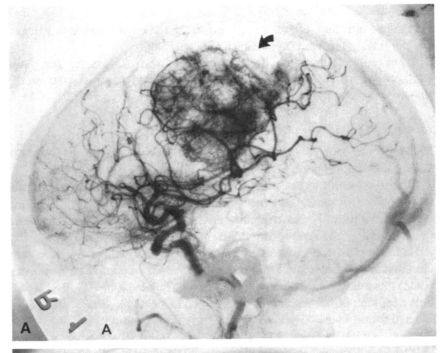

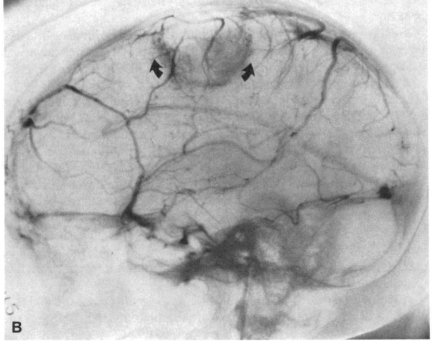

Fig. 2.17 A, B. True pial supply versus compressed parenchyma. **A** Lateral subtraction angiogram of the right internal carotid artery demonstrating pial supply to a hypervascular parietal convexity meningioma. The middle cerebral pial supply corresponds to the more central portion of the tumor. The dural supply (MMA) (not shown) corresponds to the areas of lucency in the most peripheral portion *(curved arrow)*. **B** Lateral subtraction angiogram in late venous phase in another patient demonstrates a smooth homogeneous capsular blush which represents compressed parenchyma. No pial supply was confirmed at surgery. Note, there is occlusion of the superior sagittal sinus, therefore part of the blush may represent some outflow congestion in the compressed parenchyma

to be more sensitive in the detection of the intracranial portion of meningiomas due to its ability to see Ca++ not detected by MRI. Meningiomas have a mottled appearance with a signal similar to brain on Tl (Fig. 2.13) and therefore sometimes can be indistinct from normal parenchyma, especially if no edema is present. MRI's main value seems to be in detecting vascularity within the tumor which will appear on T2 (Fig. 2.17A) as focal areas of signal void due to the flow phenomena. Relationships as well as tumor encasement of major cerebral vessels can be appreciated. In addition, it is of greater value in detecting meningiomas of the skull base [cavernous area, clivus (Fig. 2.13), foramen magnum (Fig. 2.12A), etc.] where CT may be less useful due to its inherent inability to differentiate bony structures from tumors.

The ability of MRI to demonstrate the marrow spaces of the skull may permit differentiation between diploic involvement by tumor and reactive hyperostosis.

c) Angiographic Investigation

The contributions of the angiographic investigation of meningiomas are listed in Table 2.3.

With the availability of CT and MRI scans the tumor location is usually known prior to the angiographic investigation therefore, one can plan the angiographic protocol accordingly.

The protocols of the specific regions, pedicles to be injected, and recommended projections are listed in Vol. 1, Chapters 16 and 20.

The blood supply of individual tumors will depend on the anatomical variants present, following the same principles discussed for other tumors.

Meningiomas arise from arachnoid villi in the meninges, therefore, they receive their main supply from dural branches and initially are fed exclusively by the meningeal arteries. However, as they enlarge they can acquire additional supply from pial vessels (Fig. 2.17A). The involvement of cerebral arteries however, does not necessarily mean that the brain has been invaded. In cases with dual supply the center and dural base of the tumor (site of attachment) are supplied by meningeal arteries, whereas the peripheral portion of the tumor is supplied by cerebral arteries. Therefore, there may be limitations on what we can reach for safe embolization: however, pial supply can sometimes be reached with a calibrated leak microballoon catheter (Figs. 2.3D, 2.23). It is important to differentiate true pial supply (Fig. 2.18A) from the smooth homogeneous blush of compressed parenchyma (Fig. 2.17B).

Intraventricular meningiomas are supplied by choroidal arteries, most frequently from the carotid and/or posterior cerebral circulation and for the most part are not amenable to embolization; the main thrust of angiography is to suggest the diagnosis of a curable lesion.

Table 2.3. Information provided by angiography of meningiomas

1. Arterial supply (dural and/or pial)
   Tumor vascularity
   Site of tumor attachment
   Differential diagnosis
2. Arterial displacement and relationships
3. Arterial encasement
4. Collateral circulation to the brain
5. Venous displacements
6. Cortical venous arrangement (congenital disposition or collateral venous circulation)
7. Status and patency of major sinuses
8. Possibility of endovascular embolization

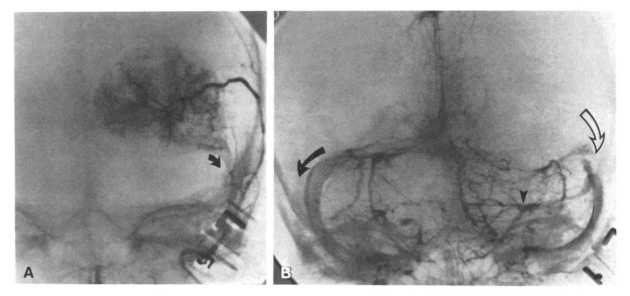

Fig. 2.18 A, B. Tumor drainage towards the sigmoid sinus. **A** Frontal subtraction angiogram of the left middle meningeal artery demonstrating a hypervascular meningioma draining towards the left sigmoid sinus and compressing the transverse sinus. **B** Frontal subtraction angiogram of the left vertebral artery in venous phase. Note, the lack of opacification of the left transverse sinus which is compressed, but not invaded by tumor. The filling defect in the proximal sigmoid sinus *(open curved arrowhead)* represents the diluted blood draining the tumor *(curved arrow* in **A**). There is good opacification of the right transverse-sigmoid sinuses *(curved arrow)*. Collateral venous circulation in the left cerebellar hemisphere is noted with primary drainage towards the superior petrosal vein *(arrowhead)*. Compare venous drainage of tumor towards the sinus with invasion of the sinus by tumor (Figs. 2.4, 2.7, and Chapter 4, Temporal Tumors)

In general, intravenous digital studies should be avoided, as they do not show the anatomical detail needed for proper analysis of a lesion or its potential for embolization. The only possible exception may be in doubtful cases of sinus occlusion where these studies may be useful. Proper arterial studies will also resolve this question (see below) Digital intravenous studies may be useful after embolization to insure that the postembolization reduction in tumor size and/or consistency have not reopened a functionally occluded sinus prior to operation.

The resectability or nonresectability of a given tumor, as predicted from CT will determine the aggressiveness of subsequent therapeutic angiography (see embolization). The angiographic evaluation may reveal features that predict a difficult surgical resection. For example evidence of carotid or other cerebral artery encasement (Fig. 2.10B) may be an indication for EC-IC bypass prior to tumor resection. Tumor supply from the cerebral arteries (Figs. 2.3B, C, 2.17A) will require close consultation between the surgeon and the surgical neuroradiologist to modify the aggressiveness during embolization (Figs. 2.3D, 2.23).

As previously alluded to (Table 2.3), proper assessment of venous anatomy and patency is of utmost importance in the planning of surgery for meningiomas that are at or near a major sinus. The venous drainage of the tumor correlated with the drainage of the normal cerebral circulation, must be assessed to determine the effects of sinus resection and ensure the safety of complete tumor removal.

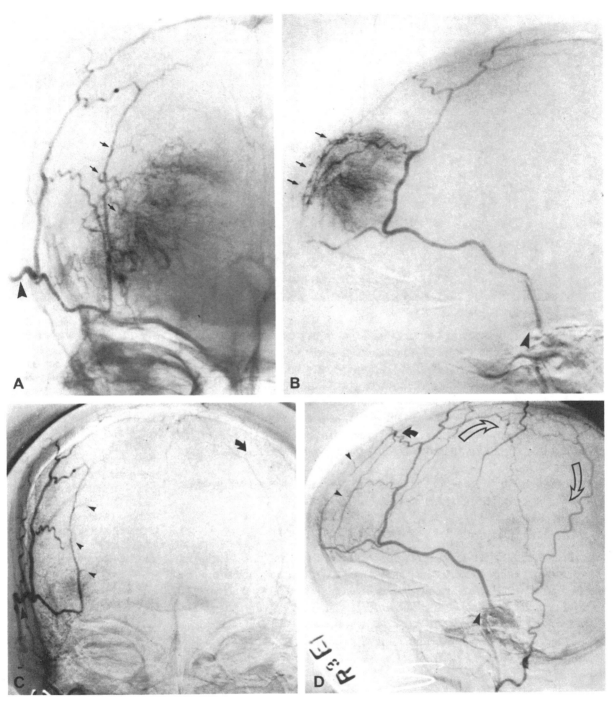

Fig. 2.19 A-D. Transosseous superficial temporal supply to a purely intracranial meningioma. **A** Frontal and **B** lateral subtraction views of the right superficial temporal artery *(arrowhead)*, supplying a frontal convexity meningioma via transosseous anastomosis *(arrows)*. The bone is not involved. **C** Frontal and **D** Lateral postembolization angiograms demonstrating the ability of flow directed diluted microparticles to reach exclusively the abnormal vessels by preferential flow, sparing normal tissue to prevent unwanted skin problems following surgical excision. The transosseous anastomosis has been blocked *(arrowheads)*. Note, excellent preservation of microanastomosis filling the contralateral superficial temporal artery *(curved arrow)* and the collateral circulation towards the posterior auricular artery *(open curved arrow* in **D**)

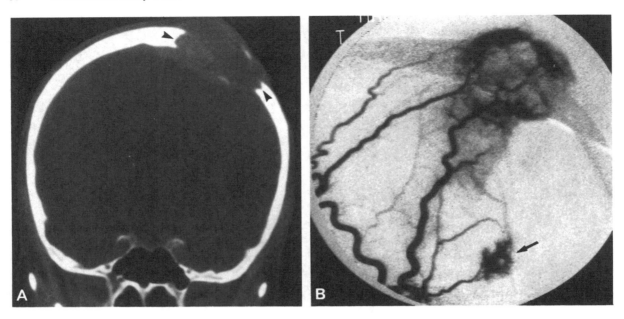

Drainage through cortical veins (Fig. 2.14) in our experience has been associated with tumors which infiltrate adjacent brain with no cleavage plane (Berenstein, Ransohoff, 1985). Drainage through diploic (Fig. 2.15) or superficial veins, may indicate bone or soft tissue involvement. Supply from the superficial temporal artery may indicate extension to extracranial soft tissues, bone or may be present via transosseous anastomoses with intracranial tumor without extracranial or bony involvement (Fig. 2.19). In this situation, significant osseous bleeding may be expected at the time of surgery.

The assessment of resectability in a given case, will depend on the skills and experience of an individual surgeon or team.

d) Differential Diagnosis

The differential diagnosis of meningiomas varies according to the location. Table 2.6 lists other tumors which may receive dural supply and therefore could be confused with meningiomas. Usually the CT appearance or multiplicity of lesions (Fig. 2.20A, B) will suggest the diagnosis.

In the parasellar region, the most important consideration is a vascular lesion, such as a giant carotid aneurysm, which is easily excluded at the time of angiography (see Fig 7.15).

Fig. 2.20 A, B. Metastatic hypernephroma. **A** Coronal CT with window level demonstrating the pathologic irregular expansion of the diploic space *(arrowheads)* with marked bone destruction and with soft tissue and intracranial extension. This appearance is more characteristic of an aggressive malignant lesion such as metastasis. **B** Coned down view of a lateral DSA demonstrating the marked tumor hypervascularity as well as a secondary metastasis *(arrow)*. This metastasis was treated by superselective ethanol infusion for palliation with good and lasting relief of pain

5. Therapeutic Strategy and Clinical Objectives

Most meningiomas are benign and curable tumors, so that every effort must be made to properly diagnose and treat them. The best available cure is offered by total surgical excision, and the surgical neuroradiologist may contribute towards this goal. There is some controversy as to the value of preoperative embolization of mengiomas of the convexity, or those in which the blood supply can be easily reached during surgery (Manelfe, 1975). The value of preoperative embolization in these situations is difficult to assess and will depend on the philosophy of the surgeon and his or her operative technique. Although it is true that ligation of the meningeal arteries as they enter the tumor would permit adequate hemostasis and proper tumor excision, some additional advantages are derived from preoperative microembolization (Berenstein, 1982) in hypervascular convexity tumors.

1. Microemboli can enter the tumor angioarchitecture and devascularize the lesion, irrespective of collateral circulation (Figs. 2.1D, 2.8C, 2.17, 2.20).
2. Bilateral dural devascularization is easy to accomplish and will obviate the need for exposure of the contralateral side during resection of tumors involving the falx or parasagittal region (Fig. 2.16).
3. Tumor necrosis will occur with a decrease in mass effect, giving more latitude during surgical manipulation (Fig. 2.8E) (Ransohoff, 1984).
4. Even with hypervascular tumors devascularization can permit the surgeon to amputate the tumor in a dry field and remove it from the inside out with minimal brain retraction.
5. The operative time is shortened.
6. Although not proven, it may theoretically reduce the chance of recurrence. Granted, a prospective long term analysis is needed to assess this statement.

In tumors of the base of the skull, preoperative embolization is most effective in controlling the supply from surgically inaccessible areas. Obvious care must be taken in embolizing skull base lesions, to avoid dangerous anastomoses and the supply to the transcranial nerves (Fig. 2.11) (Vol. 1, p. 242).

During the pretherapeutic evaluation and the planning of the angiographic and therapeutic strategy for a given meningioma, one must consider the tumor extension beyond the intracranial cavity (subtemporal, facial extension, cavernous sinus, etc., as it will require further angiographic delineation and may be an indication for a more aggressive endovascular treatment. Likewise, meningiomas presenting in patients below the age of 20 if recurrent or frankly malignant, should be treated more aggressively, in view of their poorer prognosis (see Childhood Meningiomas).

6. Technical Aspects of Embolization

Preoperative embolization of meningiomas is an easy procedure, and in our practice it is performed at the same session as the angiographic examination. In most cases, embolization is limited to the external carotid branches supplying the tumor. Midline lesions require bilateral assessment of dural supply (Fig. 2.16).

The goal of the endovascular approach will therefore be the same as in presurgical devascularization for other lesions:
1. To reach the tumor capillary bed (Fig. 2.8).
2. To desarterialize the region while preserving normal arteries, eg., those supplying the scalp (Fig. 2.19). To permit unaltered healing in the postoperative period (Ransohoff, 1985; Kerber, 1981).

At angiography, meningiomas demonstrate variable enlargement of the dural arteries with a "radial" or "sunburst" pattern of tumor vessels. Although a tumor capillary barrier does exist and no fistulization is present, early filling veins are seen in approximately 40% of cases with superselective injections, usually related to the tumor hypervascularity. The tumor vascularity may vary from one histological type to another with the highest vascularity seen in the angioblastic type of meningioma, and in the hemangiopericytoma variant (Figs. 2.3, 2.4). For the most part, the angiographic pattern is nonspecific, but can be suggestive of a more or less aggressive lesion based on the degree of vascularity, the irregularity of the tumor vessels, intensity of the blush and presence or absence of pathological venous lakes (Fig. 2.3). On the contrary, there is some controversy regarding the correlation between tumor vascularity as seen in conventional angiography and that found at surgery. We believe that a lot of this depends on the type of angiography, i.e. global vs superselective studies.

In general, the angiographic determination of tumor extent is not difficult but care must be taken in differentiating tumor invasion of muscle from the normal muscular blush seen during superselective studies (Chapter 14, Vol. 1).

Our technique consists of superselective catheterization of meningeal arteries followed by an angiographic study to look for dangerous anastomoses between the dural arteries of the internal maxillary system and the inferolateral trunk, ophthalmic, and pial arteries. The contribution of the petrosal branch of the middle meningeal artery in the supply to the VIIth cranial nerve is an important consideration, especially if liquid emboli are to be used (see Chapter 1, VI, VIII and XIII).

In the experience of both authors, when particle emboli above 140 microns in size are used, facial nerve palsies may occur but are almost always transient usually lasting only hours and seldom more than two days.

Presurgical embolization of meningiomas, we believe, should be done with the smallest possible particles that will enter the tumor bed. If in the preliminary superselective study or during the course of the embolization an important anastomosis in seen, one would change the particle size to one larger than the anastomosis. As discussed in the section on Techniques, particle embolization, and flow control, filling of an anastomosis is a function of various factors:
1. Presence or absence of the anastomosis.
2. Size of the anastomosis.
3. Pressure of injection (Fig. 2.10).
Therefore the main points of attention have to be geared to catheter position (level, wedging) and flow ("washout") (Fig. 1.30). Even if no anastomosis has been previously documented, if the washout is stagnant, it is advisable to stop the microparticle embolization as undetected anastomosis may open. It is also advisable to close the proximal middle meningeal artery with a larger particle (usually gelfoam) at the end of the embolization, to reduce bleeding at the level of the foramen spinosum during subsequent craniotomy.

When embolizing cutaneous branches of the scalp such as the superficial temporal artery, microparticles are used. In the majority of cases, the catheter tip is at a distance from the target and one should then use preferential flow to carry the particles distally. No attempt should be made to force the emboli as they may occlude normal scalp vessels and impair postoperative healing. The main trunk is left open in contrast to middle meningeal artery embolization (Fig. 2.19).

In the occipital artery two main points of caution must be considered:
1. Anastomosis with the vertebral artery at the C1 and C2 levels (see Chapter 1, Flow Control).
2. Avoid microparticles to normal cutaneous territories (see Chapter 1, Flow Control).

In the ascending pharyngeal territory, one must be careful of the collateral circulation to the vertebral system at the third cervical level or internal carotid artery at its C5 portion; as well as the supply to the IX, X, XI, and XII cranial nerves and follow a similar technique as described in the maxillary system.

Factors which limit what we can accomplish in presurgical devascularization relate to the internal carotid (C4–C5), ophthalmic, and/or cerebral arteries supplying these tumors. In general, these arteries are not embolized in benign, de novo lesions and should be only considered in special situations (see malignant meningiomas).

7. Special Considerations in Meningioma Embolization

a) Extracranial Tumor Extension (Figs. 2.1, 2.2)

These tumors, as discussed previously, usually occur in young patients and have a more aggressive behavior; therefore if de novo, microembolization with 40–140 micron particles of either PVA or gelfoam powder is suggested. The main feeding pedicle is closed with a gelfoam particle or is "pruned" and left open (Fig. 2.1C, D). In the case of tumor recurrence which in our experience is not unusual (Fig. 2.1E), or if the histological diagnosis is reported as malignant, we still have an avenue for infusion embolization with ethanol (Fig. 2.2) and/or a chemotherapeutic protocol, which, although experimental, may offer the only alternative after repeated attempted resections and/or radiotherapy have failed (Fig. 2.21).

b) Recurrent Meningiomas

This group of patients may present specific problems:
1. Altered vascular anatomy.
2. Pial recruitment of dural or cutaneous vessels which will supply normal brain and/or tumor.
3. More aggressive type of tumor.
4. Pure pial blood supply, not accessible to embolization.

The most important aspect to be recognized is the participation of dural or scalp vessels in the supply of normal brain, which carries important consequences for subsequent embolization and surgery.

A similar approach to that described for (a) is followed in these patients. It is of special importance to assess dural recruitment of pial supply to normal brain after surgery, with its obvious implications.

c) Internal Carotid Supply to Recurrent or Malignant Meningiomas after Radiation Therapy Has Failed

In these aggressive lesions the surgical neuroradiologist may be the last alternative, and therefore, the goal is different from preoperative devascularization. The need to sacrifice an ICA (Fig. 2.2) and/or ophthalmic

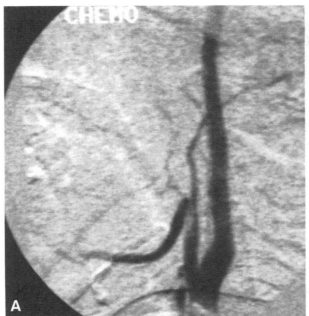

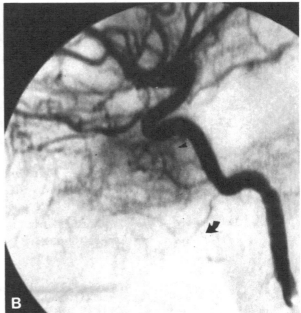

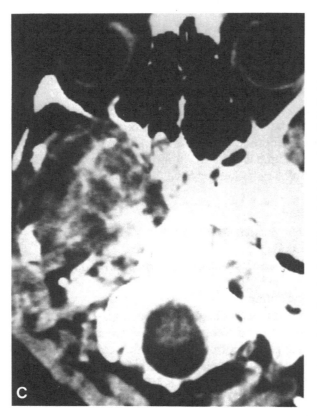

Fig. 2.21 A-C. Same patient as Fig. 2.1. Recurrent meningiosarcoma: Chemotherapeutic infusion (cisplatinum, 60 mg/mm^2) were infused superselectively in the internal maxillary artery, ascending palatine and main trunk of the external carotid artery in that order and divided in proportional doses. The superficial temporal and occipital arteries were blocked proximally with a piece of gelfoam prior to infusion to prevent alopecia. **A** Lateral DSA of the common carotid artery at the time of a second course of treatment six weeks later. The superselectively injected vessels and distal external carotid artery have thrombosed. **B** DSA of the ipsilateral *(right)* internal carotid artery at the same time as B, demonstrates no evidence of tumor reconstitution via the mandibular *(arrow)*, or ILT *(arrowhead)* branches, which did supply the tumor previously (not shown). The contralateral *(left)* sphenopalatine artery was the only minor contributor to the tumor. **C** Axial contrast enhanced CT scan at this time. Note, the multicystic lesions (compare to Fig. 2.1A , homogeneous densely enhancing mass). The only significant enhancement probably represents the supply from opposite *(left)* sphenopalatine artery. The patient has received two additional courses of intravenous chemotherapy with complete arrest in tumor growth

artery (Fig. 2.22) must be considered seriously and an assessment of the circle of Willis is therefore indicated (see Chapters 7, 8). Once this has been done, a balloon is placed distal to the tumor, to protect the brain circulation either permanently (Fig. 2.2) or temporarily to permit the use of microparticles of the smallest size available, 95% ethanol, or chemotherapeutic agents.

d) Pial Supply

Consideration of embolization of pial supply should be reserved for those cases where the preliminary study is highly suggestive of the malignant (hemangiopericytic) type of tumor or the hypervascularity of pial origin is such that surgical excision is an obvious hazard with significant morbidity and mortality (see Hemangiopericytoma). In such cases an attempt to superselectively catheterize the pial vessels with a calibrated leak microbaloon catheter (Kerber, 1976; Debrun, 1983) and to inject liquid emboli must be made. Although not always successful, as the pathological vessels are not as hypertrophied as those supplying arteriovenous malformations, it can be of significant assistance to the surgeon and to the patient (Figs. 2.3, 2.23).

e) Pre- and Postembolization Medical Management

Patients with intracranial lesions are routinely placed on corticosteroids and anticonvulsant medications (see Chapter 1, Patient Preparation).

f) Time of Operation

Although no proper studies have been done by us or others to determine the best timing for surgical removal of meningiomas (or other tumors) following embolization, it appears advisable to wait at least 12–24 hours, as further thrombosis of the embolized territory occurs during this time. CTs done within 12 hours after embolization show lucencies within the tumor bed or even a decrease in mass effect (Fig. 2.8). In our own experience preexisting neurological deficits that did not respond to corticosteroids have improved in some patients. A similar observation was reported by Didjinjian (1978) and Hieshima (1985). It is most unusual to have an increase in mass effect and/or aggravation of neurological symptoms from swelling or intratumoral hemorrhage.

On the other hand, we believe that waiting more than 7–10 days may be disadvantageous, as some recanalization and/or collateral circulation may occur.

g) Complications of Embolization

Many complications reported in the literature are related to poor technique, primarily related to reflux. Or they represent a disregard of the extracerebral-intracerebral anastomoses, and should for the most part be avoidable. In our own experience of 185 patients embolized for meningiomas we have had two permanent meningeal to ophthalmic embolizations with permanent blindness but not stroke, both at the beginning of our experience. On one patient, right hemiparesis and aphasia occurred four hours after we occluded the internal carotid artery for a recurrent angioblastic meningioma.

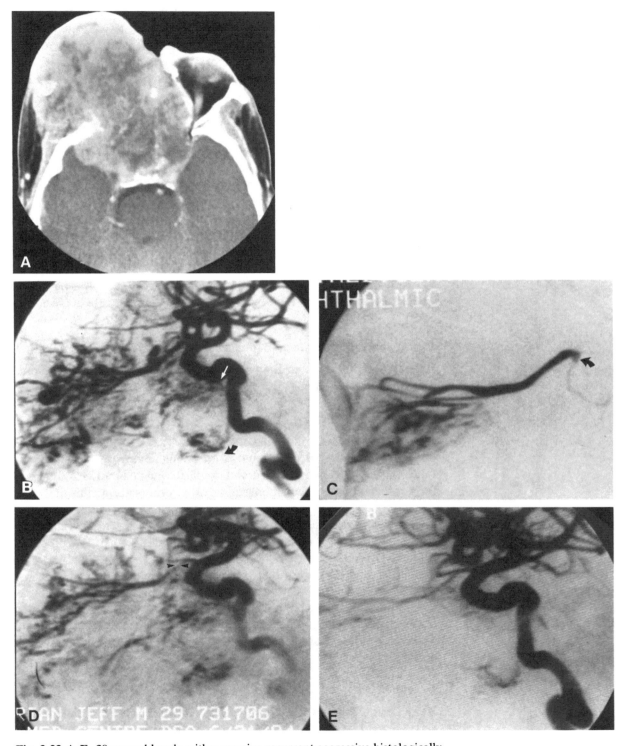

Fig. 2.22 A-E. 29 year old male with a massive recurrent aggressive histologically diagnosed esthesioneuroblastoma treated with 95% enthanol infusion. **A** Representative contrast CT demonstrates the massive enhancing tumor which is now compromising the left optic nerve. **B** Lateral DSA of the right internal carotid artery demonstrates a large hypervascular tumor which shows irregular vessels with puddling. The angiographic appearance is more that of a hemangiopericytoma or malignant type of lesion. The main vascular contribution is seen to come from the ophthalmic artery, additional supply also comes from cavernous and mandibular

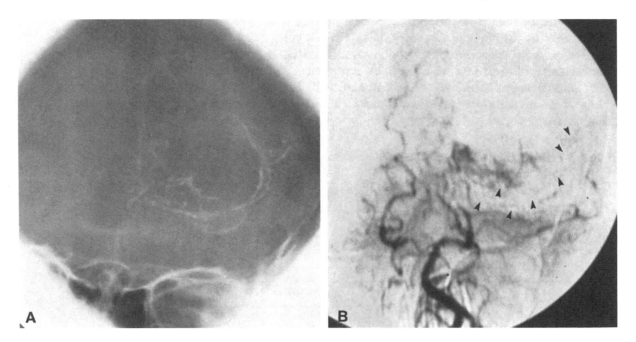

Fig. 2.23 A, B. Superselective embolization of pial vessels in a hemangiopericytoma. Same patient as Fig. 2.3. **A** Frontal 100 mm spot film of the radiopaque IBCA cast obtained after embolization of the two main posterior cerebral feeders to the tumor (compare with Fig. 2.3B). **B** Frontal subtraction angiogramm of the left vertebral artery after embolization. The arrowheads point to the subtracted cast. Note, the marked reduction in vascularity (compare to Fig. 2.3B)

◀ **Fig. 2.22** (continued)
branches. Similar supply arose from multiple branches of the internal maxillary and ascending pharyngeal arteries (not shown). **C** Superselective ophthalmic catheterization using a calibrated leak microballoon catheter *(curved arrow)*. **D** Immediate postinfusion DSA carotid angiogram. The ophthalmic infusion had to be stopped due to significant slowing in flow, to prevent reflux. There is important decrease in the vascularity as compared with **A**, the cavernous and mandibular supply is grossly unchanged. **E** Significant improvement occurred in the intervening 4 weeks. Lateral DSA a month later prior to any new infusion demonstrates a remarkable decrease in the abnormal vascularity and caliber of the ophthalmic artery. Note the significant decrease of the supply in the cavernous portion with a lesser decrease in the mandibular one. These two territories were reached via the maxillary and pharyngeal systems. The patient underwent surgical excision with plastic reconstruction. His visual loss has improved on the left side and he remains stable 18 months later

In retrospect, the ipsilateral middle cerebral artery was significantly compromised by the tumor, and a prophylactic EC-IC bypass was probably indicated prior to carotid occlusion. Five transient VIIth nerve palsies occurred and lasted less than 48 hours in all except one patient in whom it lasted three months. This patient was treated with IBCA (Fig. 2.14), whereas the remaining four were treated with PVA and/or gelfoam powder (Table 2.4).

Table 2.4. Complications of embolization of meningiomas (Berenstein's experience in 185 patients)

	Permanent	Transitory	Mortality
Cerebral	1 (0.5%)	–	
Ophthalmic	2 (1.08%)	–	
Cranial nerves	–	5 (VII nerve) 2.7%	0
Total	3 (1.6%)	5 (2.7%)	0

More recently we have seen extravasation of contrast material towards the subarachnoid space occurring in the immediate postembolization control angiogram in one patient (Fig. 2.24). The patient developed immediate focal seizures that progressed to focal status within 10 minutes, was treated with immediate intubation, i.v. barbiturates, corticosteroids, controlled, and operated upon 3 days later without sequelae. Although extravasation is unusual, it can occur in head and neck embolization, primarily with tumors such as paragangliomas. It is generally related to overembolization, and is usually of no consequence. In patients with intracranial lesions, extravasation obviously may be more significant.

Control postembolization angiograms through the embolized vessel should be compensated accordingly with the degree of flow remaining especially if the catheter is wedged in the vessel. Control angiograms through the collateral circulation, however, are done with high volume/ pressure injections.

Trismus is a relatively infrequent and transitory complaint. It is usually seen when normal branches of internal maxillary artery have been occluded and was more prevalent in our early experience; it has been reported by others (Manelfe, 1975). With superselective middle meningeal artery catheterization and occlusion of only abnormal arteries, trismus is usually avoided. Manelfe also reported in 1975 two instances of symptomatic middle cerebral arterial embolization both were felt to be due to reflux of embolic material. Other reported complications represent technical mistakes of excessive embolization or a lack of attention to extracerebral–intracerebral anastomosis.

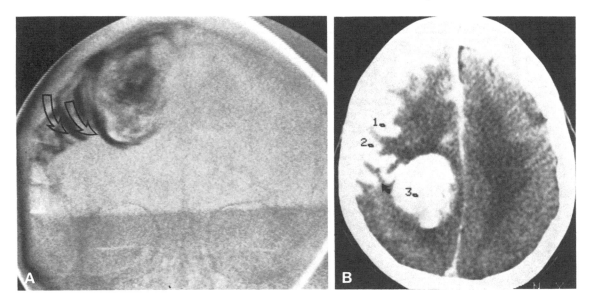

Fig. 2.24 A, B. Extravasation of contrast material during control angiography postembolization. **A** Frontal DSA late phase. Note, the extravasated contrast material following the sulcal pattern *(open curved arrows)*. The patient developed immediate focal seizures, that rapidly progressed to focal status epilepticus, despite i.v. Diazepam. Immediate intubation and deep barbiturate and i.v. Dilantin controlled the seizures. **B** CT confirmed the extravasation but no edema or increased mass effect. On the third day moderate edema was noted and surgical excision was opted for. The tumor was completely avascular and necrotic and was very easily removed without sequelae

III. Other Bony and Dural Tumors

A variety of tumors may arise or invade the bony calvarium or meninges and therefore pick up meningeal supply from the adjacent vessels (Table 2.5).

1. Cerebral Tumors

Primary cerebral tumors may penetrate the pial barrier and invade the meninges and these may appear to be of dural pial origin. They can produce a desmoplastic reaction of meningeal fibroblasts that may resemble a tumor of the meninges. Wagner (1960) found meningeal involvement by primary cerebral tumors in 10.5% of surgical specimens and in 35% of necropsy specimens. Invasion of the meninges is probably more related to the proximity of the tumor to the meninges than to histology, as it occurs with a variety of different tumors (Table 2.5). Newton states that in their experience meningeal involvement was most frequent with hemangioblastomas, but occurs only after operation. Lasjaunias (1983) has reported dural supply of a hemangioblastoma without previous surgery (Fig. 14.11, Vol. 1).

Table 2.5. Other bony tumors with invasion and/or supply from dural or scalp arteries

Cerebral tumors (intra-axial)	glioblastoma astrocytoma oligodendroglioma optic glioma oflactory neuroblastoma medulloblastoma metastatic carcinoma retinblastoma cranial nerve schwannoma melanoma pituitary adenoma ependymoma hemangioblastoma pinealoma	Melanoma	
		Chondrosarcoma	
		Fibrosarcoma	
		Plasmacytoma	
		Metastatic	carcinoid kidney thyroid adrenal carcinoma multiple myeloma prostatic
Neurinoma		Bony dysplasias	fibrodysplasia Paget's
Esthesioneuroblastoma			
Rhabdomyosarcoma		Squamous cell carcinoma	
		Giant cell tumor	
Primary neurogenic tumors	neurilemmoma ganglioneuroma ganglioblastoma neuroblastoma malignant schwannoma neurofibrosarcoma	Hemangioendothelioma	
		Chordoma	
Osteoblastoma			
Osteosarcoma			
Osteochondroma			

2. Neurinomas

Neurinomas are extra-axial tumors which are hypervascular in 68% of cases and they receive meningeal supply in up to 35% of cases as reported by Moscow (1975). Theron (1976) reported partial or complete supply by meningeal branches of the external carotid artery in each of 6 patients with acoustic neurinomas, demonstrated by superselective angiography and routine injection of the ascending pharyngeal artery.

The angioarchitecture of these tumors may be indistinguishable from meningiomas or even some intra-axial malignancies. However, some neurinomas have a dinstinctive vascular pattern which includes the presence of capsular vessels, an inhomogeneous blush characterized by interspersed areas of hypervascularity and avascularity with puddling of contrast material and persistance of the blush into the late venous phase. The feeding arteries are usually normal or only moderately enlarged. An early filling vein may occasionally be seen (King, 1974).

The embolization goals and principles are similar in these tumors to those described for meningiomas.

3. Esthesioneuroblastomas (Bataskis, 1979)

Esthesioneuroblastomas are rare neurogenic tumors of the olfactory region. They orginate from the basal cell layer of the olfactory epithelium in the upper 1/3 of the nasal septum (superior and supreme nasal turbinates of the high nasal cavity and cribiform plate), and the lateral nasal wall. There is a slight male predominance; 2/3 of the patients are between 10 and 34 years of age, but these tumors may be present from the first to the eight decades of life.

The symptoms are those of any slow growing intranasal neoplasm.

They are locally invasive and will grow into the base of the skull producing headaches, diplopia, proptosis, signs and symptoms of a frontal, extra-axial mass, or they may grow as a mass in the malar region. The neoplasms which originate from the olfactory mucosa are composed of nerve cells, either neurocytes or neuroblasts. Intracranial extension, as well as systemic metastases will invariably recur following inadequate local or block excision. Local recurrences occur in nearly 50%; distal metastasis have been reported in 20%, most frequently to lymph nodes and lung. Both the tumors and the metastasis are moderately responsive to radiation therapy with a 52% 5 year survival.

We have studied 6 such tumors by angiography; five were hypervascular with a very fine small vessel pattern, a persistant tumor blush, and no early filling veins. One recurrent massive tumor, showed some puddling, similar to that seen in hemangiopericytomas (Fig. 2.22). The goals, principles, and precautions of embolization are as described for other tumors. We have treated these recurrent tumors according to our protocol for recurrent and/ or malignant meningiomas using ethanol (Figs. 2.2, 2.22) with promising results.

Other tumors that can involve the calvarium and/or the dura with external carotid supply are listed in Table 2.5. For the most part, we are called upon to assist in the management of those in which a biopsy and/or previous intervention has demonstrated a highly vascular lesion.

Our present philosophy in cases of malignant hypervascular tumors is aggressive devascularization, usually with liquid agents such as ethanol and IBCA or superselective infusion of chemotherapeutic agents (Fig. 2.21). The goal of such embolization is to stop local growth, relieve pain or bleeding, and permit excision if possible, as cure of malignant tumors is at present beyond our reach. The endovascular route however, will offer a new horizon.

CHAPTER 3

Nasopharyngeal Tumors

I. Juvenile Angiofibromas (JAF)

Juvenile angiofibromas are benign vascular tumors which usually develop in the nasopharynx in young males around the time of puberty.

1. Macroscopic Pathology

The juvenile angiofibroma (JAF) is benign non-encapsulated fibrovascular mass lesion. It usually originates from the superolateral aspect of the choana, but may also arise more medially, near the vomer, from the pharyngeal roof where it involves the body of the sphenoid bone, or from the adjacent pterygoid plates. The tumor has a base which is attached to these osseous structures, but it does not invade the bone tissue itself. It extends submucosally into the adjacent open spaces and passages and for that reason often has a lobulated shape. Typically, the JAF is reddish-grey or red-purple in colour and has a firm rubbery consistency. Patterns of extension are illustrated in Figs. 3.1 and 3.2 and correspond to the local invasion of the tumor:

anterior	into the nasal cavity
medial	towards the contralateral nasal fossa, after progressive displacement of the septum
superior	into the sphenoid sinus and through the basal foramina or, after destruction of the greater wing of the sphenoid bone, into the middle cranial fossa.

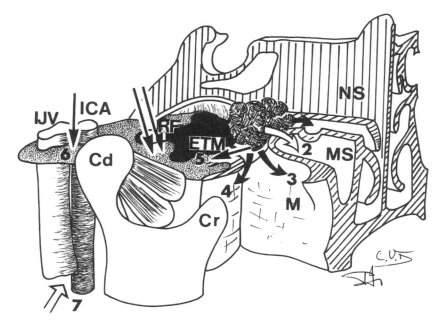

Fig. 3.1. Nasopharyngeal tumor: patterns of invasion extracranial extension. *1* Nasal; *2* sinusal (maxillary); *3* maxillo malar and facial below the inferior orbital fissure; *4* infra temporal; *5* pharyngeal and para-pharyngeal *(double arrow)*; *6* retro-pharyngeal below skull base *(arrow)*; *7* carotid. *ETM* Eustachian tube meatus; *RF* Rosenmüller fossa; *Cr* coronoid process; *Cd* condyle process; *NS* nasal septum; *M* maxillar bone; *MS* maxillary sinus

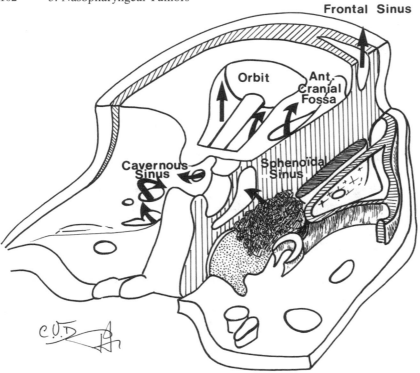

Fig. 3.2. Nasopharyngeal tumor: pattern of invasion; intracranial and orbital extensions

posterior and inferior	towards the oropharynx, displacing the soft palate and the palatine bone.
lateral	where one can identify three different patterns of extension:

1. anterolateral   into the maxillary sinus – less frequent than generally thought (Table 3.1), occurs after involvement of the pterygomaxillary fossa.

2. lateral   through the sphenopalatine foramen, either towards the infratemporal region or eventually into the orbit through the inferior orbital fissure.

3. posterolateral   into the parapharyngeal space.

Table 3.1. Patterns of extension of JAF

JAF extension	Waldman 1981 10 cases	Wilson 1969 16 cases	Hollman 1965 (not mentioned)
Nasal fossa	100%	100%	100%
Sphenoid sinus	70%	61%	68%
Pterygo-palatine and infratemporal areas	70%	89%	93%
Ethmoidal cells	40%	35%	25%
Maxillary sinus	30%	43%	62%
Intra cranial	0%	0%	37%

Fig. 3.3. 16 year old male with a recurrent JAF following surgery without embolization. Note the left exophthalmos and mass effect at the left nasal fold

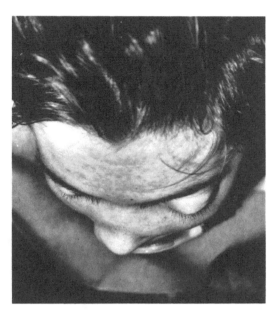

The most frequent extensions are listed in Table 3.1. Considering all the bony landmarks and barriers in the deep maxillofacial region and adjacent skull base, it is of interest to notice that the JAF's do not usually invade the bony structure, but successively displace, thin, erode and finally destroy them. These characteristics are seen best on CT axial or coronal images with bone windows at the level of the nasal septum and pterygoid plates (Fig. 3.4).

Usually, the lesions extend in continuity; multifocal tumors have never been reported. Intracranial extension is infrequent (Table 3.1) and is usually encountered in the older patients. Tumors with intracranial extension are generally those which are the most advanced, either large at the time of diagnosis or recurrent. Intracranial invasion is usually extradural, involving the parasellar (extra or intra-cavernous) or the intra-sellar area (see Vol. 1, Chapter 18). Subarachnoid spread may occur, but is seen only with recurrence. Likewise intra-orbital invasion most often remains extracapsular and extraconal for a long time (Figs. 3.1, 3.2, 3.3).

Para-nasal sinus invasion occurs frequently but must be differentiated from serous or purulent sinusitis related to occlusion of the sinus ostia by tumor in the ipsilateral nasal fossa.

Although the tumor intially arises from one of the areas mentioned above, with a topographically predictable vascular pedicle, it will recruit additional blood supply as it extends locally. The recruitment of new vascular supply is probably related to production of an angiogenetic factor (Brem, 1976); similar activity has been noted with other tumors and has been studied at angiography (see Vol. 1, Chapter 9). It is thought to express the local invasiveness of some types of juvenile angiofibroma (Schiff, 1959).

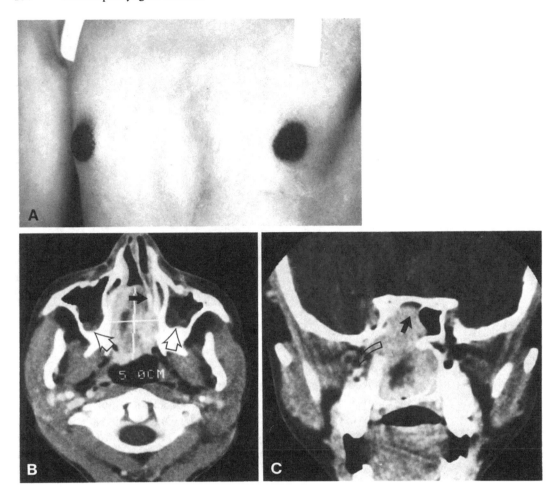

Fig. 3.4. A 14 year old boy presenting with bilateral nasal obstruction, and gynecomastia (**A**) epistaxis for four month. CT axial (**B**) and coronal (**C**) images demonstrate a typical enhancing right nasopharyngeal mass, extending into the sphenoid sinus *(solid arrow)* and the soft palate, and displacing the septum towards the opposite side. The pterygopalatine fossa is free of tumor *(open curved arrow)* and no intra cranial extension is seen. Note the non neoplastic reaction in both maxillary sinuses *(open arrow)*. The arterial supply arose exclusivly from the external carotid system (not shown)

2. Microscopic Pathology

The lesion is non-encapsulated and consists of fibro-vascular stroma. The fibrous cells correspond to a type of fibroblast (myofibroblast), which produces collagen and elastin fibres and can transform into a smooth muscle cell; it can therefore, be impossible to differentiate the stromal fibroblasts from the cells of a vascular wall. The proportion and type of fibrous tissue is variable and is probably not related to the age of the patient. It may range from an almost myxomatous fibromatosis to an erectilelike tissue (Batsakis, 1979). The vascular components, although also variable, are typically of two different types:

1. Thin-walled vascular spaces, which form endothelialized cavities without muscular layers in their walls.

2. A true arteriocapillary tree with normal muscular layers and some subintimal cushions in the vessel walls. Electron microscopy has not yet completely classified the function of the stroma. However, it has confirmed the derivation of the smooth muscle cells of the vascular walls from the fibroblasts of the stroma.

Various authors have tried to show a correlation between the spectrum of histopathologic findings and the variable clinical presentations. For example, the highly vascular tumors theoretically are more invasive and present with hemorrhage, while those which are clinically silent are more likely to have a high proportion of fibrous tissue (Batsakis, 1979).

Osborn and Friedman in 1959 and 1976, respectively, suggested that repeated hemorrhages within the tumor could stimulate the formation of granulation tissue and a fibrous reaction. This would account for some cases of so called spontaneous regression and provide some rationale for tumors seen after adolescence, which tend to have a slower rate of growth, a higher proportion of fibrous tissue and less tendency to bleed (Maurice, 1981). The relation between these evolutive forms and the sex hormones will be discussed with the physiopathology. Nevertheless, complete spontaneous regression of these tumors should not be expected and treatment should not be delayed.

JAF's do not have malignant potential, but can manifest highly aggressive behaviour. Several authors have reported cases of sarcomatous transformation, most of them following radiation therapy; Hormia in 1969 described regional lymph node invasion. Neverthless, we agree with Batsakis' statement that "this complication of angiofibroma must be considered as nearly negligible". The full potential of a given lesion is difficult to assess by histochemical methods, as it is traditionally with benign tumors; at the base of the skull they have local invasive potential, such as paraganglioma and most meningiomas. (It is of interest to recall that in 1973 Girgis and Rahny suggested that JAF may arise from non-chromaffin paraganglionic cells located at the level of the distal internal maxillary artery.) In our series, in 1980, we reported 16-year old male with a very agressive JAF and a permanent decrease of the urinary levels of 17 keto-steroids and 17 hydroxy-steroids without modification of the secondary sexual characteristics. While the behaviour of the lesion may have been related to the sex horomone level in this unusual case, it is, in general, impossible to confirm such a relationship. For the time being, there is still no biological test nor definitive angiographic pattern which allows us to predict the real aggressiveness of a given tumor (see Vol. 1, Chapter 9).

3. Epidemiology

The term "juvenile" angiofibroma has been applied because the tumor typically develops in young males at puberty. In our series, the ages ranged from 8 to 23 years with a peak at 14–17 years, identical to the figures reported by Neel (1973) and Batsakis (1979).

However, the term "juvenile" is not always appropriate, as up to 20% of the tumors are diagnosed after the age of 20 (Fu, 1974). JAFs have been reported in 49 (Goncalves, 1978) and 52 (Hiranandani, 1967) year old men. In all series, almost all patients are male but true JAFs occurring in females have been reported (Osborn, 1965; Fitzpatrick, 1970; Lasjaunias, 1980;

Ewing, 1981). Albrecht, 1959, who accumulated 452 published cases from the literature, reported that 6% of JAF's occurred in females. Although some of these patients may have had angiomatous polyps, most appear to have had true angiofibromas. Apostol and Frazel (1965) have recommended chromosome analysis in all females in whom JAF is diagnosed.

Hora (1962) found that JAF represented 0.5% of the head and neck tumors diagnosed in 6,000 admissions before 1962. Fu, in 1974, diagnosed 38 (15%) JAF among 256 non-epithelial tumors of the nasal and paranasal cavities and nasopharynx. We found no obvious geographic predominance in our series, although Batsakis mentioned a higher incidence in Egypt, India, Southeast Asia, and Kenya than in the United State and Europe. Tapia Acuna (1976), in Mexico, saw 279 cases in 22 years and 15 new cases in the first three months of 1970, suggesting the presence of an unidentified epidemiologic factor. Angiofibromas remote from the nasopharynx seem to occur in a slightly older age range with a higher percentage of females. However, most of the tumors occurring late or in females are thought to be more fibrous in type, leading to the diagnosis of either silent evolutive forms or angiomatous polyps. This differentiation does not in general seem to inferfere with the practical management of these lesions but they should be considered as separate entities (Ali 1982) (see other nasopharyngeal tumors).

4. Pathophysiology

Certain unusual characteristics of JAF (juvenile angiofibroma) have stimulated a great deal of discussion in the literature. Several aspects have to be considered:
the relationship between JAF and sex hormones;
the physiology of the nasal fossa mucosa with regard to sex hormone levels;
the effect of sex hormones on the vascular system;
a global hypothesis for the development of this tumor.

a) JAF and Sex Hormones

Johns et al. (1980) have discussed the relationship between the behavior of tumor and sex hormones. Their results can be summarized as follows:
1. Reduction in size is observed after exogenous oestrogen therapy (diethylstilbestrol 15 mg per day for one month).
2. Increase in size occurs following testosterone treatment.
3. The results of biological testing of the pituitary gonadal axis are normal.

Specific receptors for testosterone, but not for estrogen, have been demonstrated (Johns, 1980). Following diethylstilbestrol therapy, histologic examination shows partial thrombosis of the vessels as well as significant wall thickening due to an increase in the quantity of elastic and collagen fibres (Batsakis 1979). No changes seem to occur at the level of the endothelial cells, which are known to possess specific estrogen receptors. Walike and Mackay (1970), also reported the stimulation of fibrosis, leading to regression of the angiofibroma, following diethylstilbestrol treatment. Finally, it should be noted that JAF treated with exogenous hormones react in the same way as cultures of healthy tissue. Therefore, the tumoral vessels could be considered to have a normal hormonal response.

b) The Physiology and the Nasal Mucosa

The effects of sex hormone levels or cycles on the nasal mucosa are well known (Melon, 1974; Toppazada, 1981, 1982). There are interesting similarities in the histological appearances of the nasal mucosa, the genital erectile tissue, and vascular spaces of the JAF. However, most of the data concerning hormonal changes in the nasal fossa have been obtained from pregnant and non-pregnant females (Toppazada, 1981, 1982) little work has been devoted to nasal mucosal responses in males.

It is felt that nose bleeds which preceed the menses are not related to estrogen levels (which are low during that period), but to a substance called menotoxin, which is released as the estrogen level decreases. This substance shares many properties with prostaglandins of the E group, especially the inhibition of fibrinogen formation, which contributes to menstrual bleeding.

c) Hormones and the Vascular System

The action of hormones on the vascular system is complex and sometimes non specific. The following information is taken from the work of Cox (1978) and Drouet (1980) (Table 3.2).

Endogenous estrogens act in a specific manner at the endothelial cell level via specific receptors. They stimulate the synthesis of protein, particularly of prostaglandin (PG 12), an inhibitor of platelet aggregation. Their action on the smooth muscle cells is non specific and affects their multiplication; estrogens reduce the number of smooth muscle cells in the wall and thus its thickness. Their action on collagen results in a reduction in the number of fibres in the arterial wall resulting in a more compliant and elastic wall.

Androgens and testosterone appear to have opposite effects compared to those of endogenous estrogens particulary on collagen synthesis: Testosterone increases the number of collagen fibres in the vascular wall. Exogenous estrogens and progesterone also have opposite effects to those of endogenous estrogens: they increase the fiber content of the arterial wall but in addition increase the number of smooth muscle cells, producing a hypertrophic pattern. Finally, they act at the level of the endothelial cells to increase their number and reduce synthesis, of proteins, particulary prostacyclin.

Table 3.2. Effects of sex hormones on the normal vascular wall (Cox 1978, Drouet 1980, Schiff 1959, Johns 1980, Lasjaunias 1980)

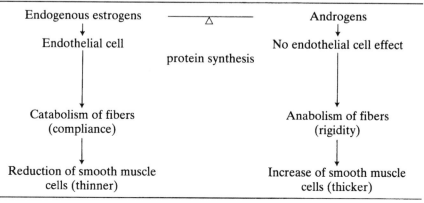

d) Global Hypothesis for the Development of JAF

Martin in 1948 and 1954 stated that development of a JAF could be related to a deficiency in androgens with an over-activity of estrogens. Schiff, 1959, proposed that the tumor growth should be related to the vascular component while the connective tissue content would correspond to the activity of the sex hormone sensitive tissue, following a disturbance of pituitary activity (Table 3.3). In fact, most apparently contradictory explanations are not mutually exclusive since they focus either on the vascular aspect of the lesion or on its fibrous component. Johns, MacLeod et al. in 1980 introduced the notion of target cells, located in the nasopharynx and dormant before puberty. These testosterone-sensitive cells would become activated with the maturation of the pituitary-gonadal axis at puberty. Maurice, in 1981, from pathological studies of JAF tumors and penile-cavernous tissue, found enough similarities to support the concept that ectopic genital erectile tissue in the choanal region represented the same target cells. The muscularized vascular channels would be the remnant of the original erectile tissue giving rise to the tumor, while the thin walled non-vascularized vascular spaces would result from the formation of granulation tissue around hemorrhages. Therefore, one has to suggest that simultaneously, testosterone stimulation and estrogenic hypersensitivity

Table 3.3. Pathophysiological hypothesis for JAF development

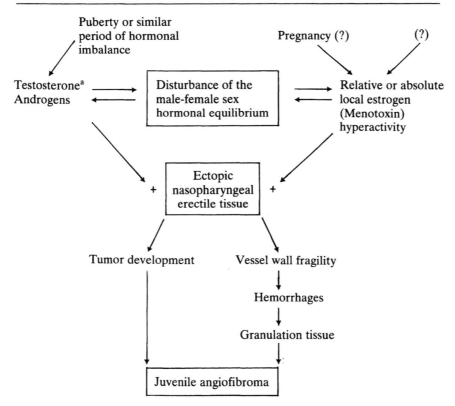

[a] Systemic hormone levels may be inferior to usual normal values, but local levels may be high enough to produce the adverse effect (i. e. proximity of the venous system of the pituitary gland to the nasopharynx ?).

(direct or via menotoxin) could stimulate this erectile genital nasopharyngeal tissue and, following estrogen induced bleeding, would transform its original pure erectile aspect into a combination of erectile and granulation fibrous tissue. It is impossible to know whether this dual hyperactivity is simultaneous or if a primary phenomenon secondarily induces the other. However, it seems to provide a satisfactory explanation for most of the hormonal effects observed, if we recall that exogenous estrogens have vascular effects antagonistic to endogenous estrogens. In practice, most of the cases reported have not been studied in enough detail to support this pathophysiological hypothesis. Three of our own cases were especially peculiar, emphasizing the dual hormonal background in which some JAF are diagnosed:

1. In one female, the JAF was discovered during the last trimester of her second pregnancy.
2. A young male had an exceptionally agressive JAF with permanent decrease in the urinary levels of 17-keto and 17-hydroxy-steroids (see Vol. 1, Fig. 9.17).
3. A young male presented with a typical JAF and gynecomastia (Fig. 3.4).

5. Clinical Findings

The symptomatology of a JAF is related to its size and direction of extension. The most constant presenting symtoms are nasal obstruction and epistaxis.

Nasal obstruction is usually the first symptom to appear and frequently produces serous sinusitis by obstruction of the ostia of the ethmoidal, sphenoidal and maxillary sinuses and less frequently can produce otitis by obstruction of the eustachian tube meatus. Infection then leads to intermittent purulent rhinorrhea and/or otorrhea and systemic manifestations of infection. Decreased hearing may result from long standing otitis (serous or purulent) and is usually preceeded by ipsilateral tinnitus. Further superior extension produces anosmia, usually associated with bilateral nasal obstruction and a nasal voice.

Recurrent hemorrhage is a constant symptom of JAF.

Moderate spontaneous epistaxis may even occur at night and can lead to anemia.

Life threatening massive hemorrhage can occur, and is usually incompletely controlled by nasal packing; it requires an early diagnosis of the source of hemorrhage in addition to compensation for blood loss. Emergency ligation of the distal internal maxillary artery or other branch of the external carotid artery should be avoided as it will compromise the definitive treatment of the tumor. Facial (Fig. 3.3) or temporal swelling, proptosis, extra-oculomotor nerve palsy usually indicates infratemporal, temporal, orbital or cavernous extension of the tumor (see Figs. 3.1, 3.2). However, these extensions may also exist without obvious clinical manifestations. On the other hand, over-estimation of the sub-clinical extension of the tumor may suggest incorrectly that the lesion is non-resectable. Therefore, accurate topographic analysis of the tumor extent must be performed with the best available tools.

The clinical examination of the cavum usually reveals a redish or greyish tumor bulging into the nasopharynx, sometimes inferiorly or even displacing the soft palate. The tumor may bleed on contact; there is usually no ulceration and the surrounding areas do not show any evidence of malignancy (biopsy should be avoided, as the clinical history and the appearance of the tumor should be sufficient to make the diagnosis).

Further detailed examination should be directed to sex hormone deficits, and signs of secondary sex organ development (Fig. 3.4).

In practice, the diagnosis of JAF is simple, even if one considers it a rare tumor.

6. Natural History

The natural history of these tumors is controversial; as already discussed above, spontaneous stabilization of the lesion cannot be expected on the basis that JAF observed in older patients are rare and less aggressive. At least, in our experience, a significant regression from an aggressive to a stable form has not been demonstrated. On the contrary, spontaneous extension in the adjacent areas is to be expected more or less rapidly depending on the tumor. Delay in treatment should be avoided since true sub-clinical intracranial extension may occur during the period of observation transforming what was an easily curable JAF into an inoperable one. The possibility of malignancy has been discussed, but it should be remembered that most cases reported in the literature were secondary to radiation therapy.

7. Pretherapeutic Evaluation

α) **CT** examination should be performed with proper soft tissue and bone windows, before and after adequate bolus contrast administration, in axial and coronal planes. Direct coronal imaging following contrast enhancement provides the best anatomic information, especially regarding bone involvement at the cranial base and intracranial extension. Computer reformatted images made from axial sections are inadequate due to their suboptimal spacial resolution. Plain skull radiographs and complex motion tomography do not provide further useful information although if they are obtained early in the evaluation of the patient, they help to distinguish between the benign category of tumor including JAF, which typically thins and displaces bony structures such as the pterygoid plates, and the malignant tumors which are common in children, such as rhabdomyosarcoma, which typically destroy adjacent bone.

MRI imaging at this time does not offer a significant advantage compared to CT, and may be less valuable, as it less well demonstrates the osseous changes. Before the extend of tumor can be categorized and a therapeutic strategy proposed, two problems must be resolved:
- differentiation between sinus extension and sinusitus
- intracranial extension

The differentiation between sinusitus and tumor involvement of the paranasal sinuses is usually not difficult. In the presence of sinusitis, contrast enhanced CT images typically show a fluid level or, if the sinus is filled with soft tissue, peripheral mucosal enhancement without bone expansion or destruction (Fig. 3.4). Diffuse or patchy enhancement of the soft tissue, sinus expansion or bone destruction should suggest tumor extension. In addition, the last phase of an angiographic study will only show a blush in the presence of tumor invasion.

CT is presently the most accurate modality in the assessment of intracranial tumor extension, especially for subclinical cavernous invasion as emphasized above, contrast enhanced high quality direct coronal images are necessary. False intracranial extension has been described by angiography, but is due to incorrect interpretation of tumor vascular recruitment. This type of misinterpretation has far-reaching consequences, as it can lead to the diagnosis of a non-operable lesion. Global arterial or intravenous angiographic studies should be avoided as they frequently lead to inaccurate interpretation.

β) **Angiography.** *True intracranial extension:* At angiography, intracranial extension corresponds to a blush projecting above the base of the skull on A.P. and/or lateral views. This blush is seen during internal carotid, ascending pharyngeal, or proximal internal maxillary artery injections. It may be present but not seen on the internal carotid artery injection, in specific anatomic dispositions. A frontal view, in transorbital projection permits differentiation between, intra-sellar, intra-cavernous and extra-cavernous extension. Subarachnoid extension typically recruits arterial supply from cerebral arteries, and therefore, is easily diagnosed. The late phase of the internal carotid angiogram verifies the patency of the cavernous venous plexus and completes the study of the para-sellar area (see Vol. 1, Figs. 18.3, 18.4).

False intracranial extension: Its recognition is extremely important so that potentially curative surgery is not incorrectly rejected (see Vol. 1, Figs. 14.12, 14.16, 18.1, 18.2). The false diagnosis of intracranial tumor extension is usually based on the visualization of a blush during selective internal carotid angiography. Careful examination of the films reveals that this blush projects outside of the cranial cavity. It is produced by tumoral supply from extradural internal carotid artery branches (intrapetrous or intra cavernous) which leave the cranial cavity via their respective foramina and supply the tumor which is adjacent to the skull base but is extracranial. The cavernous sinus venous plexus is normal in these cases, if the cerebral venous anatomic disposition permits its visualization on the late phase of the internal carotid angiogram. Similarly, false angiographic intra-orbital extension may be diagnosed. This corresponds to tumor invasion of posterior ethmoidal cells which are superimposed on the orbit in the lateral projection. A frontal view (in Caldwell projection) will definitely exclude orbital tumor infiltration. When present orbital involvement is usually clinically evident and proper CT examination gives a very accurate analysis of its extent (see Vol. 1, Chapter 18).

Recognition of these arterial characteristics is important, as they affect surgical resectability. However, these territories are supplied by branches of the internal carotid arteries as well as the internal maxillary and ascending pharyngeal arteries which may be used for embolotherapy. Sacrifice of the internal carotid artery to reach the portion of tumor supplied by siphon branches may be considered if it permits radical removal of a large tumor; it requires proper functional testing (Fig. 3.5) (see tolerance test, Chapter 1; and special considerations in meningioma embolization, Chapter 2). Two surgical classifications have been proposed

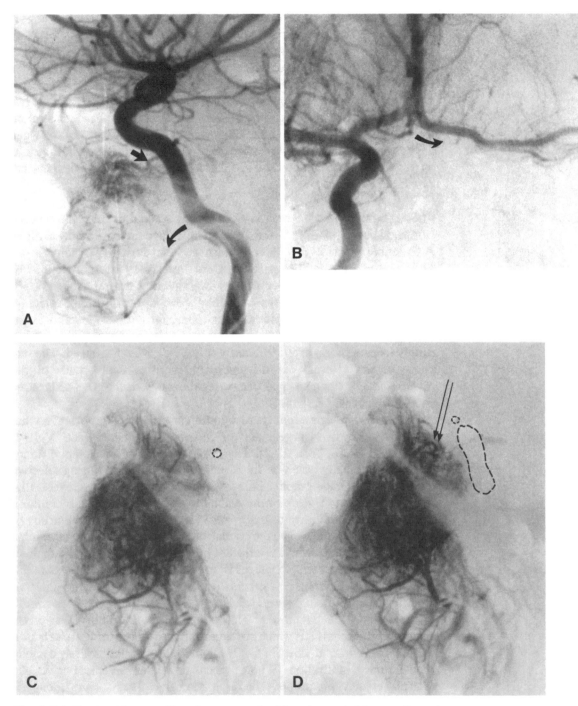

Fig. 3.5 A-R. An 18 year old male presented with a 1 month history of nasal obstruction and epistaxis. Extracavernous middle cranial fossa tumor extension is primarily supplied by the ILT *(arrow)* from the left internal carotid artery siphon **(A)**. The mandibular artery *(curved arrow)* arises from the intrapetrous portion of the same internal carotid artery **(A)** and vascularizes the nasopharyngeal portion of the lesion. In an attempt to preserve the internal carotid artery we tried to reach the intracranial extension via its external carotid supply, by occluding transiently the internal carotid artery at the level of the ILT and mandibular artery. Morphological **(B)** and functional testing of the circle of Willis was first carried out under neurolept analgesia, and successively the left accessory meningeal artery **(C, D)** distal internal maxillary artery **(E, F)** and the anterior branch of the ascending pharyngeal artery

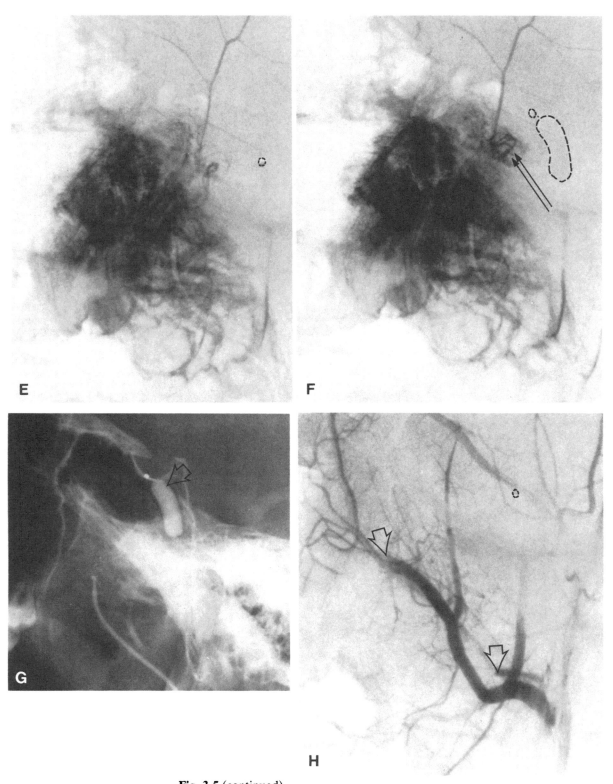

Fig. 3.5 (continued)
(**J, K**) were injected with the balloon inflated and then deflated in the siphon. Although changes in the quantity of intra cranial tumor supplied by the external carotid artery supply were minimal *(double arrow)*, embolization of these arteries was carried out with 140 PVA with the balloon inflated in the internal carotid artery siphon *(open arrow, dotted lines* around balloon)

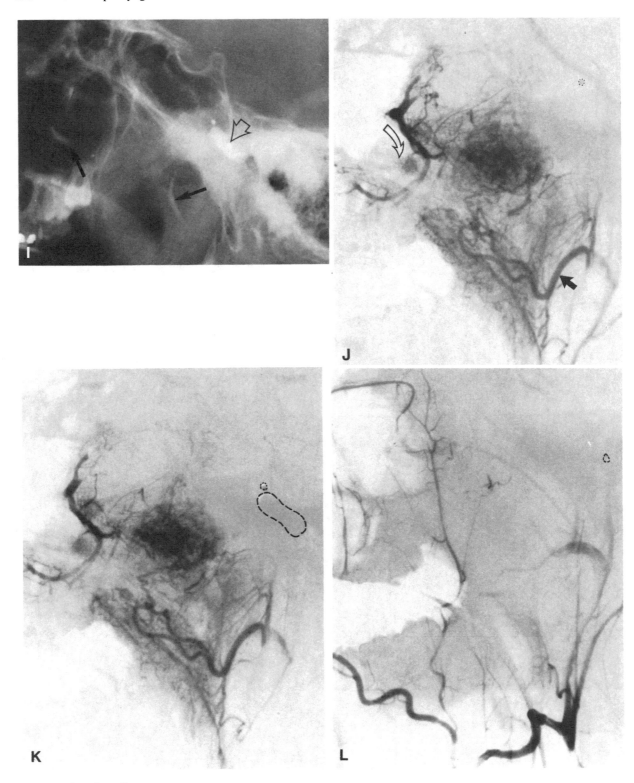

Fig. 3.5. (continued)
Control angiograms performed in the external carotid systems following each
embolization (**H** and **L**) showed satisfactory occlusion of the tumoral feeders.
Stagnation of contrast material in the embolized vessels *(arrow)* was seen on plain
skull X-rays (**I, G**). However, the supply from the internal carotid artery persisted
and had even increased slightly (**M**) only the mandibular artery territory appeared

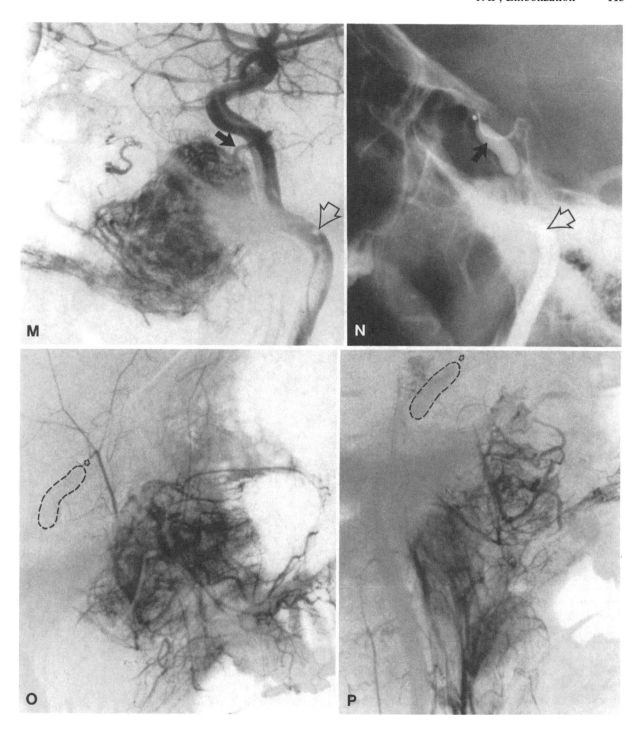

Fig. 3.5 (continued)
to have been controlled. As the morphological and functional patency of the circle
of Willis had been tested previously, the siphon was occluded by means of a
detachable latex balloon (Debrun's type, No. 16 Ingenor), below the ipsilateral
ophtalmic artery (**N,** *arrow*); a second one was detached at the level of the origin of
the mandibular artery (**N,** *arrowhead)*. Contralateral distal internal maxillary (**O**)
and ascending pharyngeal (**P**) arteries were then embolized

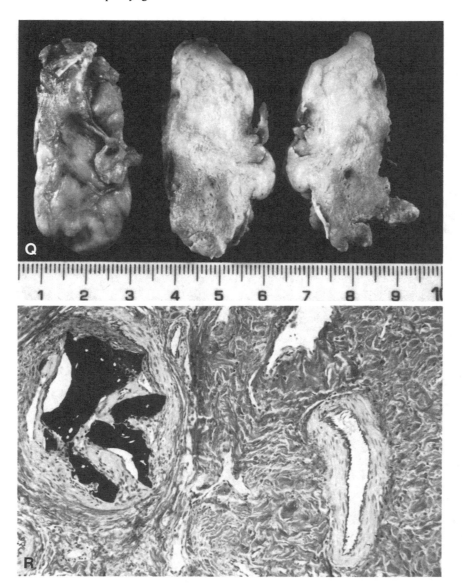

Fig. 3.5. (continued)
One week later, the tumor was removed, en bloc (**Q**) with minimal blood loss.
Emboli can be seen within the tumor specimen (**R**). In this particular case, careful
attention should be paid to the opening of the internal maxillary artery-ophthalmic
anastomosis, following internal carotid artery balloon occlusion before and during
embolization. As already pointed out in the text, the blood pressure and fluid
balance must be monitored in the hours following embolization to avoid any
hypovolemia or hypotension which would change the status of the circle of Willis
from that was tested, with a high risk of stroke

to stage the various patterns of tumor extension and predict the surgical
resectability (Table 3.4). Other purely morphological classification,
incompletely related to therapeutic strategy have been proposed, but are
less useful.

Table 3.4. Topographical classification of juvenile angiofibromas (comments in the text)

	Type I	Type II	Type III	Type IV
Sessions R.B. 1981	A. Nasal cavity B. Paranasal sinus extension	A. Pterygopalatine fossa B. Pterygomaxillary fissure C. Infratemporal fossa	Intracranial extension	
	Class I	Class II	Class III	Class IV
U. Fisch 1984	Nasopharynx and nasal cavity no bone destruction	Pterygopalatine fossa, and paranasal sinuses with bone destruction	Infra temporal, orbit and extra cavernous intra-cranial extensions	Cavernous sinus pituitary fossa optic chiasm

8. Therapeutic Goals

The therapeutic goal for JAF should be the eradication of the tumor. Surgical removal of the lesion still represents the best avaliable technique; however two factors may limit the resection: intra-operative bleeding and the size of the tumor.

Three modalities may help in diminishing these two factors:

1. Embolization carried out in a rational fashion with a proper protocol by a fully trained surgical angiographic team carries no significant morbidity nor mortality. Reported complications or unsatisfactory results are probably related to insufficient training or knowledge or poor judgement during the procedure itself. Over a five-year period, we have found this technique to be safe and helpful in the presurgical tumor devascularization (Table 3.5).

2. Radiation therapy. Although radiation therapy can routinely be expected to produce at least a partial regression in an angiofibroma, the functional morbidity, as well as the significant long term hazard of

Table 3.5. Effect of Embolization on intraoperative blood loss. From Waldman (1981)

Series		Number of cases	E°	Average blood replacement in ml
Conley	1968	34	–	1,850
Jafek	1973	34	–	2,700
Christiansen	1974	29	–	1,700
Ward	1974	12	–	1,300
Fletcher	1975	16 7	– +	2,387 1,177
Roberson	1979	12	+	800
Lasjaunias	1980	53	+	<1,000
Waldman	1981	10	+	775

secondary neoplastic induction, place this form of treatment in an adjunctive role, if indicated (Batsakis 1955). Radiation has no demonstrable effect on the cellular portion of this benign tumor, its effect is felt to be secondary to post-radiation vasculitis.

3. Estrogens have produced interesting effects on the operative bleeding. However, the morbidity caused by the dosage required for a clinically significant effect, is particularly important considering we are dealing with adolescent males. Testosterone has been proposed by Aubin (1933), but his results are extremely controversial. The effects of estrogens were confirmed at pathology by Delarue (1956). The side effects of this type of treatment on gonadal development and function, given the population involved, make it undesirable as well.

Cummings in 1980 analyzed the relative risk factors in the treatment of JAF. Although no reference is made to proper embolization nor to the respective efficacy of the available therapeutic modalities the author demonstrated that surgery and radiation therapy carried the same risks of fatal iatrogenic complications (1%). The results of surgery alone are a function of the technical skills of the surgeon and, therefore, it is difficult to predict the results possible in each medical center. Based on Fisch's classification, most surgeons in the international literature agree to operate on stages I and II, some on stage III, and a few on stage IV.

The overall mortality is thought to be 3% (Batsakis, 1979) and the rate of recurrence between 30% to 50% depending on the series.

Our own strategy, therefore, systematically favours presurgical embolization and embolization alone (or associated with estrogens) if the lesion is not surgically resectable; sacrifice of the internal carotid artery should be discussed individually, in patients with intracavernous extension (Fig. 3.5). Radiation therapy should be reserved for bilateral cavernous sinus involvement, failure of embolization, and for the situation where adequate surgical

Table 3.6. Primary treatment of JAF

Series Type of treatment combined	Number of cases treated	Number of recurrences	Number of recurrences following repeated treatment
Surgery alone (Sergent 1968; Muller 1971)	49	21	11
Surgery alone (Biller 1974)	43	16	Not mentioned
Embolization and surgery (Lasjaunias 1980) Group II	41	3	1
Embolization and surgery (Waldman 1981)	10	0	0
Radiation therapy and surgery (Cummings 1984)	55	11	2

or therapeutic angiographic teams are not available in a given geographic location.

Radiation Therapy: The results of radiation therapy as the primary treatment of JAF by radiation therapy were reviewed by Cummings in 1984. In over 55 patients followed from 3 to 26 years, the overall results were considered to be very good. Eighty percent had "tumor control"; however, 20% (11 patients) presented with recurrence following radiation, of which 8 patients were re-irradiated with good results. Although these figures may appear to be satisfactory, two patients developed malignant tumors (thyroid and skin). Two cataracts (one in the patient presenting with the skin cancer), and one case of clinical hypopituitarism were also noted. Most patients developed mucositis during the radiation therapy.

One can then consider the results of radiation therapy alone, or associated with surgery, to be almost as good as those of embolization and surgery in comparable series. However, the 5% morbidity of the former includes induced cancer, the latter has no associated late morbidity. Therefore, our preference is embolization combined with surgery each time both teams are available in a given place (Table 3.6).

9. Technical Aspects of Embolization

Presurgical embolization of a JAF is a simple procedure in most cases; the tumor is supplied exclusively by the external carotid artery most of the time, via branches which are easily catheterized.

The goals of the endovascular approach will, therefore, be:
1. to reach the capillary bed (it is a tumor).
2. to devascularize the region.

Angiographic patterns are predictable in most cases. The location of the arterial feeders depend upon the site of origin of the lesion; they are usually only moderately enlarged. The parenchymal blush is intense, with no arteriovenous shunting, nor early venous return (Fig. 3.5).

Several specific characteristics may make the procedure difficult: anastomoses between branches of the internal maxillary and ascending pharyngeal arteries and the intracranial or intra-orbital arteries, and internal carotid artery supply to the tumor (see Vol. 1, Fig. 18.2).

In general, JAF differs from other lesions, in demonstrating a strong correlation between the angiographic blush and the true extent of the tumor. Therefore, the angiographic appearance following embolization is a reliable indication of the adequacy of the procedure.

As a general philosophy, the limiting factors are sought first: internal carotid artery supply, in particular. Therefore we start with angiography of the opposite internal carotid artery with cross compression in the A.P. projection (Caldwell), followed by ipsilateral internal carotid artery injection in the lateral projection (with or without Caldwell view, if necessary). These injections will demonstrate existing ethmoidal, sphenoidal, and middle cranial fossa extensions (see Vol. 1, Figs. 18.3, 18.4).

The next step will be the successive catheterization and embolization of the external carotid artery feeders to the tumor. All extracranial feeders can be predicted accurately from the CT examination if one has a clear understanding of territorial vascular anatomy. In general, the distal internal maxillary arterial branches, accessory meningeal artery, superior pharyngeal division of the ascending pharyngeal artery and ascending palatine artery (or its equivalent) are the most constant supplies to JAF and must be reached consecutively (Fig. 3.5).

We prefer to perform the selective catherization and embolization using a specific sequence. If one has to embolize several branches of the external carotid artery, one should always try to embolize the most distal one first, to avoid later loss of access due to spasm. The second or next artery to be catheterized should control the quality of the embolization achieved; it should, therefore, be one of the possible sources of collateral circulation to the region embolized, providing an alternate route to reach the territory, in case the first embolization was too proximal, or if spasm had compromised its accessability (see Chapter 1).

By personal choice, we start by the ipsilateral distal internal maxillary artery, followed by the accessory meningeal, the ascending pharyngeal, and the ascending palatine arteries. On a given side, the final control angiogram will be performed in the facial artery. Sequential catheterization and embolization of feeding vessels from the opposite side should be carried out in almost all cases, in the same order. However, it may require a less aggressive approach than the dominant side, depending on the midline extension, and controlateral collateral circulation.

Angiographic series will be made to confirm the tumoral blush, and more specifically to demonstrate dangerous vessels prior to embolization. Any visible anastomosis between the external carotid branches and the intracranial system will in general contraindicate the use of microparticles smaller than 100 μ or liquid agents. However, in selected cases, flow control may provide the necessary security to use these agents in certain specific anatomic situations.

For many years, we have used 140 μ PVA (polyvinyl alcohol) particles to embolize the tumoral bed. Smaller particles may be used if the selective catheterization of the tumoral feeders can be achieved and if no anastomosis is demonstrated before or during the procedure. We usually complete the small particle embolization of the tumor bed by an injection of two or three large pieces of gelfoam (3 mm in calibre, 1 cm in length). The objective of this secondary embolization is to produce a transient devascularization of the region adjacent to the tumor, as well as augmentation of the distal thrombosis within the tumor itself. This technique is used in all of the feeders, and bilaterally if neccessary. Our preference leans towards the use of small catheters – 4 French or smaller – as they allow comfortable catheterization of small arteries and the delivery of all the types of emboli neccessary for this type of lesion. 5 French catheters can be used but to be complete, the procedure must adequately study the ascending pharyngeal and ascending palatine arteries, and this is more difficult with too large catheters. Following the procedure, one of us (P.L.) routinely administers steroids (Decadron 4 mg three times per day for two to five days), up to the day of surgery.

The management of intracranial extension or large nonresectable tumors may require the use of:

1. Fluid agents (IBCA, alcohol or others) with flow control in the internal maxillary or ascending pharyngeal branches (see Vol. 1, Fig. 11.4), and/ or:

2. Transient or definitive occlusion of the internal carotid artery siphon (see Chapters 1, 2; Fig. 3.5).

Each of these two modalities of embolization carries its own risks which must be carefully analyzed before they are undertaken (Table 3.7). Cerebral functional testing should always be carried out before sacrifice of the

Table 3.7. Hazards of embolization of specific vessels

Distal internal maxillary artery:	Orbital and cavernous ICA anastomoses.
Accessory meningeal artery	Intracavernous ICA anastomoses and cranial nerve blood supply
Ascending pharyngeal	Intrapetrous and intracavernous ICA anastomoses, cranial nerves, and vertebral artery anastomoses.

internal carotid artery (see tolerance test, Chapter 1). Usually within 12 hours following the embolization, shrinking of the tumor is observed both radiologically and clinically (breathing is improved often with return of nasal patency). The epidural base of the skull and ethmoidal or sphenoidal tumor extensions can be removed by an exocranial approach if this decrease in size produces sufficient retraction from the skull base. Using our technique, the effect of embolization on the ease of surgical resection is consistently excellent, and justifies, for us, the rejection of more aggressive embolic agents in most patient. To our knowledge, the use of intra-arterial injection of sex hormones or cytotoxic drugs in nonsurgical cases has not yet been reported. However this approach may be considered in very specific situations, in which surgery is impossible without or with aggressive embolization.

10. Tumor Recurrence

The rate of recurrence varies in the literature, but is generally above 30%, following surgery alone, in non selected series. Symptomatic recurrence usually occurs in the first 12 months but may occur after up to 5 years, with an average of 2.5 years in 19 patients. This relatively high recurrence rate usually represents incomplete removal of the lesion. We were confronted with this problem in our review in 1980. However, the surgical team involved in group I, was able to cure every patient with recurrence by additional surgery, preceeded by embolization (Table 3.8). The embolization in these cases can be carried out if no surgical ligature has been

Table 3.8. Results of embolization in JAF. From Lasjaunias (1980)

	Number of presurgical E°	Number of recurrence	Number of Re E°	Cures
Group 1[a] 11 cases	11	9 (72%) in 8 patients	9	11 (100%)
Group 2 42 cases	36[b]	3 (12%)	3	35[c] (97%)

[a] Group 1 and group 2 are different in by the surgical team involved.
[b] 5 patients operated without pre-surgical E° (felt not needed)
   1 patient considered as non surgical and treated with radiotherapy.
[c] 1 recurrence with intracranial extension, radiotherapy (stabilized) (1 year follow up)

performed during the previous intervention. In practice, most of the recurrences we encountered followed surgery without embolization and some had undergone intra-operative arterial ligation for control of bleeding. Some of them had also received radiotherapy.

In these instances, knowledge of collateral circulation in the head and neck areas is particularly important and helpful. A lesion still accessible to embolization may require the use of liquid agents (see Vol. 1, Fig. 11.4) or microparticles smaller than 100 microns. With these embolic agents, it is possible to traverse narrowed arterial segments or small collaterals. Some recurrences may be asymptomatic and discovered during a late follow up or during a CT examination for some other reason. The therapeutic strategy then will depend on the experience of the team. We would still recommend removal of the recurrent tumor, if possible, as future growth is unpredictable and further subclinal extension is possible.

II. Other Nasopharyngeal Tumors

The angiographic and therapeutic protocols described for JAF's are readily applicable to other benign hypervascular tumors of this region. Embolization with particles usually does not sufficiently alter the tumor architecture to exclude a histologic diagnosis. Therefore we feel comfortable using this type of embolization prior to diagnostic biopsy or radical removal.

In young patients, we have had the opportunity of embolizing hemangiomas (Fig. 3.6) and hemangiopericytomas of this region (Fig. 3.7). One of the latter involved the pterygo-palatine fossa in a 13 year old girl who presented with a facial mass and oral bleeding, 2 months after a local dental procedure. The lesion was embolized and resected, and has not recurred after 2 years (see Vol. 1, Fig. 19.1). We have also embolized benign lesions in the adjacent frontal, ethmoidal and maxillary osseous structures preoperatively with good results (see vascular lesions).

In the adult population (Table 3.9) benign nasopharyngeal tumors are less common than malignant ones. Malignant nasopharyngeal tumors are discussed in another chapter. Paragangliomas may occur in this region. Clinically they may simulate malignant lesions (see Vol. 1, Fig. 18.5). Although they are hypervascular and invasive, they are benign lesions and are not sensitive to radiation therapy. Therefore they should benefit greatly from the embolotherapeutic protocol described for JAF. Begnin vascular lesions which can occur in the nasal fossa include neuroblastomas, esthesioneuroepitheliomas, hemangiopericytomas, hemangioendotheliomas (most of which are considered malignant), and what Aufdemorte (1981) named hemangiopericytoma-like-tumors. This separate entity is encountered in adults between the ages of 14 and 79 years with a mean age of 53 years (Compagno, 1976). The benign course of the lesion, following surgery, is remarkable compared to its local invasiveness (25% to 50% recurrence), and to the potential for metastasis (12% to 60% of hemangiopericytomas in general) (Enzinger 1976). More recently, Batsakis (1983), reported an electron microscopic study of the biological and histological low-grade character of hemangiopericytomas in the nasal cavity. He outlined the difference between the low-grade true hemangiopericytoma and the hemangiopericytoma-like-tumors (see Vol. 1,

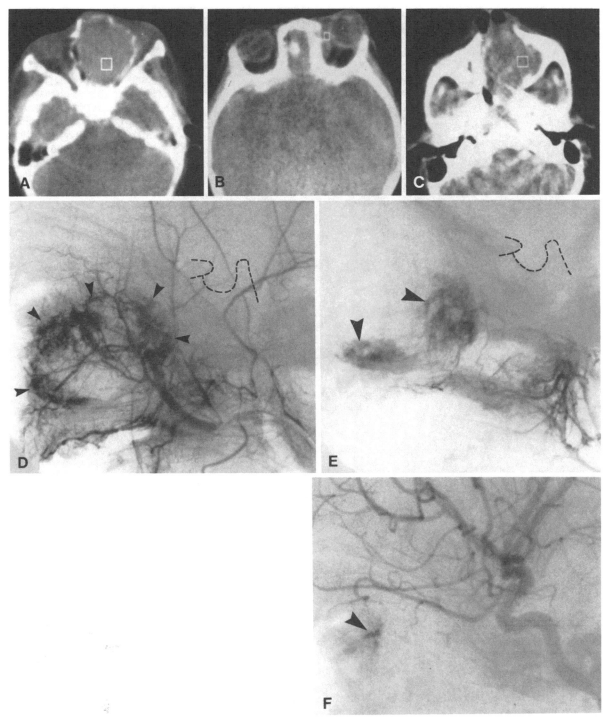

Fig. 3.6 A-F. A four-month old boy had surgery at the age of one month for epistaxis of tumoral origin. Removal, at that time, was incomplete, due to profuse intra-operative bleeding. The diagnosis of potentially involutive hemangioma was made. Rapid recurrence developed within a few month with hypertelorism and proptosis as seen on CT (**A, B** and **C**). Selective catheterization embolization of the left distal internal maxillary artery (**D**) and anterior branches of the ascending pharyngeal artery (**E**) achieved occlusion of 90% of the tumoral bed *(arrowheads)*. Tumoral shrinking was observed a few hours following embolization. Three days later, surgical control of the left anterior ethmoidal supply (**F**) through an orbital approach immediately prior to the surgical removal of the nasal tumor, completed the devascularization of the lesion. The hemangioma was entirely removed with almost no blood loss

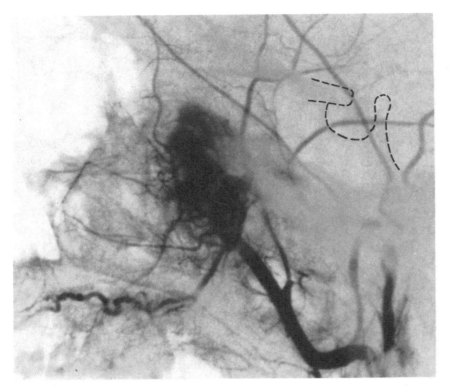

Fig. 3.7. 14 year old female presenting with epistaxis. Rhinoscopy disclosed a redish tumor. Distal internal maxillary angiogram demonstrates tumoral parenchymography fed by the sphenopalatine branches. Ipsilateral facial, internal carotid and controlateral internal maxillary artery angiograms (not shown) were normal. Although rare in females the presurgical diagnosis of JAF was maintained. The lesion was further embolized and the patient's tumor removed. Pathological diagnosis was hemangiopercytoma

Table 3.9. Nasopharyngeal and paranasal tumorous conditions. Modified from Whelan (1984)

Benign	*Malignant*
Angiofibroma	Carcinoma
Hemangioma	Sarcoma
Inverted papilloma	Malignant histiocytoma
Benign adenoma	Hemangiopericytoma
Lymphangioma	Esthesioneuroblastoma
Hystiocytosis	Malignant tumor of salivary origin
Neurogenic tumor	Lymphoma
Hemangioericytoma-like (pediatric form)	Metastatic carcinoma
Chondroma	Hemangioendothelioma
Nasopharyngeal ecchinococosis	Hemangiosarcoma
Osteoma	
Reparative granuloma	
Fibromatosis and fibromyoxoma	
Extra cranial meningioma	
Vascular malformation	
Mucocele	
Teratoma	
Angiomatous polyp	

Fig. 19.1). Similarly, Cole (1982) collected 14 cases of hemangioendotheliomas of the nose and nasal cavity and paranasal sinuses. The ages of the patients ranged from three months to 71 years of age. Four of them were in the pediatric group. The mean age was 42 years for the males and 40 for the females. Only three of them died from their disease, nine are still alive (eight without recurrence) and two were lost to follow up. These tumors are all highly vascular and in this specific area have a relatively benign course. We feel that they should undergo radical surgery whenever possible and therefore, benefit from pre-surgical embolization.

Extracranial meningiomas are rare in this region and usually develop in the parapharyngeal space. They represent only 1% of overall meningiomas (Geoffray, 1983) (see Chapter 2).

In her review, Geoffray, 1983, collected 94 cases of meningioma involving the head and neck: 39 in the paranasal sinuses and the naso-oral cavity of which 15 had documented intracranial extension. In addition to these, 19 were in the para and retro-pharyngeal space.

Tumors developing in the parapharyngeal space were reveiwed by Work (1974) who reported over 40 cases, of which 80% were benign. The lesions (benign and malignant) were distributed as follows:

Salivary	48%
Neurogenic	32%
Vascular	5%
Miscellaneous	6%

In other series, neurogenic tumors were the most frequent benign lesions encountered in the parapharyngeal space (Conley, 1978; Ferlito, 1984). Schwannomas are encountered in the nasal fossa and the paranasal sinuses (Khalifa, 1981; Mahe, 1983); maxillary sinus (Agarwall, 1980); and sphenoid sinus (Calcaterra, 1974).

The angiomatous polyp is a rare benign lesion. Som et al (1982) described 5 cases of which 3 were biopsy proven. These lesions have histologic findings similar to JAF and may bleed profusely at the time of biopsy. Most patients with these lesions present in a similar fashion to those with JAF, and therefore are referred for pre-surgical angiography and embolization. At angiography, they are less vascular than the typical JAF probably because they contain more fibrous tissue, but because they have a high potential for intra-operative hemorrhage, they benefit equally from preoperative embolization.

In 1982, Ali reported a 28 year old woman with an "extra-nasopharyngeal" angiofibroma in the tonsilar area and reviewed the literature extensively. Over 36 cases have been reported since 1936, with a mean age of 22 years (Ali 1982, Neel 1973). Among these 36 cases of extra-nasopharyngeal angiofibromas, 44% were between 10 and 20 years of age at the time of the discovery of the lesion, compared to 80% of patients with nasopharyngeal JAF.

Thirty-one percent of the extra nasopharyngeal angiofibromas occured in females. Because of these differences in site of origin, sex ratio and age, Lucas in 1976 and Ali in 1982 felt that although the structural aspect and clinical presentation and benign course are idential, extranasopharyngeal angiofibromas and the usual type of juvenile nasopharyngeal angiofibromas should be considered as two different entities.

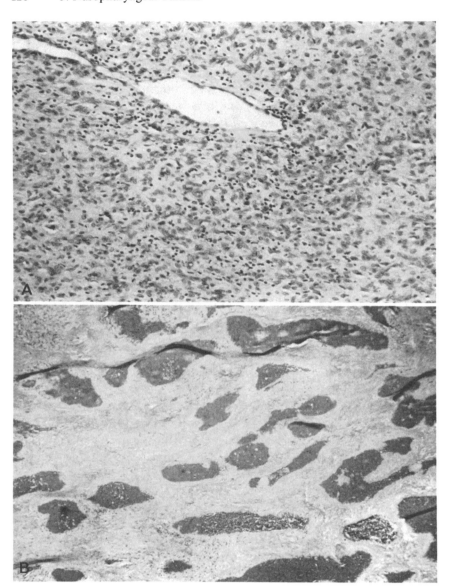

Fig. 3.8 A, B. 16 year old male presenting with a nasopharyngeal juvenile angiofibroma. **A** Pathological specimen from surgery performed a few days following gelfoam embolization. Note the intense cellularity. **B** Pathological specimen following second surgery for recurrence of the tumor 8 month later. Silicone fluid embolization was performed few weeks before this resection. Note the fibrotic transformation of the tumor and the organized thrombi into the vascular lumen; no recurrence with 11 years follow up

III. Conclusion

We feel that benign vascular tumours such as JAFs, angiomatous polyps, extranasopharyngeal angiofibromas, nasal, paranasal and naso-pharyngeal paragangliomas, meningiomas, hemangiomas, hemangiopericytomas, esthesioneuroblastomas, and hemangioendotheliomas can benefit from preoperative embolization. Their location, at the base of the skull, the frequence of recurrence following incomplete surgery, and the controversial effects of radiation therapy on the tumoral cells, are all factors which support the use of embolotherapy prior to their removal, and endovascular control of the tumor growth in the recurrent or non surgical forms (Fig. 3.8).

CHAPTER 4

Temporal and Cervical Tumors

Branchial Paragangliomas

1. Introduction

Paragangliomas occur in a variety of sites in the head and neck with almost one half arising in the temporal bone (Tables 4.1, 4.2). Although tumors of the middle ear occur infrequently, paragangliomas are the most common in this location.

If one considers all tumors of the temporal bone, paragangliomas are second in frequency to neurogenic tumors (Spector, 1973).

Paragangliomas best represent the multidisciplinary therapeutic strategy and technical aspects involved in the treatment of benign neoplasms of the cervical and temporal regions.

The considerable interest generated by these lesions is apparent from the 2000 cases reported in the literature, compared to the fact that they represent only 0.012% of tumors in the pathology files of large centers (Lack, 1977).

The interesting features of paragangliomas include their multicentricity and their frequent association with other neural crest tumors.

Table 4.1. Neural crest derivatives. Modified from Turpin (1978)

Mesenchymal cells	Ectodermal cells	Ectomesenchymal cells after endodermic settlement (Argentaffin cells)
Muscular, osseous Cartilaginous, etc. Structures of the head and neck	Ganglion cells (autonomic nervous system; cranial and spinal nerves)	
Odontoblasts	Neural coverings and stroma (microglia leptomeninges)	
	Secretory cells • Chromaffin cells • "non-chromaffin" paraganglions (brachial etc.) • melanoblasts • hypothalamic cells • pineal cells	Compact endocrine system (thyroid, pituitary; parathyroid) Disseminated endocrine system (pancreas) Diffuse endocrine system (g. i. tract)

Cells of the APUD system are included in the box.

Table 4.2. Locations of head and neck paragangliomas in order of frequence. From Zak (1982)

Temporal { Tympanic	Temporalis muscle
Temporal {	Buccal mucosa
{ Jugular	Tongue
Carotid	Soft palate
Vagal	Pterygopalatine fossa
Laryngeal	Mandible
Orbital	Nasal fossa
Nasopharyngeal	Cervical oesophagus
Thyroid, parathyroid	Intracranial (sphenoid sinus, para-
Face, ear, submastoid area, parotid	sellar region, intrasellar, epithalmic)

Glomic tumors, chemodectoma, non-chromaffin paraganglioma, and neurocristopathic tumor are the most of common names given to the benign neuroendocrine neoplasms which arise from the neural crest derivatives.

2. Embryology

The neural crest gives rise to three types of cells (Table 4.1; Rosenwasser, 1968; Louvel, 1979): mesenchymal, ectomesenchymal, and ectodermal.

Ectomesenchymal: these cells migrate to colonise the endodermal derivatives (hypophysis, thyroid gland, thymus, digestive tract), they belong to the so-called argentaffin cell group (from which the serotonin secreting carcinoid tumors develop). Argentaffin cell derivatives are further categorized into two subgroups depending on their chromaffin reaction: those that react positively are termed enterochromaffin cells while those with a negative reaction are argyrophilic cells. The argyrophilic cells are very different from the cells giving rise to the paragangliomas, and although they can both release serotonin, their initial embryonic pattern of migration results in different patterns of differentiation.

Ectodermal: this group gives rise to the leptomeningeal cells, the microglial cells, ganglion cells (for the spinal nerves, autonomic nervous system, and sensory cranial nerves) and special secretory cells. The secretory cells are divided into two subgroups depending on the chromaffin reaction. The chromaffin-positive subgroup includes the cells of the adrenal medulla (pheochromocytes, adrenalin secreting) and the para-aortic cells (chromaffin paraganglion cells which release noradrenalin). The non-chromaffin cells extend throughout most of the body, where they have both receptive and secretory functions. The hormones released includes catecholamines, serotonin and glomine, with no relation to cellular topography. Some groups of cells are, however, more consistently located in the same areas: branchial and aortic, for example.

In the past few years, Glenner and Grimley, and Zak and Lawson (1982) have emphasized that the chromaffin reaction of the cells may not be a satisfactory test to differentiate among these subgroups.

For example, catecholamine secretion by both extraadrenal chromaffin tumors and adrenal nonchromaffin tumors has been described. Therefore, the term *branchial paraganglion* most appropriately describes the specific group of neural crest cells in the head and neck regions which give rise to the tumors to be described below: *the paragangliomas* (Table 4.2).

The use of the name "glomus tumor" should be reserved for those tumors which actually develop in the glomus of Masson, a vascular structure located in the finger tips. These glomi have two types of cells – endothelial cells and pericytes, with smooth muscle cells and amyelinic nerve fibres. The tumors developing from the glomus of Masson are painful benign neoplasms which occur in young patients and have the potential to transform into hemangiopericytomas.

The term Apudoma refers to the neoplasms which are derived from the APUD system described by Pearse (1977) (APUD = Amine Precursor Uptake and Decarboxylation).

They consist of cells which can produce polypeptides and fluorogenic amines (catecholamines, serotonines, etc.). This category includes the cells of the ectomesenchymal and ectodermal groups, both of which have endocrine activity regardless of their chromaffin response.

Branchial paragangliomas also belong to this group as do tumors which release: calcitonin, MSH, ACTH, parathormone (compact endocrine system); insulin, glucagon, gastrin, somatostatin, thymin (disseminated endocrine system); secretin, enteroglucagon, motilin, pneumokinin (diffuse endocrine system).

This embryologic over-view supports three possible conclusions.

A dysgenetic lesion derived from the neural crest can include several cells of the same subgroup or of different subgroups of the APUD system with the potential for multifocality and polymorphism. Clinical manifestations are illustrated by the association of single or multiple unilateral tumors or bilateral paragangliomas, other tumors such as abdominal pheochromocytoma.

The neural crest cells carry the potential of producing different types of polypeptides; therefore, a clone of tumor cells within a paraganglioma may mature towards cells which release a different hormone (single paraganglioma with polymorphic secretory activity). This characteristic is illustrated in the case reported by Farrior in 1980, of a carcinoid tumor within a temporal paraganglioma.

The early polymorphic potentiality of each cell is preserved until migration is complete.

Therefore, ectopic tumors and hormonal release can be found. Most of the ectopic paragangliomas reported are located in the head and neck areas. One important fact is that most of the head and neck paragangliomas in the usual location develop from a pre-existing normal paraganglion (Table 4.2). However, head and neck paragangliomas have been reported to occur in areas where normal paraganglions have not been observed, and these should be considered ectopic tumors.

3. Epidemiology

One of the unique features of paragangliomas is the fact that the tumor which brings the patient to the physician may be part of a complex disease (neurocristopathy). Therefore, epidemiology of the sole paraganglioma may appear too restrictive.

For practical purposes we shall consider that the most common branchial paragangliomas can be differentiated by their location: tympanic, jugular, carotid, vagal, laryngeal, nasopharyngeal, and orbital. In fact, pure tympanic and pure jugular paragangliomas are not frequent; also, since their clinical manifestations are similar, they are usually classified as a single entity: temporal paragangliomas.

Table 4.3. Epidemiology of paragangliomas. From Zak (1982)

Location	Number of patients	Benign tumors			Malignant tumors		
		Age range	mean age (yrs)	Female (%)	Total (%)	mean age (yrs)	Female (%)
Temporal	507	18–85	(46)	71	3	(45)	70
Carotid body	370	5–89	(44)	52	10–15	(32)	59
Vagal	115	18–79	(48)	72	10	(45)	81
Laryngeal	34	14–71	(47)	55	18	(58)	83
Orbit	17	3–69	(44)	52	3 reported cases		
Nose and pharynx	16	8–92	(44,5)	75	none reported		
Total	1059						

Zak and Lawson in 1982 in their book reviewed about 2000 cases and discussed the problems arising from paragangliomas in the head and neck territory.

Table 4.3 displays the age and sex distribution of the paragangliomas. One can note that two groups are present: the branchial paraganglioma with a female dominance of 2.5 to 1 (temporal, vagal, nasal and nasopharyngeal) and the branchial paraganglioma with no sex dominance (carotid, laryngeal, orbit). For almost all locations, the mean age is in the fifth decade, with a range from six month in (Wosnessenski, 1923), to 89 years (Besznyak, 1959). The youngest and oldest patients both had carotid body tumors. There is no significant relationship between sex hormones and the clinical presentation or evolution of the tumor in any of the groups mentioned above, although rare cases have shown some symptomatic changes during menses or pregnancy (Mirizzi, 1935). The duration of symptoms before diagnosis, is related to the medical environment and cultural habits of the patient. Branchial paragangliomas are usually considered to be slowly growing benign neoplasms, but in younger patients they may develop rapidly and tend to be larger and more endocrinologically active and to produce more rapid cranial nerve impairment. There is no definitive racial nor geographic distribution, but Saldana in 1973 found that branchial paragangliomas (carotid) were ten times more frequent in high altitude (2500 to 4500 meters) dwellers in the Peruvian Andes than in sea-level residents. Hypoxia, present from birth, was thought to be the stimulating factor for chronic hyperplasia leading to further tumoral development. These observations were confirmed by a few other reports but were not supported by large series. Our review of personal cases did not disclose any patient of this group.

Although paragangliomas appear to be neoplasms, there is evidence of a familial distribution which is not restricted exclusively to branchial paragangliomas tumors but to all apudomas. In familial cases the inheritance is autosomal dominant with strong penetrance, but variable expression. Each offspring carries the disorder, but the disease may not be revealed in a given patient. Thirty percent of patients with familial forms have multicentric disease; this multicentricity has the same epidemiologic distribution as the multicentricity encountered in the spontaneous form.

Multicentricity can be expressed in many ways, including bilateral and unilateral multiple lesions and multiple lesions in the same tumoral mass (Zak, 1982; Moret, 1981). Vagal and carotid paragangliomas are more

Table 4.4. Multicentricity of paragangliomas

Topography	Incidence (%)
Carotid	15
Jugular	2
Vagal	10
Number of tumors	
2 tumors	84%
3 tumors	13%
4 tumors	2%
5 tumors	1%

likely to be multifocal than those in other locations (Table 4.4). The number of tumors and the possible endocrine activity are also variable. Among non familial cases, tumors are bilateral in 2.8% and multifocal in 10%. In a series of over 2000 patients Zak estimated that 1% had tumors with secretory activity. This subgroup had no sex dominance, but 40% were below 25 years of age. (Only 15% to 20% of patients with secretory paragangliomas are below 25 years of age). Multicentricity and secretory activity can be observed with malignant paragangliomas (Strauss, 1983). The malignant character of the lesion is difficult to assess at pathology (see below) and only lymph node involvment or metastasis can be considered reliable indicators. The incidence of malignant forms are probably under-estimated.

Vagal, carotid and laryngeal paragangliomas have a malignant potential estimated at between 10% and 18%, while those in the temporal region have a lower incidence at 3% (Table 4.3).

4. Pathology

The *macroscopic* appearance of branchial paragangliomas is usually typical. The tumor is encapsulated, polypoid, brown or frankly purple, with an inflammatory appearance. Depending on the location, the tumor may be lobulated or oval in shape. At histology, the findings are those of a paraganglion with epithelial cells and a highly vascular stroma. Usually, the lesions appear to be true neoplasms showing no normal relationship between the nerve fibres and the cells, unlike either a hyperplasia or a hamartoma. The degree of vascularity is variable; the most vascular lesions may be almost cavernous including fenestrated endothelium. The epithelial cells have clear cytoplasma with eosinophilic granules. Unfortunately, it is impossible to correlate the histologic differences, the clinical symptoms, the catecholamine storage or the type of secretion, with the appearance or the number of granules seen in electron microscopic studies. Neurons and ganglion cells can also be seen within the tumor, with no particular significance.

The *histologic* diagnosis of malignancy is not definitive, but the following minor findings may cause suspicion of malignancy in any given branchial paraganglioma; rupture or absence of the capsule, invasion of vessel wall by tumor cells, vacuolization of the cytoplasm, and increased mitotic activity. Although mitotic activity is usually minimal, variations in its appearance may be related to changes induced by therapy.

The differential diagnosis of the histologic findings includes hemangiopericytomas, carcinoid tumors, alveolar sarcomas, metastatized thyroid carcinomas, some neurogenic tumors, and granular cell myoblastomas.

Ectopic paragangliomas, especially intracranial ones represent a diagnostic challenge. Some meningiomas labelled angioblastic, transitional or neuroepithelial, often show "glomic" patterns and may be mislabelled, (Zak, 1982); more rarely, cerebellar hemangioblastomas, pineal tumors, metastatic hypernephromas and cauda equina tumors may be misdiagnosed as paragangliomas.

Vascular architecture. Small arteries are present in the capsules and septa of branchial paragangliomas; the stroma as mentioned above contains sinusoidal spaces. These spaces, in some areas, appear to be all that separates the tumor cells from the blood stream (Pettet, 1953). Willis and Birell in 1955 showed a complex arterial arrangement within carotid body tumors with a centropetal distribution: the arteries often have a normal proximal calibre of about 90 microns and enlarge deep within the tumor where they may reach a calibre of 300 to 600 microns. These vessels, called paracapillaries, metacapillaries and medium calibre vessels, have anastomoses with each other as well as with the veins and the sinusoids.

From these observations and the angiographic findings in branchial paragangliomas the following remarks can be made.

Moret (1986), describing lesions in the temporal region and in the cervical area, show the compartmental arrangements of paragangliomas in which an artery, super-selectively injected, will opacify a segment of the lesion with a specific venous drainage. The tumor can therefore, be rebuilt like pieces of a puzzle. Two types of puzzles can be identified: unicompartmental masses (with only one "puzzle piece") and multicompartmental masses (with two or more "puzzle pieces"); each puzzle piece can be visualized by the injection of one or more than one artery.

This analysis has theoretical and practical implications multricentric lesions can be bilateral or unilateral and can be close together. Therefore, multicompartmental masses could, theoretically, constitute multiple adjacent tumors which are macroscopically not separable. The second implication of this theoretical analysis is practical. The existence of a capillary bed and of arteriovenous communications explains the rapid venous filling seen on angiographic studies and the efficiency of small particle embolization.

Two characteristic patterns of involvement of the large vessels of the neck by branchial paragangliomas should be emphasized. The development of the jugular paraganglioma within the lumen of the jugular vein is a very specific feature compared to the extrinsic vascular compression produced by other branchial paragangliomas and other cervical masses.

The irregular narrowing of the internal carotid artery seen in some cervical paragangliomas is similar to encasement by tumors, and is probably not specific.

The role of the vascular system in the development of branchial paragangliomas is very interesting. Spector in 1973 pointed out the possible role played by neovascularization, preceding tumor invasion regardless of its site. This concept is supported by the work of Folkman on the tumoral angiogenetic factor (TAF). We have observed this phenomenon twice and will discuss it further with the pretherapeutic evaluation.

Finally, the angiographic analysis of the vascular architecture of these branchial paragangliomas provides some additional insight into their pathology. Clinically, tympanic and jugular paragangliomas are seldom multifocal (2% versus 15% for other locations). Analysis of the surgical results of large paragangliomas (Fisch types C2 and D2) of the temporal bone (Table 4.8), shows the following:

In *Type C2* (petrous extension) their carotid arteries is sacrifized or repaired in 10% of cases and all of the lower cranial nerves remain intact.

In *Type D2* (intradural extension larger than 2cm) although the carotid artery is preserved in 100% of cases, the lower cranial nerves are constantly impaired.

These two groups seem to represent the extreme forms of two different branchial paragangliomas. The C-Type appears to be the evolution of a tympanic paraganglioma, and the D-Type that of a jugular one. Coexistence of both types raises the possibility of multicentricity within the temporal bone itself. Angiographic analysis supports this theory. Typically because they are encapsulated, branchial paragangliomas do not recruit arterial feeders from adjacent territories like other types of invasive or nonencapsulated tumors. For example, the jugular paraganglioma which extends within the jugular vein occupies an angiographically isolated compartment which can only be occupied by the neuromeningeal branch of the ascending pharyngeal artery. In our experience large paragangliomas of the temporal bone which extend into the tympanic cavity and the jugular vein do not correspond to a single vascular territory but to two, fed by the tympanic arteries and the jugular branch of the neuromeningeal division of the ascending pharyngeal artery. We feel that even though grossly these lesions appear to be a single mass, they may actually represent two separate tumors. Lack of appreciation of the significance of the pattern of vascular supply underlines the past underestimation of the multicentricity of the tympanic and jugular paragangliomas (Fig. 4.1).

Several authors have reported surgical evidence of separate tumours within the temporal bone further supporting the possibility of multicentricity in the tympanic-jugular location (Berg, 1950; Buckingham, 1959; Samy, 1962; Rosenwasser, 1968, 1974).

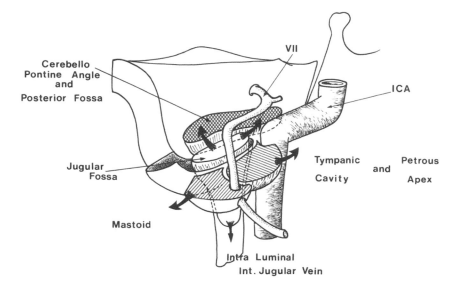

Fig. 4.1. Tympano jugular paraganglioma: patterns of invasion

Retrospective analysis of the origin of tumors reported before the mid 1970's is difficult, as the lesions tended to be diagnosed after they were advanced, and as the radiologic techniques used were not sufficiently sophisticated to provide the answers to the questions asked now.

The ascending pharyngeal artery is a unique link between paragangliomas in the tympanic, jugular, vagal, carotid and laryngeal locations, as each of these territories is supplied by a different branch of this artery.

Other branchial arteries, the internal maxillary artery more rostrally and the superior and inferior laryngeal arteries more caudally primarily supply paragangliomas which develop in their respective territories.

5. Natural History

Spontaneous regression of paragangliomas has never been reported. The growth is generaly slow, but it can be rapid or associated with additional tumours in other territories.

The therapeutic strategy will also be based on the answers to the following questions: is the lesion malignant? can a paraganglioma become malignant?

If the staged classification of Alford (1962) is true, any paraganglioma (Table 4.5) will eventually become malignant (stage 4), if its local invasion does not compromise the life of the patient first.

Table 4.5. Evolutive classification of temporal paragangliomas. From Alford and Guilford (1962)

	Presenting symptoms	Additional clinical findings
Stage 0	Hearing loss and/or pulsatile tinnitus.	Discolored tympanic membrane conductive hearing loss
Stage 1	+ discharge (otorrhea (ottorrhagia	+ Bulging or polypoid mass in the EAC.
Stage 2	+ VII – aural pain	+ perceptive hearing loss
Stage 3	+ IX nerve neuralgia	+ palsy IX, X, XII, ± XI
Stage 4	+ intra cranial symptoms (ataxia)	+ complete cranial nerve paralysis from III to XII. • papilledema • metastasis

Comments: Metastasis is presented as a predictable evolution of the tumors. Could they be malignant at stage 1 or 2? Could they remain benign? EAC, external auditory canal.

Table 4.6. Life expectancy of patients with temporal paragangliomas. From Harrison (1974) (personal survival statistics)

71% of patients alive and well at 5 years
29% of patients alive and well at 10 years
17% of patients alive and well at 15 years
10% of patients alive and well at 20 years

According to Harrison's (1974) series of paragangliomas of the temporal area (Table 4.6), the mean age of the patients presenting with this "benign" tumor is 45 years (see Epidemiology), and his life expectancy is 34 more years or a little less depending on the sex: it is impressive to note that only 10% of patients presenting with a temporal paraganglioma are alive and well 20 years after the discovery of their tumors.

Therefore, since we consider that lymph node invasion and metastasis are the only manifestations of malignancy, every reasonable attempt to totally remove the lesion should be made and any incomplete treatment be discouraged.

Delay in radical treatment while waiting for symptoms such as cranial nerve involvement to justify an aggressive approach should be avoided.

Our pre-therapeutic evaluation will endeavour to find the safest way to cure the patient of his tumor, and to disclose an already existing but asymptomatic associated lesion.

6. Clinical Aspects

Two clinical aspects of branchial paragangliomas should be considered: the tumor itself and the neurocristopathy.

The symptoms of paragangliomas are related to the primary location of *the tumor*. Schematically, three syndromes can be described: tympanic, jugular and caroticovagal. The symtomatology (mass, bruit, cranial nerve palsies, pain), is usually progressive (typically neoplastic) but may be fluctuating, acute or even regressive (pseudovascular). Gaillard (1978) related this phenomenon to possible intratumoral hemorrhage or peritumoral inflammatory reaction.

a) Tympanic Paragangliomas

have often been considered as an unique entity because they are usually already large at the time of diagnosis (Tables 4.7, 4.8). However, specific features can be recognized.

The most prominent symptom is the presence of pulsatile tinnitus which usually increases during effort, and often decreases with the Valsalva maneuver or cervical vascular compression. It is present early in the history of the disease because of bone conduction at the promotory; it may be intermittent but progressively more intense and intolerable. Typically unilateral, it is always related to the arterial pulsation. Tinnitus is usually not associated with headaches.

Any subjective bruit described as a "buzzing" or "roaring" is unlikely due to a tympanic paraganglioma. In the evolution of the tumor the disappearance of tinnitus indicates cochlear destruction.

Conductive hearing loss, otorrhagia, VIIth nerve palsy and reddish or bluish bulging of the tympanic membrane, complete the typical presentation of a tympanic paraganglioma.

In 30% of cases, VIIth nerve palsies occur acutely (Spector, 1976). They can regress spontaneously, thus leading to the incorrect diagnosis of Bell's palsy. They are though to be related to transient arterial "steal" following activation of arteriovenous shunt within the tumor. Further growth of the tumor will lead to its extension towards the mastoid cells, with reto-

Table 4.7. Temporal paragangliomas: presenting symptoms

Hearing loss (perceptive or conductive)	Vertigo
Pulsatile tinnitus	Hemorrhage (otorrhagia)
VIIth nerve palsy	Lower cranial nerve palsy
Discharge	Mass effect (EAC, pharyngeal, mastoid)
Pain	

Table 4.8. Classification of temporal paragangliomas (72 patients over 12 years). From Fisch (1982) and Valavanis (1983)

Type A 6 (8%)	Tumor limited to the middle ear cavity	Surgery (tympanoplastic techniques)
Type B mastoid 16 (22%)	Tumor limited to the tympano mastoid (without infra labyrinthic extension)	Surgery (tympanoplastic techniques)
Type C Petrous pyramid extensions 33 (47%)	C1 and C2 destroy the jugular foramen and ascending portion of carotid canal C3 extension to the petrous pyramid.	Surgery (infratemporal techniques). ICA: 10% suture or ligature 90% intact Lower cranial nerves: IX lost in CI IX, X lost in C2 IX, X, XI lost in C3

Type D
Intra cranial
Intra dural
17 (23%)
	D1 < 2 cm
	D2 > 2 cm
	D3 inoperable intra-
	        cranial
	        Extension (?)
		Surgery (infra temporal)
		± Neurosurgery
		ICA: 100% intact
		Lower cranial nerves:
		IX, X, XI lost

Comments:	– Extradural extension although intracranial do not affect the classification. – No reference is made to: exocranial extension, jugular vein occlusion and lateral sinus patency, false intracranial extensions.	

auricular pain, and mass effect in the external auditory canal, parapharyngeal space and petrous apex.

Medial extension towards the inner ear will cause additional symptoms such as perceptive deafness and vertigo. Posteromedial growth towards the jugular bulb and pars nervosa will produce other cranial nerve manifestations. In general, when one considers the diagnosis, tympanic paragangliomas can be recognized and treated at an early stage when the tumor is still small, resulting in preservetion of hearing function.

b) Jugular Paragangliomas

They typically present with a jugular foramen syndrome (Vernet's syndrome) which includes paralysis of the IXth, Xth, and XIth cranial nerves. At this stage, they are already large tumors.

Jugular paragangliomas can, over a long period produce minimal symptoms like hypoglossal neuralgia (sore throat without infection). Intermitent pulsatile tinnitus is often neglected, even at the stage of cranial nerve involvement, but is recalled by the patient following embolization, when it disappears and is replaced by what is described as complete silence. The tinnitus may be non pulsatile and is, probably related to slighly turbulent jugular vein circulation from the intraluminal tumoral extension. Retroauricular pain can also be encountered when lateral expansion of the tumors occurs. Later, when the lower cranial nerves are impaired, cough due to aspiration, hoarseness, uvular displacement and sternocleidomastoid and trapezoid muscle paralysis will be noted.

The venous occlusion of the internal jugular vein and retrograde adjacent extension in its tributaries either by the tumor or induced thrombosis, usually have no specific clinical manifestations. However, vertigo and hearing loss may occur without obvious inner ear extension of the tumor.

A XIIth nerve palsy is usually combined with facial nerve involvement, following progressing tumor growth, but it may occur before the XIth nerve palsy. In our experience, function of the XIth nerve is often preserved for a long time.

In this location, further extension occurs towards the tympanic cavity (i. e. local multicentricity) and intracranially. Although they usually remain extradural for a long time, large jugular paragangliomas have also been reported in the intradural cerebellopontine angle (D type of Fisch's classification). Where they produce cerebellar symptoms and increased intracranial pressure. Forty percent of jugular paragangliomas were thought by Glenner in 1973 to have an intracranial extension. Only one of over 37 patients in our experience had intracranial extension; however four had either a false angiographic extension or strictly extradural spread (see Fig. 4.2). Compression of the motor pathwasys in the posterior fossa and subarachnoid hemorrhage occur rarely (Moody, 1976).

c) Cervical Paragangliomas

Cervical paragangliomas have in common a cervical mass effect, but some specific findings can help to differentiate the vagal from the carotid forms (Fig. 4.3).

Carotid paragangliomas present as pulsatile expansile masses and when they occur as single, isolated lesions, are usually associated with few other symptoms. However, although the mass is typically cervical, it may extend into the parapharyngeal space (10% in Zak's review) (Table 4.9) or even into the oral cavity or larynx. This apparently contradictory behavior, extensive regional spread at the time of diagnosis of a slow growing lesion, may be explained by multicentric origin of the various components of the mass.

Cranial nerve involvement is rare with isolated carotid paragangliomas, and has been reported in patients with large (or multicentric) lesions. Typically the superior laryngeal nerve (leading to hoarseness which is perceived by the patient) and the descending branch of the XIIth nerve are affected. The unilateral hemiaotrophy and tongue fasciculation produced by the involvement of the XIIth nerve are generally not noticed by the patient.

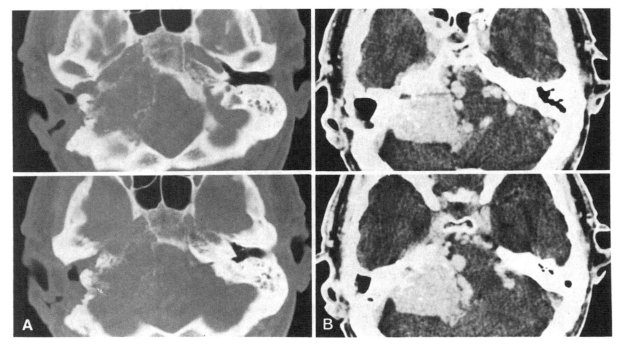

Fig. 4.2 A, B

Horner's syndrome and cerebral infarction may result from local invasion, the latter caused by internal carotid artery occlusion following tumor extension into the arterial wall.

Vagal paragangliomas demonstrate some characteristic features related to the site of origin of the mass within the neurovascular bundle of the neck, adjacent to the pharyngeal wall and high in the cervical space. The most frequent presenting symptom is a mass in the cervical (78%) or pharyngeal (44%) spaces (Fig. 4.4).

Thirty percent of patients have cranial nerve impairment (Table 4.10) which frequently manifests by neck hypoesthesia and pharyngeal pain. The high incidence of symptoms of peripheral cranial nerve involvement is probably related to the tight neurovascular compartment in which the tumor arises.

In our experience, a female in her forties with a painful pharyngeal mass, associated with Xth and XIIth nerve impairment has a very high likelyhood of having a vagal paraganglioma; tumors in this location and population are more likely to be malignant (3/37 vagal tumors in our series were malignant; all were in females; 16, 40 and 45 years of age) (Fig. 4.4).

Vagal paragangliomas may arise from paraganglions in two locations; intravagal at or below the ganglion nodose and extravagal. Those arising from intravagal paraganglions produce rapid vagal nerve impairment and generally do not permit preservation of the nerve during tumor resection. With tumors arising from extravagal paraganglions, the vagal nerve can often be preserved even when the tumor is large. As with paragangliomas in other locations, further growth results in extension to the base of the skull or intracranial contents, again, it is difficult to know whether this pattern reflects multicentric origin or malignant expression, as classical for jugular tumors with destruction of the base of the skull (Rosenwasser 1958).

Fig. 4.2 A-D. 56 years old male presenting a right recurrent jugular paraganglioma, and complaining of VIIth to XIIth cranial nerve palsies and long tract deficits (motor and cerebellar). Note on the CT sections (**A** and **B**) the bone destructions and cerebral venous drainage. On the right vertebral angiogram (**C** and **D**) note the extra dural extension fed by the odontoid arterial arch *(arrow)* and the occipital branches (proximally ligated during the previous surgical attempt) *(open arrow)*. The cerebello pontine extension recrutes intradural supply from AICA displaced superiorly *(arrowheads)*, and PICA inferiorly *(double arrowhead)*. Note the bilateral venous drainage of the tumor *(curved arrows)*, and the upper venous ectasia *(arrowhead)*

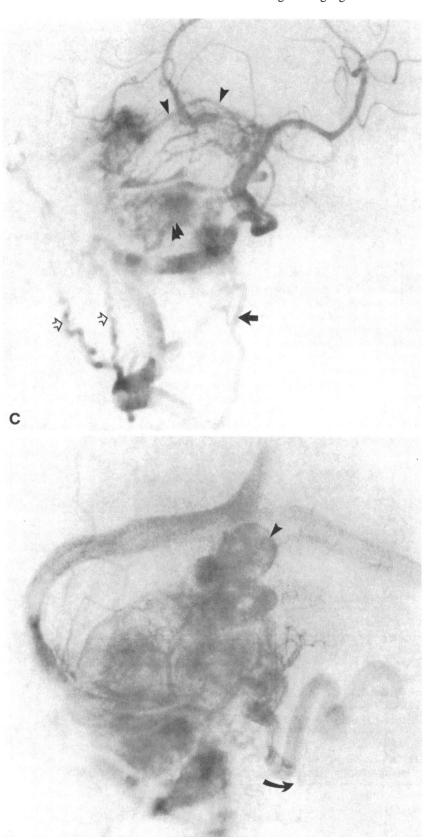

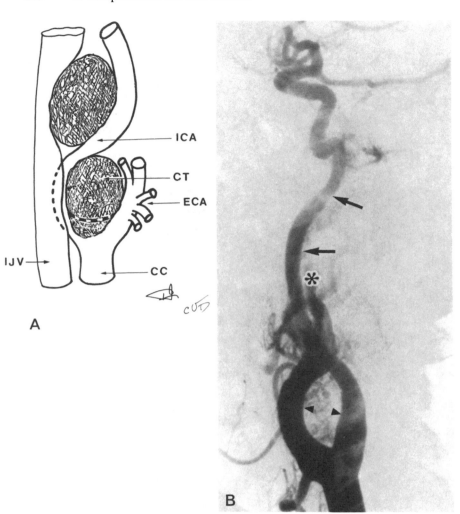

Fig. 4.3. A Diagrammatic illustration of the relationship between vagal *(VT)* and carotid *(CT)* tumors, and the large vessels of the neck. (*CC* = common carotid artery; *ECA* = external carotid artery; *ICA* = internal carotid artery; *IJV* = internal jugular vein). **B** Left carotid angiogram in a 50 year old female with a left temporo-jugular, vagal and carotid body paraganglioma following PVA embolization of the external carotid branches *(asterisk)*. Note the displacement of the vessels related to the vagal *(arrows)* and carotid *(arrowheads)* tumors

Table 4.9. Carotid paragangliomas: Clinical presentation in over 254 patients. From Zak (1982)

Symptoms	
Pain	19%
Dysphagia	11%
Syncope	9%
Hoarseness	8%
Horner's syndrome	7%
XIIth nerve deficit	2%

Table 4.10. Vagal paragangliomas: peripheral nervous system involvement

X	24%
XII	14%
IX	11%
XI	8%
Horner's syndrome	11%

Fig. 4.4. 16 year old female presenting with a left cervical mass (**A**) and ipsilateral XIIth nerve palsy (**B**). A vagal paraganglioma was embolized (see Fig. 17.4, Vol. 1) and removed entirely. However 6 month later, the patient was readmitted for progressive paraplegia. Spinal angiography (**C** to **G**) demonstrates metastases in the low thoracic spine (**C**), mid thoracic epidural space (**D**), cervical space (**E**) and para spinal tissue (**F**)

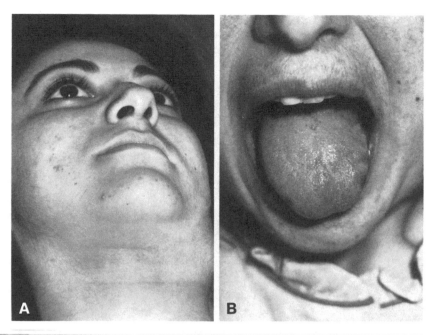

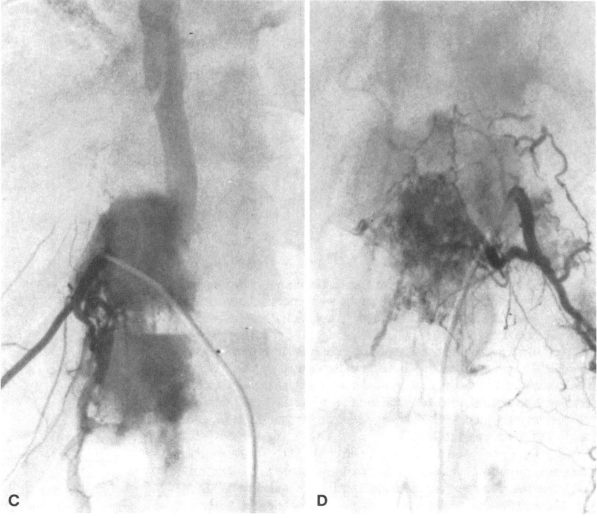

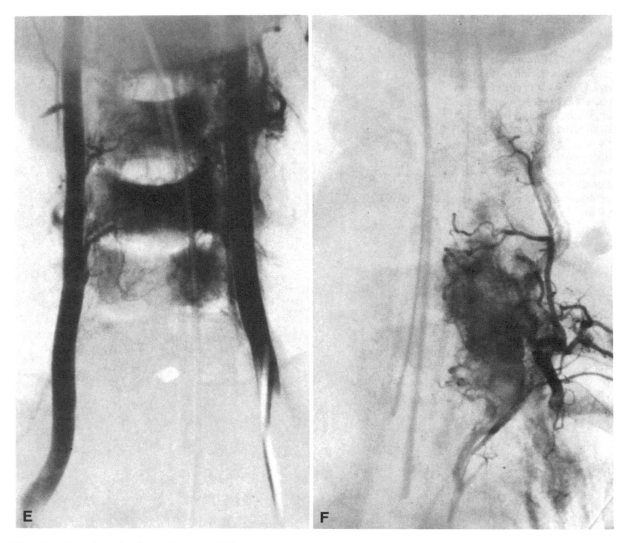

Fig. 4.4 (continued) (legend see p. 141)

d) Paragangliomas in Other Locations

Paragangliomas which arise in atypical locations within the head and neck regions are much more difficult to diagnose and generaly require biopsy. Delay in specific diagnosis, unfortunately, frequently leads to delay in appropriate treatment.

Those which present in the nasopharynx are frequently misdiagnose as pharyngeal carcinomas, as they develop in the same age group. Unfortunately, some may even be irradiated without a diagnostic biopsy. These lesions are infrequent, so it is difficult to characterize their clinical features; our patient presented with diplopia, painful hypoesthesia of V_3 cranial nerve; and serous otitis (Fig. 4.5).

Prabhaker (1984) reported a seven year old girl with a sellar paraganglioma who presented with a hemibase syndrome involving most of the left cranial nerves, and recurrent episodic reversible ophtalmoplegia. The CT findings were those of a solid mass containing a cystic (or necrotic) lucency (Fig. 4.6).

Fig. 4.4. G shows displacement ▶
of the artery of Adamkiewitz
due to an intraspinal metastasis
as well as extraspinal disease

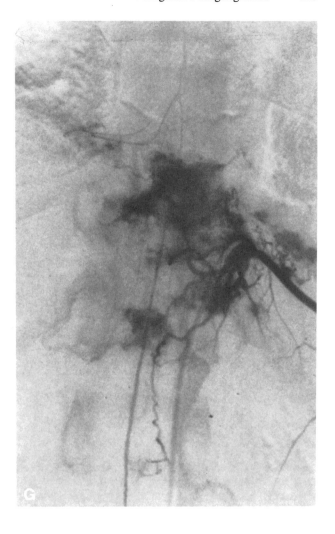

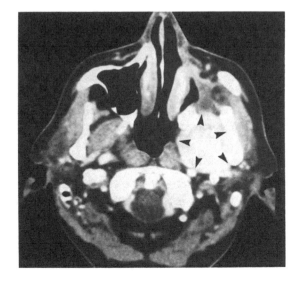

Fig. 4.5. Enhanced axial CT
examination in a patient with a
left sided paraganglioma of the
cavum. Note the highly enhanced tumor *(arrowheads)*
(see also Vol. 1, Fig. 18.5)

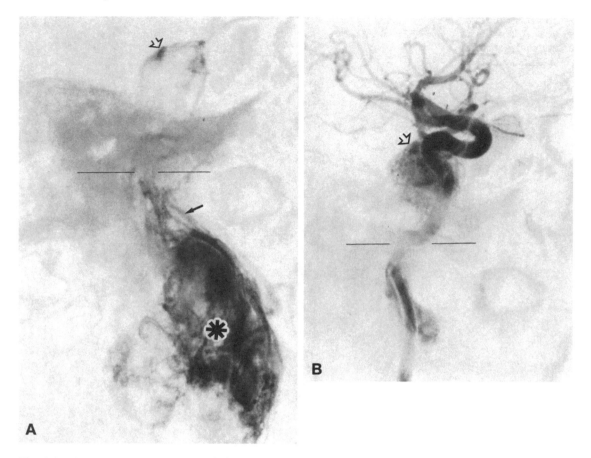

Fig. 4.6. Right ascending pharyngeal (**A**) and internal carotid (**B**) angiograms, in a 65 year old patient complaining of a moderately painful chronic parapharyngeal mass. A large vagal paraganglioma *(asterisks)* was associated with an asymptomatic clival localization *(open arrow)*. Note the normal appearance of the pharyngeal artery *(arrow)* and the discontinuity between the extra and intracranial tumor masses

Laryngeal paragangliomas are also rare, but can be diagnosed early due to their localizing symptomatology; hoarseness (70%), dyspnea (43%) and pain. Like other paragangliomas, they can be endocrinologically active, multicentric and malignant (see Chapter 5).

Orbital paragangliomas are intraconical and present with non pulsatile proptosis and decreased vision. Unfortunately they produce no specific symptoms which allow differentiation from other orbital tumors, and require histologic examination or diagnosis. Zak, after analyzing the cases reported in the literature, emphasized the local invasiveness of orbital paragangliomas, and their tendency to recur and metastasize.

e) Secretory Paragangliomas

The endocrine activity of some paragangliomas may produce additional symptoms, but this occurs relatively infrequently, in 5% of patients if minor manifestations are taken into account (Table 4.11). It is often difficult to confirm by laboratory essays, and is usually diagnosed retrospectively when manifestations are relieved following embolization and/or surgical removal of the tumor (see Vol. 1, Fig. 17.2).

Table 4.11. Secretory activity: clinical manifestations

Headache
Hypertension
Palpitation
Diaphoresis
Anxiety

Manipulation of some secretory tumors, either by massage or during surgery, may produce hypertensive crisis requiring the pre- and intraoperative use of alpha-adrenergic receptor blocking agents and/or nitroprusside (Strauss, 1983). Elders in 1962 reported a 12 year old boy with a carotid body paraganglioma in whom massage of the tumor produced hypertension, sweating and pallor. Its removal resulted in intractable hypotention and death.

Less commonly, tumor manipulation may result in hypotension, with black-out spells (Strauss, 1983). Although we have noted no evidence of release of catecholamines or serotonin during pre surgical embolization procedures, blood pressure fluctuations usually stop once the devascularization of the tumor is completed. In our experience, systolic blood pressure frequently decreases by 20 mmHg following embolization, even when no evidence of secretory activity was noted prior to treatment.

Hypertensive crises have been reported to occur during angiography of secretory paragangliomas, and require urgent therapy. This complication may be secondary to hypertonic contrast agents. If possible, secretory activity should be assessed prior to angiography and embolization, and appropriate anti-hypertensive agents should be readily available. One of us (PL) performs nearly all of those procedures under general anesthesia, uses non-ionic contrast material, and has not experienced this complication.

Twenty functional paragangliomas included in Zak's series were distributed as follows: carotid (5), temporal (7) laryngeal (1), vagal (1) and ectopic (6). At histochemical examination, twelve were non chomaffin and three were chromaffin tumors. High level of the following substances were detected in samples of blood, urine or tumor: total catecholamines, normetanephrin and homovanilic acid.

Strauss (1983) pointed out that malignant carotid and laryngal paragangliomas were more likely *to have endocrine* manifestations. Unfortunately, in this series, only metastatic tumors were included so that the relationship between secretion and malignancy cannot be accurately assessed.

We have observed three patients with hypertension suggesting endocrine activity in whom biological evidence could not be obtained by laboratory assays. In one of these, a 20 year old female with episodes of Bouveret tachycardia a surgical attempt at removal of a carotid paraganglioma had to be interrupted because of fluctuating blood pressure. She then underwent embolization and reoperation with complete removal of the tumor, with no additional hemodynamic manifestations (see Vol. 1, Fig. 17.2).

We have wondered about a possible relationship between endocrine activity and the influence of a local angiogenetic factor on the development of the tumors. However, in two patients who demonstrated a peritumoral "blush" at angiography. We were not able to confirm the presence of a true abnormality underlying the blush, either at the time of post operative control angiography in one patient or at histologic examination in the other (see Vol. 1, p. 366).

f) Associated Lesions

Theoretically, numerous syndromes can be distinguished, depending upon the combination of paraganglioma and other tumors involving the cells of the APUD system.

Carcinoid tumors, pheochromocytomas, pituitary adenomas thyroid carcinomas, other secretory tumors and neurofibromatosis have all been reported to occur in association with paragangliomas.

Albores (1968) pointed out an analogy between the association between carotid paragangliomas and thyroid adenomas and papillary or follicular carcinomas and the more classical association between medullary thyroid carcinoma and pheochromocytoma.

In individual patients, these associations do not alter the diagnostic or therapeutic approach to the paraganglioma. They do, however, emphasized the need to consider all of the possible causes of symptoms in individuals with these tumors, and the need to thoroughly investigate these patients prior to treatment. Regardless of the presence of additional lesions, radical surgical removal (following embolization) of the paraganglioma is still the treatment of choice.

7. Differential Diagnosis

The differential diagnosis of the symptoms and/or mass aspect of paragangliomas includes a variety non- surgical and *non-neoplastic diseases,* listed in Tables 4.12 and 4.13.

Non surgical lesions include normal anatomic vascular variants, such as aberrant internal carotid flow in the tympanic cavity (see Vol. 1, Chapter 2) persistent stapedial artery and ectopic jugular bulb.

A dominant jugular bulb may produce pulsatile tinnitus, partly because it receives a normally pulsating venous flow from the inferior petrosal tributaries which drain the cavernous sinus (Buckenwalter, 1983). Aside from this entity, all other causes of objective pulsatile tinnitus are produced by arterial flow (Noyek).

Table 4.12. Differential diagnosis of jugular-tympanic paraganglioma. Modified from Zak (1982)

Prominent jugular bulb
Intratympanic course of internal carotid circulation
Stapedial artery persistance
Granuloma (tympanic)
Neurogenic tumor (cochlear nerve, Jacobson's nerve)
Meningiomas (temporal bone)
Metastasis (jugular foramen)
Hemangiomas (osseous, tympanic)

Table 4.13. Differential diagnosis of carotid paragangliomas. Modified from Zak (1982)

Lymphadenitits
Branchial cleft cyst
Metastasis (Thyroid cancer[a], lymphoma, or Hodgkin's disease)
Neurogenic tumors
Aneurysms
Dolicocarotid sinus

[a] Thyroid carcinoma can be associated with carotid body paragangliomas whereas medullary cancer of the thyroid is associated with pheochromocytoma.

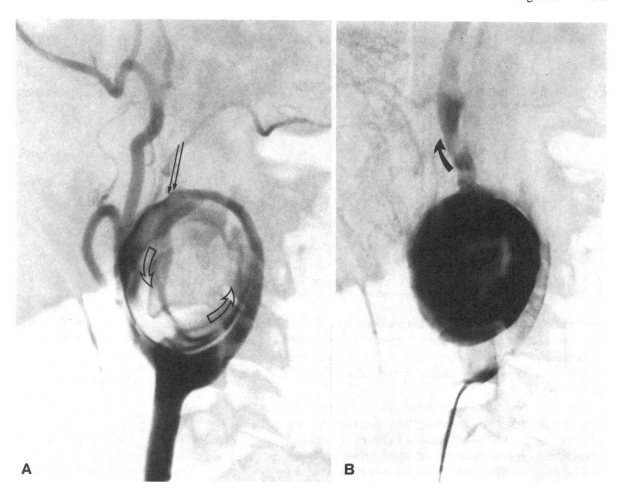

A   B

Fig. 4.7. Left common carotid angiogram (**A**) early and (**B**) late phases, in a 32 year old female presenting with a painful cervical pulsatile mass, thought to be a carotid body tumor. Note the giant aneurysm of the cervical internal carotid body *(double arrow).* Turbulent flow in the pouch *(open curved arrow)* is followed by filling of the distal cervical internal carotid artery *(curved arrow)*

Moderate ectasia of the internal carotid bulb or dolicho carotid artery may be associated with local pain, parapharyngeal mass effect and even lower cranial nerve palsies, and may be mistaken for small carotid body tumors. Likewise, internal carotid artery aneurysms may simulate carotid, vagal or tympanic paragangliomas by producing dysphagia, mass effect, cranial nerve palsies and pulsatile tinnitus (Margolis, 1972). Among 20 patients with aneurysms of the internal carotid artery reported by Margolis (1972) five were atherosclerotic, 7 were congenital, 6 were traumatic and two were secondary to local infection (mycotic). They may be associated with other aneurysms or vascular lesions, and the associated lesions may be the underlying cause of the symptoms (subarachnoid, hemorrhage, traumatic carotid cavernous fistulae, etc.). Their management requires a multidisciplinary approach and often benefits from the use of endovascular techniques (see Chapter 8) (Fig. 4.7).

Postoperative symptomatic scar tissue, which is difficult to diagnose, may stimulate recurrence. Lastly, non neoplastic lesions, such as enlarged lymph nodes or branchial cysts may transmit carotid pulsations, simulating pulsatile tinnitus.

The congenital vascular anomalies can be assessed or predicted from a careful study of the foramena using CT high quality, angiography with proper analysis of the venous phase. The carotid and dominant vertebral

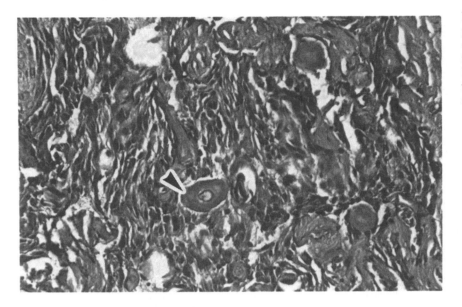

Fig. 4.8. A 48 year old female presented with progressive deafness related to a strictly intratympanic meningioma. Note on the pathological section the typical psamoma *(arrowhead)*

artery injections provide definitive confirmation of any of the congenital or aquired vascular causes of tinnitus (see Vol. 1, Chapter 2).

Because of the importance of establishing the correct diagnosis, we think that there is no place for mediocre vascular studies, such as intravenous or global arterial injection.

The discovery of a congenital anatomic variant or other vascular abnormality during the investigation of a symptomatic patient, in whom one has anticipated the presence of a surgically treatable tumor, often leads to confusion regarding the most appropriate management. One must be careful to avoid the temptation of overly agressive treatment.

Other tumors which enter the differential diagnosis of paragangliomas are listed in Tables 4.14 and 4.15. The final diagnosis rests with the histologic findings in the surgical specimen.

Metastatic disease involving the jugular and carotid lymph nodes may simulate paragangliomas, especially when they are hypervascular at angiography and the primary tumor is not appreciated.

Meningiomas which are purely tympanic in location may be mistaken, even at histologic examination, for paragangliomas, but can be distinguished from them at angiography. On the other hand, their therapeutic management is the same with embolization followed by surgical resection (Fig. 4.8).

Neurogenic tumors are fairly common in the parapharyngeal space (see Nasopharynx); less commonly they may occurr at the jugular or hypoglossal foramena. In the few cases we studied, the tumors were all supplied by the ascending pharyngeal artery but were less vascular than most paragangliomas. The clinical features may be helpful in distinguishing these lesions, as they tend to have neurological deficits early (Crumley, 1984; Fujiwara, 1980; Chang, 1984). Similarities to cervical paragangliomas include hoarsness dysphagia, and pulsation. These tumors may be malignant and are radioresistant, so their management also includes embolization and surgical resection (Fig. 4.9).

Primary malignant tumors or metastases can be highly vascularized and a specific diagnosis by angiography may not be possible. Cerebellopontine

Fig. 4.9. 55 year old female presenting with progressive deafness of the right ear, related to an intratympanic neurofibroma involving Jacobson's nerve. Note the cutaneous manifestations of von Recklinghausen's disease (Neurofibromatosis)

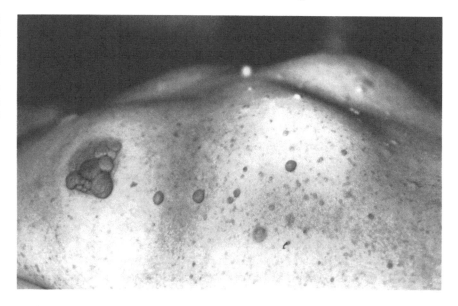

angle tumors such as acoustic neurinomas and hemangioblastomas may be supplied by the external carotid artery, but generally have a different angiographic blush compared to paragangliomas (see Vol. 1, Figs. 14.11, 16.1; and Vol. 2, Figs. 2.4, 2.11).

One of our patients was referred to us with the diagnosis of tympano-jugular paraganglioma on the basis of lower cranial nerve palsies and low cerebellopontine angle tumor associated with bluish discoloration of the tympanic membrane. Increased intracranial pressure due to the size of the mass led to ventricular shunting. Pulsatile tinnitus could not be expected since the patient had perceptive deafness related to the cerebellopontine angle lesion. Clinical examination revealed a bluish discoloration of the external ear including the helix and external auditory canal. Aside from the last findings, the features were felt to be consistent with the diagnosis of a branchial paraganglioma. However, tympanic tumors do not produce discoloration of the helix and this abnormality was found to be due to a venous vascular malformation, present since birth. The cerebellopontine angle tumor was a malignant melanoma (see Vol. 1, Fig. 16.1).

Most bone tumors have CT findings which distinguish them from paragangliomas, although vascular malformations involving the bone may have some features in common (Glassock, 1984).

Table 4.14. Primary lesions involving the petrous apex. From Flood (1984)

Epidermoid cyst
Mesenchymal tumor
Eosinophilic granuloma
Primary mucocele

Table 4.15. Secondary lesions involving the petrous apex. From Flood (1984)

Osteomyelitis	Secondary to mastoiditis Secondary to malignant external otitis
Direct tumor Spread	Nasopharyngeal carcinoma of the clivus. Paraganglioma Neurogenic tumors (V to XII) Meningioma
Erosion by disseminated tumor	Metastatic carcinoma Lymphoma
Other osteolytic process	Sphenoid mucocele Aneurysm of the internal carotid artery

Ascending pharyngeal angiography will nearly always confirm or rule out the diagnosis of a suspected branchial paraganglioma. Absence of the typical appearance of the tumor blush seen with paragangliomas essentially excludes that diagnosis. Other branchial lesions, which may occur in order of decreasing angiographic tumor vascularity, include metastases, hemangiomas, meningiomas, neurogenic tumors, and lymphatic neoplasia.

8. Pretherapeutic Evaluation

Although the clinical presentation is often stongly suggestive of the diagnosis of a branchial paraganglioma, CT examination is useful and necessary in demonstrating or ruling out vascular variants which may simulate paragangliomas and in demonstrating the topography of large masses (Figs. 4.2, 4.10). As with other mass lesions the examination should be performed without and with contrast enhancement, and should be filmed or at least viewed at bone as well at soft tissue windows. Direct coronal images are indispensable in the presence of cervical or base of the skull mass lesions, and thin (1.0–3.0 mm) sections are necessary to evaluate the petrous temporal bones. The following structures should be specifically examined: the carotid canal, inner and middle ear, cerebellopontine angle, mastoid process, cervical vessels and pterygoid muscles, as involvement of these structures will modify the surgical and embolization approaches (Figs. 4.2, 4.10).

Supraselective angiography remains the most specific diagnostic technique and if a paraganglioma is suspected, it should always be performed before biopsy is attempted.

a) Angiographic Protocol

The arterial feeders which should be selectively catheterized can usually be predicted from the topography of the mass demonstrated on the CT examination. Embolization is performed at the time of diagnostic angiography.

The typical angiographic features of paragangliomas include moderate enlargement of the feeding arteries, an early, intense parenchymal blush, and rapid venous filling. As previously discussed, some tumors are opacified by a single feeding artery, while others are supplied by several. After all possible arterial supply has been studied, the most efficatious and safest route for embolization can be selected.

The arteries which should be studied in each region are described in Vol. 1, Chapters 15–21.

b) Temporal Paragangliomas: Specific Features (Fig. 4.11)

The arteries which should be studied selectively include the ipsilateral vertebral, internal carotid, distal external carotid, posterior auricular and occipital arteries and the ascending pharyngeal artery bilaterally (ipsilateral neuromeningeal and inferior tympanic branches). The late phase of the dominant vertebral artery injection is also necessary, for visualization of the venous flow pattern. Jugular vein occlusion will be demonstrated and the collateral venous drainage outlined. However, a larger arteriovenous shunt within a tumor draining into the internal jugular vein may produce a

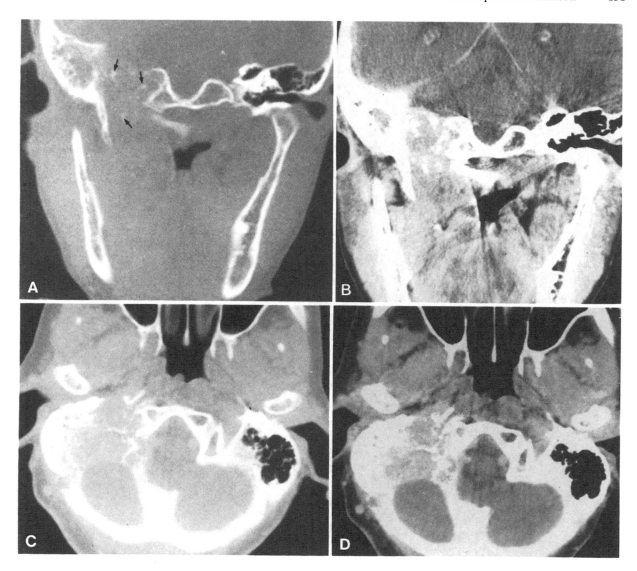

Fig. 4.10 A-D. CT Examination of a 82 year old female presenting with an intensive subjective and objective pulsatile bruit of the right ear caused by a large jugular paraganglioma. Surgical resection of the lesion was not considered. Embolization with PVA was undergone. Note on the direct coronal (**A** and **B**) and axial (**C** and **D**) CT images after the treatment, the radio opaque emboli *(arrow)* and the minimal contrast enhancement of the lesion. Clinically, the bruit diminished to a tolerable level, and the result remains stable with 3 year follow-up

"wash-out" of contrast within this vein, and lead to the erroneous diagnosis of venous occlusion. In the presence of true tumor invasion, a discrete intraluminal filling defect will be seen on the venous phase, and selective arterial injections will demonstrate a tumor blush within the vein. In patients where the jugular vein was not well seen due to "wash-out", its patency should be confirmed by repeat vertebral angiography following embolization (Fig. 4.12). Jugular venography, for the most part is unnecessary.

α) Intradural posterior fossa extension (Fig. 4.2) must be carefully distinguished from extradural or extracranial tumor, in order to avoid misinterpretation which could result in avoidance of surgery in potentially resectable lesions. A tumor blush is frequently seen at or caudal to the level of the temporal bone on vertebral angiograms, but in most instances it originates from the extradural branches of the vertebral artery at CI, C2 or C3, and represents extradural tumor. True intradural tumor spread is best confirmed or ruled out by careful analysis of the ipsilateral A.I.C.A. and

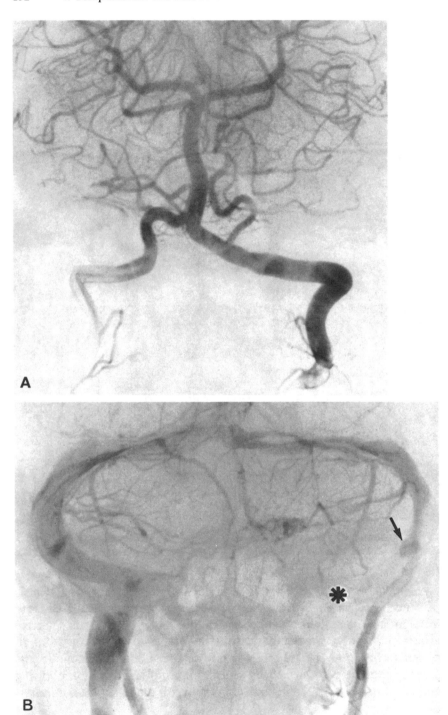

Fig. 4.11. 40 year old male presenting with pulsatile bruit in the left ear and ipsilateral lower cranial nerve palsies (**A**) early and (**B**) late phase of the dominant (left) vertebral. Note the absence of CP angle arterial supply, the occlusion of the left jugular foramen *(asterisk)* and the venous collateral circulation via the mastoid foramen *(arrow)*

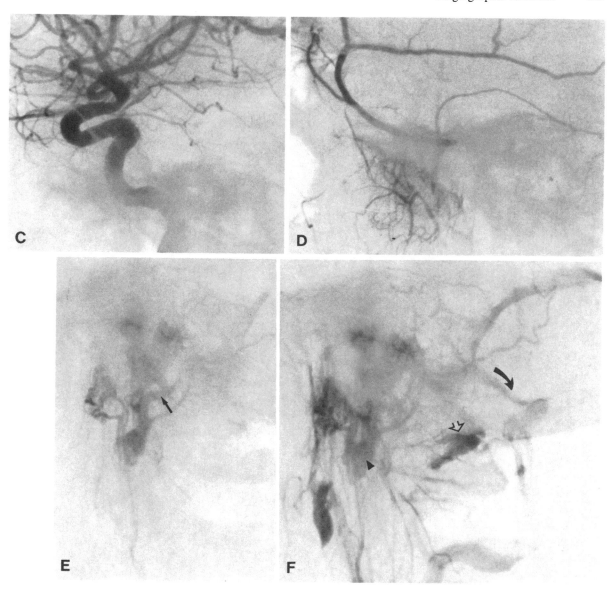

Fig. 4.11 (continued)
Normal left internal carotid (**C**) and middle meningeal artery (**D**) angiograms.
Selective injection in the auricular branch of an occipito auricular trunk (**E** and **F**)
shows arterial supply to the tumor via the stylomastoid artery *(straight arrow)* and
venous drainage via the mastoid *(curved arrow)* and posterior condyloid *(open
arrow)* canals

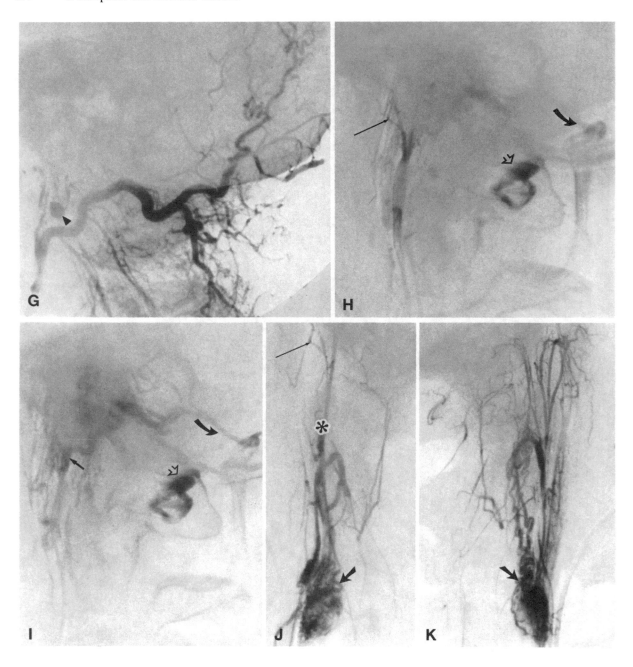

Fig. 4.11 (continued)
G Post embolization injections in the proximal occipito-auricular trunk and proximal ascending pharyngeal artery (**H**). Note the pharyngeal branch *(arrow)* and the venous drainage of the tumor into the mastoid *(curved arrow)* and the posterior condyloid *(open arrow)* veins. **I** Selective injection of the posterior branch of the ascending pharyngeal artery *(arrow)*. **J** Control in the pharyngeal artery after the embolization of the posterior branch *(asterisk)*. Note the patency of the pharyngeal branch *(arrow)* and the additional tumoral stain proximal on the artery *(solid arrow)*. **K** Injection in the ascending pharyngeal artery on the opposite side shows the same type of proximal stain *(solid arrow)*

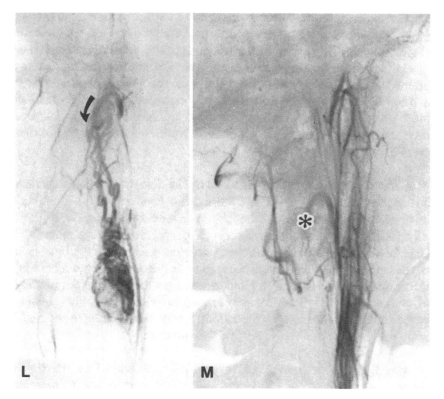

Fig. 4.11. (continued)
L Selective injection of the musculo spinal artery, and the control study of the ascending pharyngeal trunk (**M**) shows satisfactory occlusion of the feeder *(asterisk)*. The three lesions were removed in one surgical session. The temporal lesion was a typical tympano-jugular paraganglioma whereas both cervical ones were lymph nodes metastates

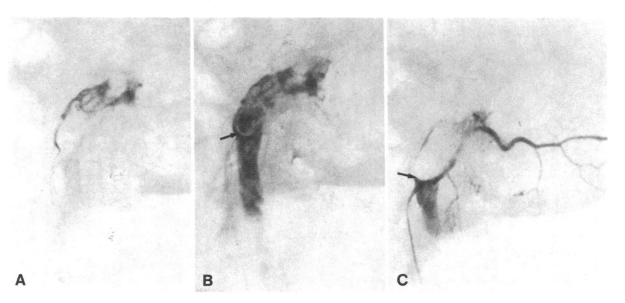

Fig. 4.12. Jugular paraganglioma (**A**) early and (**B**) late phases of the ascending pharyngeal artery injection. **C** Ipsilateral occipital artery angiogram. Note how the intra luminal jugular vein tumor delineates the lower extension of the lesion. Distal jugular vein injection is obtained through the tumoral arteriovenous shunt, which shadows the inferior convex margin of the paraganglioma *(arrows)*

P.I.C.A. territories in Townes' projection, as intradural tumor will be supplied by branches of these arteries. Comparison of the vertebral angiographic findings with those from the ipsilateral selective occipital and ascending pharyngeal injections usually permits an accurate assessment of tumor extent. Misinterpretation of the tumor blush produced by the extradural vertebral artery branches may account for the high incidence (40%) of intracranial extension reported by Farrior (1980). The same problem has already been seen with 36% erroneous JAF extension to the cranial cavity (Holman, 1985).

β) **Carotid canal invasion** is diagnosed by the detection of soft tissue mass and bone destruction involving the carotid canal on CT examination, associated with narrowing of the intra petrous carotid artery at angiography. Arterial supply to the tumor (e.g. tympanic paraganglioma) by branches of the internal carotid artery does not necessarily signify invasion of the carotid canal. The internal carotid artery constantly has a branch to the tympanic cavity through a small foramen posterior to the petrous angle of the vessel. The Stenvers projection, in which the X-ray beam is perpendicular to the intrapetrous carotid artery, best demonstrates the free bony margin between the vessel and the tumor blush.

γ) **Angiographic blush** in the region of the petrous bone adjacent to the soft tissue mass outlined on CT examination may correspond to increased vascularity of healthy tissue, probably the result of stimulation by an angiogenetic factor (see Vol. 1, Fig. 9.18) or pretumoral stage.

Fig. 4.13 A, B

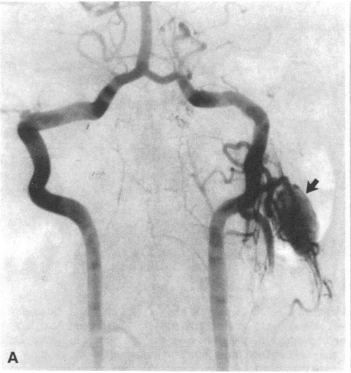 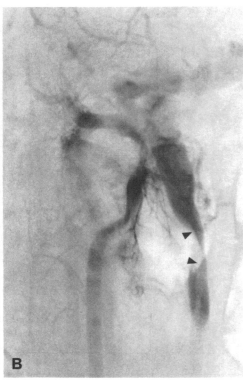

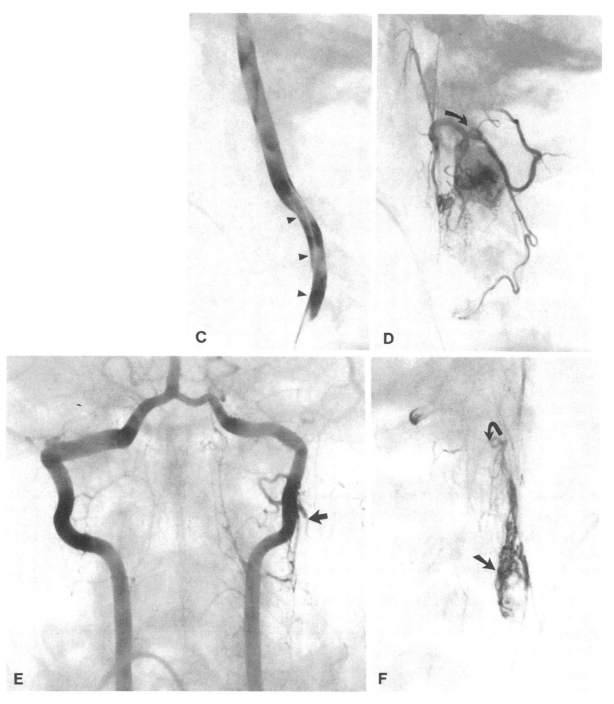

Fig. 4.13. 15 year old female presenting with a left cervical mass (**A**) early and (**B**) late phases of the dominant left vertebral artery injection demonstrates a vagal paraganglioma *(arrow)* and the extrinsic indentation of the jugular vein *(arrowheads)*. **C** Left internal carotid injection shows posterior displacement by the tumor *(arrowheads)*. **D** Selective injection of the pharyngeal artery demonstrates the tumoral supply via the musculo spinal artery *(curved arrow)*. **E** Vertebral artery angiogram after embolization of the sole supply from the ascending pharyngeal artery fails to demonstrate the tumoral blush *(arrow)*. **F** Opposite ascending pharyngeal angiogram discloses an additional lesion *(arrow)* fed by the musculo spinal artery *(broken arrow)*. The tumors were removed in two surgical sessions and were found to be typical bilateral left vagal and right carotid paragangliomas

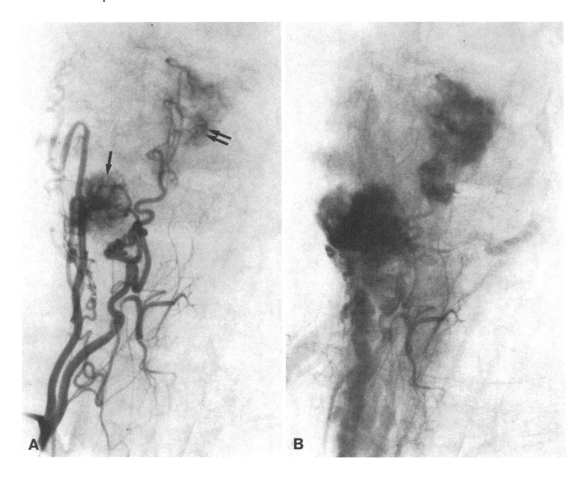

c) Cervical Paragangliomas: Specific Features

The arteries which should be selectively injected in the investigation of a suspected cervical paraganglioma include the following: ipsilateral vertebral, proximal internal carotid, facial, lingual, superior laryngeal, carotid body artery, ascending cervical, inferior laryngeal and bilateral ascending pharyngeal arteries (Figs. 4.13, 4.14).

Cervical paragangliomas frequently compress the internal jugular vein without parietal invasion. Unfortunately, true tumor involvement of the adventia of the internal carotid artery is not rare. The pattern of vessel displacement is a useful distinguishing feature, as vagal paragangliomas typically displace the interal carotid artery anteriorly and medially, whereas carotid paragangliomas displace the internal carotid artery laterally and posteriorly (Fig. 4.3).

Bilateral disease can be effectively diagnosed or ruled out by selective contrast injection in the contralateral ascending pharyngeal artery, which is generally the first part of our angiographic study. Each of the 95 branchial paragangliomas which we have studied was supplied at least partially by the ascending pharyngeal artery, and 20% of them received their blood supply exclusively from this vessel. Therefore, a normal contralateral ascending pharyngeal arteriogram eliminates the possibility of bilateral cervical paragangliomas. Only laryngeal and orbital lesions are supplied by other vessels (Figs. 4.11, 4.13).

Fig. 4.14. Inferior thyroidal artery injection early (**A**) and late (**B**) phases. Right anterior oblique projection in a patient with a large carotid body paraganglioma. Note the laryngeal extension *(double arrow)* and the lymph node invasion *(arrow)*

Angiographic features which suggest malignancy include arterial invasion and indistinctness of the tumor margins (after the entire "puzzle" reconstruction is complete).

Metastases have the same angiographic features as primary paragangliomas so that for those lesions which present in unusual locations in the head and neck it may be impossible to distinguish between ectopic or metastatic tumors.

In conclusion, angiography is presently the diagnostic procedure of choice in the delineation of tumor extent but is still imprecise in distinguishing malignant from multicentric disease (Figs. 4.11, 4.13, 4.14).

9. Therapeutic Strategies

Like the treatment of other complex lesions of the head and neck area, optimal therapy requires a multidisciplinary approach but will vary between different centers depending upon the skills of the available individuals.

Interpretation of the results of various therapeutic modalitites reported in the literature is difficult. In particular, it is almost impossible to distinguish between recurrence, metastasis and late manifestation of multicentricity.

The efficacy of radiotherapy in the treatment of paragangliomas differs greatly in different series in the literature. Doses above or equal to 40 Grays have been reported to result in tumor control in over 90% of patients (Cummings, 1984), whereas two surgical series found only a 25% cure rate using radiotherapy (Ogura, 1978, Spector 1973). It is recognized that the tumor cells are not radiosensitive, and the predominant effects of radiation are via the secondary vascular arteritis and fibrosis. Late complications such as brain necrosis are being recognized more frequently since CT has become available (Sharma, 1984).

We feel that the treatment of choice is complete removal of the tumor whenever possible, and this opinion is shared by many others in different centers (House and Glassock, 1974; Spector, 1973; Ogura, 1978, Fisch, 1982).

Although in use for over 12 years, embolization is still underutilized in the management of paragangliomas. This is a safe and efficient method to devascularize these tumors and it can be used as the sole therapy for inoperable tumors, where the objective is the stabilization of growth.

There is electron microscopic evidence (Bosq, 1983, unpublished data) that presurgical embolization with particles produces cellular damage, which can be irreversible and related to ischemia. Necrosis and fibrotic transformation of the tumor can also be observed. Therefore if an active agent can be safely delivered into the tumor bed, one can expect complete control of the lesion with regression of some of the symptoms (Figs. 4.16, 4.17).

Aggressive embolization can be expected to have similar beneficial effects compared to radiotherapy, without the complications.

Preoperative embolization allows easier resection of the lesion, and may allow resection of a tumor initially felt to be inoperable.

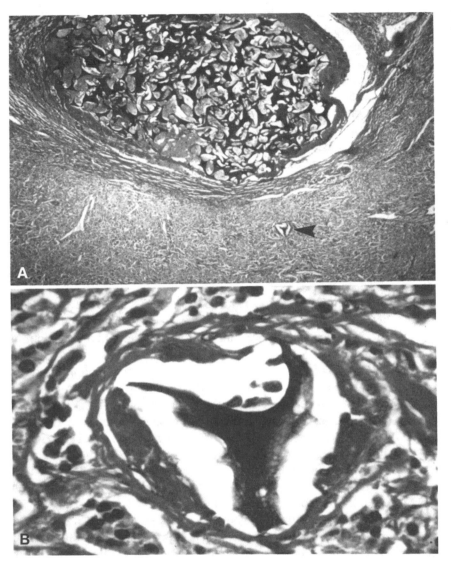

Fig. 4.15. A Pathological section of a cervical paraganglioma. Note the large vessel occlusion and the PVA particle in a small artery *(arrowhead)*. **B** Pathological section in a case of paraganglioma, intra luminal PVA particle (250 microns)

10. Technical Aspects of Embolization

In most cases, embolization is performed prior to surgical resection, so that PVA particles of 140–250 microns diameter are sufficient. The capillaries within the tumor measure 200 microns in diameter. Liquid embolic agents should be used only in the treatment of inoperable tumors, and only when optimal flow control can be achieved. As with other tumors, there is no indication for the use of larger particles.

The embolization techniques which we use are similar to those described in the treatment of other benign craniofacial tumors. Individual feeding arteries are selectively catheterized and embolized with PVA particles, and then the same arteries are occluded proximally by strips of gelfoam. This proximal gelfoam occlusion helps to promote the distal thrombosis induced by the small particles (Fig. 4.15).

Special attention must be paid to the intracranial and orbital anastomoses whenever the middle meningeal or occipital arteries are embolized.

Fig. 4.16. Electron microscopy of two paragangliomas, one which has not been embolized (**A**) and one post embolization (**B**). Note the swelling of mitochondria (*M*) and lipoid vacuolization of the cytoplasm (*LV*) on the embolized lesion (*N* nucleus) (Bosq, non-published data; Institut Gustave Roussy, France)

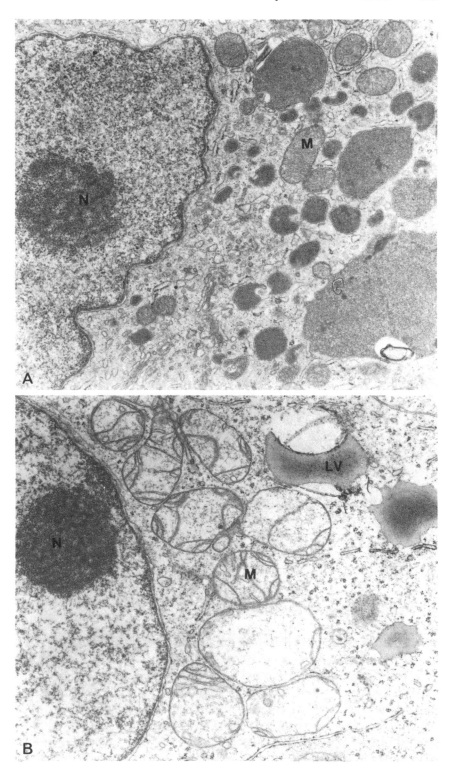

Angiographic series may be necessary during embolization in the ascending pharyngeal artery, if the quality of the fluoroscopic image is not satisfactory to confirm the preferential flow towards the tumor.

The ascending cervical and inferior laryngeal arteries can safely be embolized in most cases of large vagal or carotid lesions, but one must be

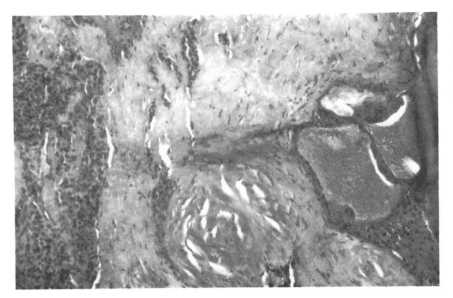

Fig. 4.17. Pathological section of a vagal paraganglioma embolized with PVA (160 microns particules) one year prior to its removal. Note the fibrotic transformation of most of the tumor

aware of and avoid the possibility of flow toward the spinal artery and reflux into the vertebral artery.

In specific cases in which a compartment has to be reached more effectively (common compartment with the internal carotid artery, or vertebral artery branches) microparticles, fluid material or cytotoxic agents may be used (Figs. 4.16, 4.17).

However, in Fisch's classification, two challenging stages represent difficult situations for embolization. The D3 type, in which the AICA or the PICA supply the lesion are almost never amenable to embolization. The C3 type, with petrous apex involvement, on the other hand, can be controlled by sacrificing the internal carotid artery, and proximal embolization.

In exeptional cases, selective catheterization and embolization of the carotico tympanic artery has been performed (Manelfe, 1983). We do not recommand this technique before first attempting to reach the same territory via the ascending pharyngeal artery, with or without flow control.

11. Complications of Embolization of Paragangliomas

In our series reported in 1983, we noted minor complications.

In two patients, extravasation of contrast medium below the tumor occurred during embolization and was probably related to the high pressure of injection of embolic material. This problem involved catheterization of the inferior tympanic artery and embolization with particles in both cases, and has not occurred again in the past eight years.

One patient developed a transient facial nerve palsy following embolization of a large tympanomastoid paraganglioma which involved the third portion of the facial nerve.

Finally, embolization of the ascending pharyngeal artery with fluid agents may produce a lower cranial nerve palsy, regardless of the skill of the angiographer. Therefore, the patient should always be warned in advance of this potential complication. The use of provocative tests (see Chapter 1.XIII) is recommended prior to liquid embolization in these territories.

CHAPTER 5

Other Craniofacial Tumors

I. Thyrolaryngeal Tumors

Most thyrolaryngeal tumors are malignant although they are usually highly vascularized (Zachrisson, 1976), surgical resection is generally not limited by intra-operative bleeding, and they are not referred for either diagnostic or therapeutic angiography.

We have used embolization to treat patients with the following lesions:

cavernous hemangiomas (supraglottic in adults)

capillary hemangiomas [subglottic in children (see Vol. 1, Fig. 21.2)]

pharyngeal paragangliomas (see Vol. 1, Fig. 21.5)

thyroidal paragangliomas (Fig. 5.1)

malignant synovialomas (see Vol. 1, Fig. 21.4)

parathyroid adenomas (Fig. 5.2 and Vol. 1, Fig. 6.6)

Most of these are benign lesions and their management has been discussed elsewhere (Vol. 1, Chapter 21).

Pretherapeutic evaluation of thyrolaryngeal tumors (Noyek et al. 1983) includes conventional radiograms, CT, ultrasound and radionuclide scanning. It is well recognized that CT is limited in the specific diagnosis of these tumors (Lacourreye et al. 1983); particularly in malignant ones.

Thyrolaryngeal lesions illustrate the usefulness of angiographic protocols and also the hazards related to this specific territory; arterial supply to the laryngeal nerve, tracheal cartilages, etc. To our knowledge thyroid gland dysfunction has not been reported following embolization.

Highly vascularized tumors of this area usually require embolization of the superior and inferior thyroidal arteries bilateraly.

Paragangliomas of the larynx, thyroid, or ectopic carotid body tumors (Zak 1982, Ali 1983, Marks 1983) are rare. Their association with neuroendocrine tumors has been discussed in the section on temporal and parapharyngeal lesions. Because paragangliomas are uncommon in this location, simultaneous parapharyngeal and thyroid tumors are usually related to thyroid malignancy or metastasis from pharyngeal carcinoma (Fig. 5.4, see also Vol. 1, Fig. 21.3).

Hemangiopericytomas (Pesavento and Ferlito 1982, Hertzanu 1982) or other highly vascularized locally malignant lesions (Geachan et al. 1983) in particular, benefit from presurgical embolization. They are considered to be radioresistant or poorly radiosensitive.

In spite of the fact that primary tumors of the thyrolaryngeal area are rarely treated by embolization; the thyroidal arteries are frequently used in endovascular techniques. They constitute one of the major sources of collateral circulation to the floor of the mouth and the carotid region, and therefore may be occluded during the embolization of lesion which arise in those territories.

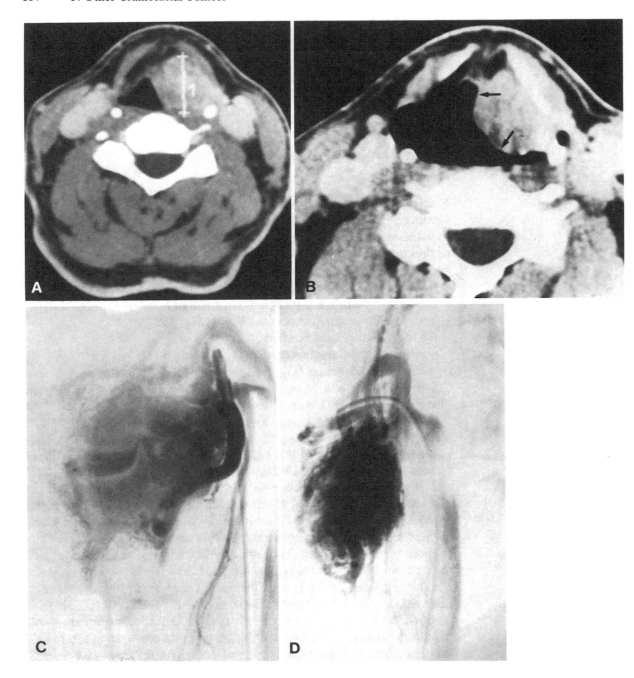

Fig. 5.1 A-D. 55 year old male presenting with progressive dysphonia. Laryngo-
scopy shows a tumoral mass on the left subglottic pharyngolaryngeal wall. No other
lesions (mass or adenopathy) were found at clinical or CT examination (**A, B**). **C**
Pretherapeutic evaluation shows a well demarcated enhancing mass, highly vascularized, fed mainly by the superior laryngeal artery; it also received some supply
from the opposite superior laryngeal and ipsilateral inferior laryngeal arteries (not
shown). Presurgical embolization with PVA (160 microns) allowed total resection
of a laryngeal paraganglioma. Swallowing was normal 3 weeks after surgery

Fig. 5.2. Selective injection of ▶ the thymic branch of the right internal mammary artery in a 26 year old patient presenting with adenomatous hypercalcemia. Selective injection demonstrates the upper mediastinal adenoma *(double arrow)*. Contrast material ablation was selected in this case, with excellent results. After 5 years, the result remained stable. No surgery has been done

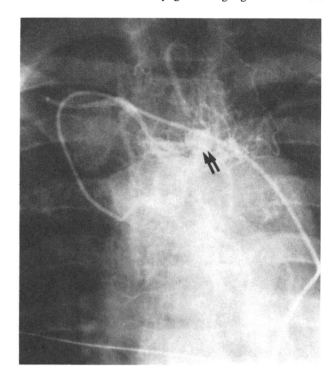

Fig. 5.3. Left (**A**) and right (**B**) superior thyroidal angiograms in a patient presenting with a goitre and thyrotoxicosis. Note the hypervascularization of the thyroid tissue and the role played by the marginal arcade in the supply to the pyramid. Early venous filling was observed without evidence of AV fistulas

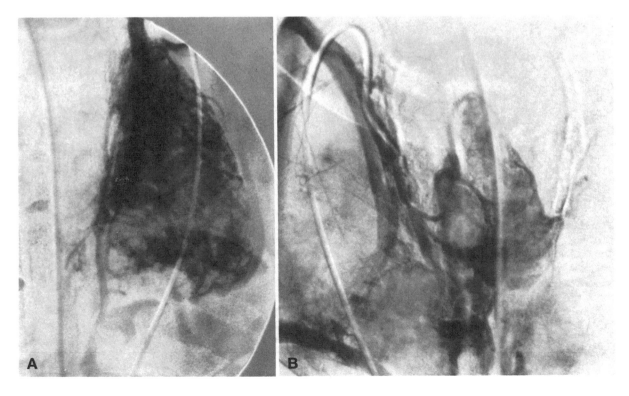

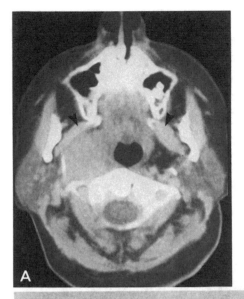

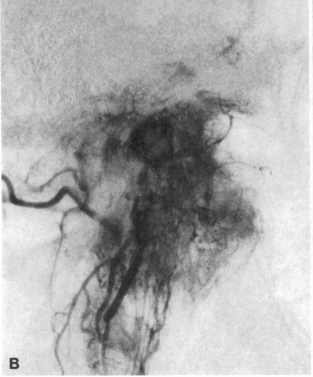
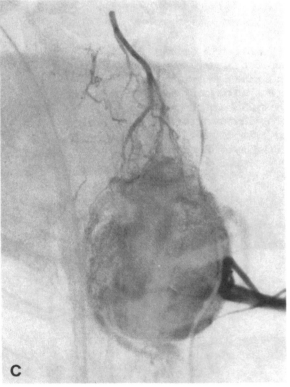

Fig. 5.4 A-C. 50 year old female presenting with multiple painful subcutaneous nodules, paralysis of the IXth and Xth cranial nerves and hypersecretion of thyrocalcitonin, without elevated carcinoembryonic antigen levels. One mass was prominent in the parapharyngeal space. No tumor could be palpated in the thyroid area. Histologic examination of one of the nodules was consistent with a metastasis from an undifferentiated carcinoma, but certain staining characteristics were suggestive of a neuroendocrine tumor such as paraganglioma. This hypothesis was reinforced by the thyroid scintigram which showed a non functioning area within the left lobe. The final diagnosis following further surgery was a typical medullary thyroid carcinoma with cutaneous lymph node and parapharyngeal metastasis

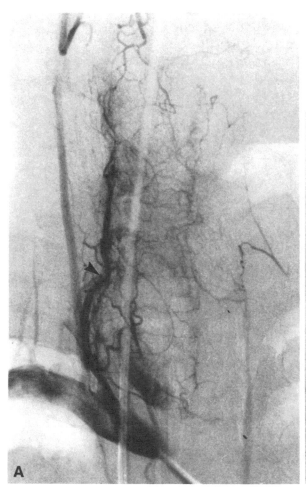

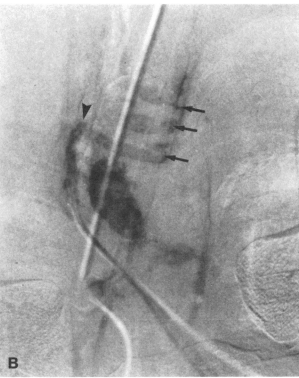

Fig. 5.5. Selective injection of the inferior laryngeal artery in a patient with a parathyroid adenoma before (**A**) and after (**B**) therapeutic angiography. Two surgical procedures in this patient have modified the initial anatomical patterns, since the 4 thyroid arteries were ligated. Only the right laryngeal arcade persisted, and this permitted retrograde opacification of the ventral branch of the superior laryngeal artery, which originates from the ascending pharyngeal artery. Note that the tracheal rings *(arrows)* are opacified following infusion of the contrast material

In presence of previous proximal ligation of the linguofacial system, the thyroidal channels represent the only access to the floor of the mouth (see Vol. 1, Chapter 12).

Parathyroid adenomas still represent a diagnostic challenge with the exception of very large tumors; the available non invasive techniques can rarely document the location of the hormone secreting lesion (Wolverson et al. 1981, Obley et al. 1984, Adams et al. 1981, Stark 1983, Stock et al. 1981). Since Doppman's (1980) contribution to the angiographic approach to parathyroid adenomas and Dunlop's (1980) review of venous sampling little attention has been devoted to angiographic studies in this disease.

However, the endovascular techniques in the treatment of parathyroid adenomas differ from those used to treat other masses in the head and neck. They include the superselective injection of 2 to 30 ml of contrast material (Doppman 1980, 1982) with a higher dose of iodine than that used for diagnostic angiography (Fig. 5.5, and Vol. 1, Fig. 6.6). The damage produced in the secreting lesion is illustrated by the persistance of the parenchymal stain for hours or days. A decrease in blood calcium levels usually occurs rapidly following an initial moderate increase related to the liberation of granules contained in the cells. The stability of the results depends upon the amount of the lesion treated and the irreversibility of the cellular damage produced. Classical embolization of this type of tumor without surgical excision is always potentially incomplete. In the experience of Doppman, and ourselves parathyroid adenomas treated by particle embolization alone usually recur (Fig. 5.5). Tumor infusion with cytotoxic agents such as ethanol is atractive, but has not been used yet.

The embolization of subglottic hemangiomas is described in the chapter on vascular lesions (see Vol. 1, Fig. 21.2).

II. Craniofacial Malignant Lesions

Therapeutic angiography in malignant lesions of the head and neck should be discussed separately for two different groups:
1. Malignant or locally invasive lesions which have recurred following incomplete surgery. Some have been already illustrated or described in the chapters dealing with lesions of the scalp, vault meninges, nasopharynx, temporal and laryngeal regions.
2. Primary malignant lesions or metastasis in the head and neck area (Figs. 5.6, 5.7).

The latter group does not represent an important part of the present practice of embolization. Ischemic damage is still the main effect that endovascular treatment can achieve. As a unique treatment embolization should be reserved for nonsurgical lesions (see Chapter 1).

Certain techniques may maximize the effect of particle embolization, in particular the rearrangement of the vascular supply to the lesion. In large

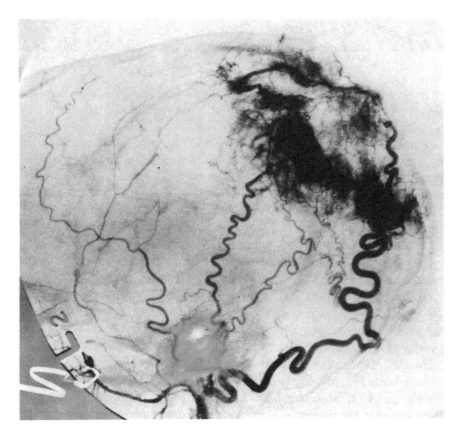

Fig. 5.6. Selective external carotid angiogram in a case of metastatic adrenal carcinoma. Note the highly vascularized aspect of the lesion which can easily be reached by endovascular approach. The patient was treated with 95% ethanol with good paliation

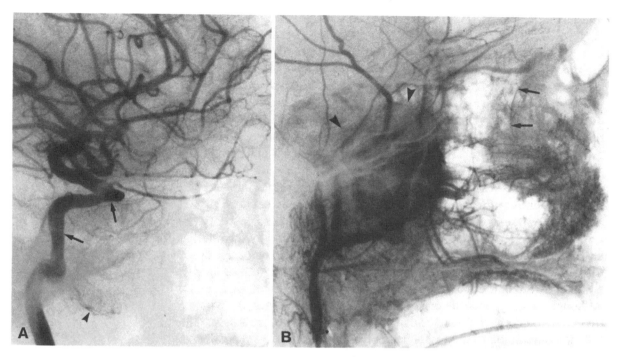

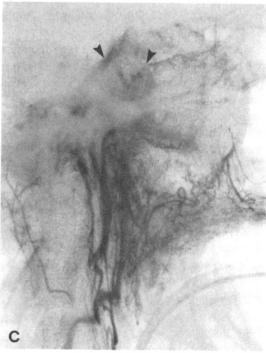

Fig. 5.7 A-C. Tumor of the base of the skull in a 46 year old female who had been treated for breast cancer. An attempt to biopsy it led to profuse bleeding. No conclusive pathological diagnosis could be made. Internal carotid injection (**A**) shows a cavernous extension which is probably extradural *(arrows)* from an extracranial tumor. Note the mandibular remnant *(arrowhead)*. Distal external carotid angiogram (**B**) shows a capillary enhancement of the tumor which occupies the base of the skull and extends to the cavum as well as to the intradural region *(arrowhead)*. Note the choroidal crescent visualized through a middle meningeal-ophthalmic artery anastomosis. **C** Selective injection of the ascending pharyngeal artery showing posterior extension of the lesion and inferior part of its nasopharyngeal portion. Control of the supply to the area was achieved by particle embolization, the packing was removed and biopsy and surgical resection were achieved later. Pathology concluded to breast cancer metastais

tumors of the base of the skull and nasal fossa, the goal may be to reach as much of the tumor as possible with minimal side effects. The internal maxillary, ascending pharyngeal and internal carotid siphon bilaterally are theoritically involved in the supply to the naso-pharynx. In our cases, the lesions were slightly lateralized and we decided to increase the role of one feeder to the territory; sacrifice of the ipsilateral internal carotid is only undertaken after proper functional testing. Embolization of the controlateral branches of the internal maxillary and ascending pharyngeal arteries can then be achieved. Depending on the anatomic disposition of the patient, accessibility of the vessels and collateral circulation to the orbit, either the ipsilateral ascending pharyngeal or the internal maxillary artery is then embolized with particles. The remaining feeder is deliberately left open. A few weeks later repeat angiography is performed to verify the stability of the results and to assess the territory supplied by the internal maxillary or the ascending pharyngeal artery which has been left open. Catheterization of this branch then allows the use of agressive agents: powder, cytotoxics, ethanol, loaded microcapsules, etc. (see Chapter 1). Although we have had little experience with these techniques, the patients treated this way showed spectacular decrease in the size of their mass. The use of manipulation of the vascular supply in this fashion could possibly in the future be combined with embolization of the chemotherapeutic agents in the form of long acting microcapsules, maintaining patency of the arterial route for multiple courses.

One specific hazard related to this technique is the hypotensive effect of certain drugs (*cis*-platinum); it carries the risk of stroke if, the circle of Willis is inadequate, in the presence of decreased blood pressure to maintain cerebral perfusion after sacrifice of one ICA.

Embolization is also used in two other situations in patient with malignant lesions:

1. before a diagnostic biopsy where hemorrhagic complications are anticipated (particles should be used to preserve tissue diagnosis; Fig. 5.7).
2. To treat complications of the disease or its treatment. Our experience in this latter situation has concerned three types of symptoms: pain, hemorrhage and mass effect.

Malignant lesions always respond dramatically to particle embolization probably because they are already in a subischemic state as illustrated by intralesional necrosis often seen in pathology.

Embolization usually produces an important necrosis and decrease in the mass effect in few days. Pain related either to the volume of the mass or to "congestion" of the sourrounding structures is poorly understood (Fig. 5.8).

Pain relief after embolization of a cavernous sinus meningiomas (retroorbital) or vertebral hemangiomas (localised without fracture) without change in the volume of the mass supports the hypothesis that the congestion of normal tissues may be contributing factor. The stability of the relief of pain depends as with other symptoms on the type of damage accomplished within the lesion.

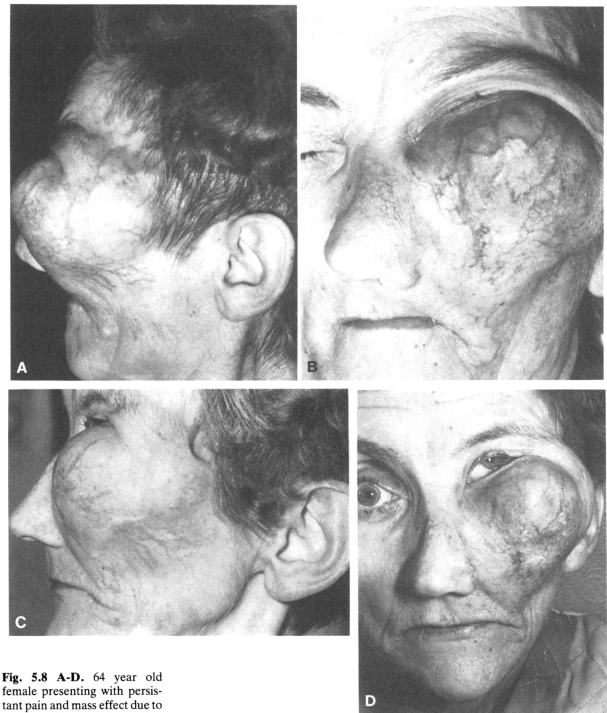

Fig. 5.8 A-D. 64 year old female presenting with persistant pain and mass effect due to a progressively growing orbital and facial metastasis from thyroid carcinoma. Surgery, radiation therapy and biological agents were either rejected or ineffective. PVA embolization of the left distal external carotid and facial arteries was carried out. The ophthalmic artery also supplied the lesion and the eye was thought to be non functional. No attempt was made to occlude this system although catheterization of the ophthalmic artery could have been achieved. **A** Lateral and **B** frontal view of the lesion before embolization. **C, D** Four days after the embolization almost 30% of the mass was evacuated through the left nasal fossa without any bleeding. The pain disappeared simultaneously. The patient could see with the left eye although she had diplopia. 3 years later this metastasis had not recurred again, but the patient died from metastasis in other localizations

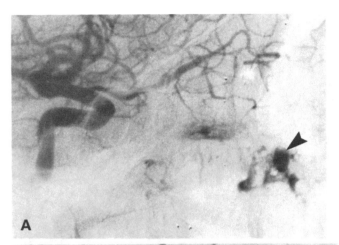

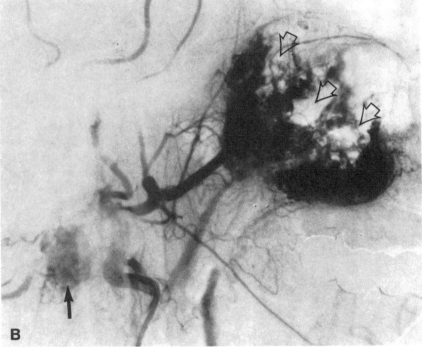

Fig. 5.9. Selective ICA (**A**) and ipsilateral (**B**) and opposite (**C**, p. 173) distal external carotid arteries injections. A 56 year old male presented with significant spontaneous epistaxis which required packing and transfusion. Clinical examination showed a tumor to be the source of the nose bleed and biopsy confirmed its metastatic nature. Embolization was performed to stabilize the bleeding and to facilitate the surgical resection. Notice the nonheterogenous appearance of the blush which was related to intratumoral necrosis and multicompartmental vascular arrangements: ethmoidal *(arrowhead)*, and distal internal maxillary arterial *(open arrows)* territories. The absence of supply from the septal branches of the contralateral internal maxillary artery *(small arrowheads)* and of cross filling of greater palatine artery collaterals *(curved arrows)* from the opposite side is unusual. Note the incidental discovery of an additional metastasis in the mastoid region (**B** *solid arrow*)

Fig. 5.9 C

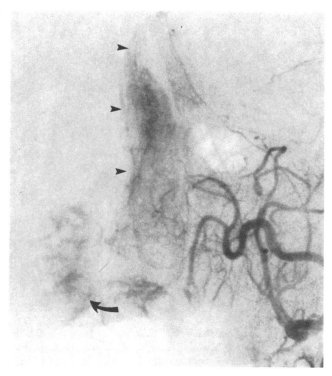

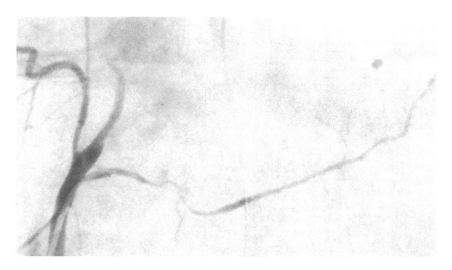

Fig. 5.10. Proximal injection in the external carotid artery in a patient presenting with cancer of the base of the tongue extending to the floor of the mouth. Previous surgery, radiation therapy and chemotherapy had stabilized this extensive lesion for a short period of time. The patient was referred as an emergency with acute intraoral hemorrhage. Cutaneous changes and post radiation therapy trismus made surgical control and analysis of the bleeding site extremely difficult. Note the changes involving the proximal lingual artery. Embolization successfully controlled the bleeding

Hemorrhages due to arterial ulceration result from either tumor invasion or from post radiation necrosis. In both situations control of the bleeding depends upon accessibility. Arterial changes following radiation may compromise intravascular navigation. Surgical control of these hemorrhages is usually very difficult. In the presence of intraoral bleeding due to lingual ulceration associated post radiation trismus, even local compression of the involved area is difficult. Embolization may be useful in controlling acute and chronic bleeding due to neoplastic ulceration (Figs. 5.9–5.12).

The overall prognosis of the tumor is obviously not significantly modified by embolization; however, the quality of the remaining life is sometimes dramatically improved.

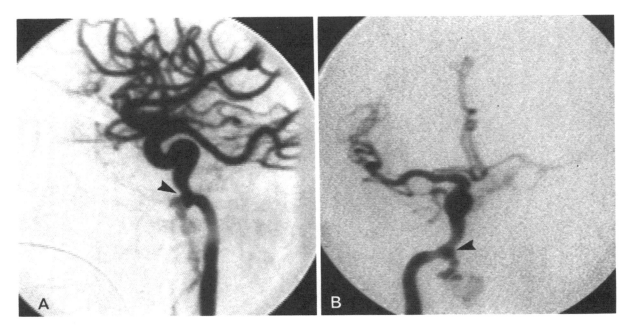

Fig. 5.11 A, B. Selective internal carotid angiogram. **A** Lateral and **B** AP views in a patient presenting acutely with a post radiation arterial ulceration. Note the false aneurysm of the internal carotid artery at the level of the foramen lacerum with extravasation into the pharyngeal region

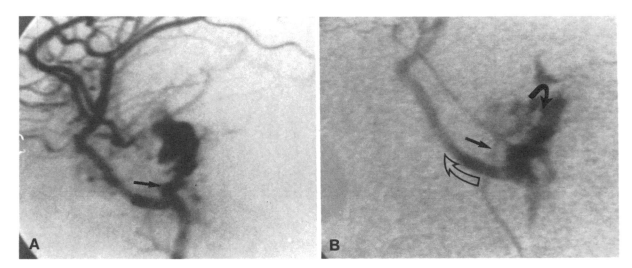

Fig. 5.12 A, B. 23 year old female presenting with a chondrosarcoma, radiated 4 years before this examination for significant recurrence. (Same patient as Fig. 2.2.) A fistula has developed between the tumor and the internal carotid and middle meningeal arteries secondary to tumor invasion of the arteries. **A** DSA of the left internal carotid artery demonstrates a fistula between the internal carotid and the tumor *(arrow)*. **B** DSA control angiogram following embolization with 7 ccs of ethanol through the middle meningeal artery *(arrow* points to the tip the catheter). The contrast injection has opacified the tumor fistula *(curved arrow)*, and secondarily the internal carotid artery *(open curved arrow)*. In embolization for malignant invasion of major arteries the outmost care must be taken to prevent cerebral embolization via these most unusual intratumoral anastomosis

CHAPTER 6

Arteriovenous Fistulas (AVFs)

I. Introduction

Arteriovenous fistulas (AVFs) (Table 6.1) represent an abnormal communication between an artery and a vein secondary to vessel laceration. Therefore, it may be only part of a more complex clinical situation where other structures such as soft tissues, bone, brain, cranial, or peripheral nerves may also be injured. Some fistulas may be part of other vascular abnormalities such as pre-existing developmental aneurysms or angiodysplasias. In addition, there are predetermined sites where fistulas occur because the anatomical relationship between an artery and an adjacent or surrounding vein makes it possible for a ruptured or lacerated artery to communicate directly with a vein. The consequences of this acute hemodynamic change can be at the site of the fistula, distal to the fistula, systemic, or secondary to venous hypertension.

Locally, secondary to venous dilatation and high flow, a pulsatile mass with a thrill may be apparent and a variable pitch bruit can be heard at the site of fistula. A bruit can also be heard at other locations depending on the venous drainage, and this can be a useful sign to assist in the clinical localization of fistulas in deep, nonpalpable locations or when bony structures surround the fistula. A pulsatile bruit is sometimes heard by the patient more frequently in traumatic arteriovenous fistulas than in vascular malformations, or dural arteriovenous malformations (DAVMs).

A sudden deprivation of arterial blood flow in the territories neighboring or distal to the fistula can produce ischemia. If the arterial "steal" is severe enough, neurologic changes can occur that may vary from mild transient insufficiency syndromes, such as dizziness, unsteadiness, or other vertebrobasilary insufficiencies, to more severe permanent insults including stroke.

Abrupt venous hypertension, that may vary from mild to severe, can produce reversal of flow in the venous system. This in turn may produce symptoms of mass effect, or venous congestion, which includes secondary

Table 6.1. Arteriovenous fistulas etiologies

I. Traumatic	II. Spontaneous
A. Blunt	A. Congenital
B. Penetrating	B. Acquired
C. Iatrogenic	a) Secondary to a preceding thrombosis?
	b) Secondary to a ruptured aneurysm?
	c) Associated to an angiodysplasia
	1. FMD
	2. Neurofibromatosis
	3. Ehlers Danlos syndrome
	4. Other dysplasias

glaucoma, hydrocephalus, or engorgement of cortical cerebral veins. The potential risk of cerebral hemorrhages exist, with cortical venous drainage although not as in dural AVMs (see Chapter 8). Possible explanations on the rarity of hemorrhagic episodes secondary to cortical venous rerouting in traumatic arteriovenous fistulas, as opposed to dural AVMs, could be explained by the multiplicity of venous outflow channels from the cavernous sinus and the pre-existing normal venous system in traumatic fistulas versus a pre-existing venous pathology in dural AVMS.

Frequently, a delay between the vascular traumatic insult and the clinical manifestations is seen, and related to the development of a false aneurysm and/or a tamponade effect from the hematoma. Only after repture of the pseudoaneurysm, or lysis of the hematoma, do the symptoms of the abnormal arteriovenous communication become apparent.

Systemic manifestations of these high flow fistulas such as high-output failure are unusual and may be seen in friable debilitated patients with a pre-existing insufficiency of the cardiovascular system (see Figs. 6.40, 6.45). Older children or young adults are usually asymptomatic, although some degree of left ventricular hypertrophy and/or cardiomegaly may be detected. Cardiac failure is unusual; when present, it is usually associated with the congenital type AVFs (Fig. 8.7) (Norman, 1950).

II. Carotid Cavernous Fistulas (CCFs)

In the craniofacial area the most frequent type of arteriovenous fistulas are the traumatic ones and of these, CCFs are by far the more common. They occur secondary to laceration of the internal carotid siphon, or from rupture of its intracavernous branches.

On occasion, the ruptured C4 and/or C5 branches may only be injected from the external carotid system. DAVMs of the cavernous sinus constitute a different entity and are discussed in the chapter on DAVMs.

We will study in detail these lesions, as they best illustrate the clinical syndromes produced by high flow traumatic arteriovenous fistulas.

To properly understand these fistulas a thorough knowledge of the vascular anatomy of the base of the skull is necessary (see Vol. 1, Chapter 2, 3, 15 and 16).

The vascular arrangement in the parasellar region is unique with the internal carotid artery surrounded by the venous plexus that constitutes the cavernous sinus (see Vol. 1, Chapter 1 and 15).

1. Anatomo-Clinical Features

The cavernous portion of the internal carotid artery is fixed to the surrounding dura at the base of the skull. Thus, it is exposed to shearing stresses as well as penetrating injuries such as stab wounds, blunt instrument, or gunshot wounds. When there is a laceration of this artery or one of its branches, and subsequent AVF, the venous drainage into the cavernous sinus is reversed. The drainage can be multidirectional and manifest itself in various manners. By far the most important presenting problems are those affecting the orbit (Fig. 6.1, Table 6.2).

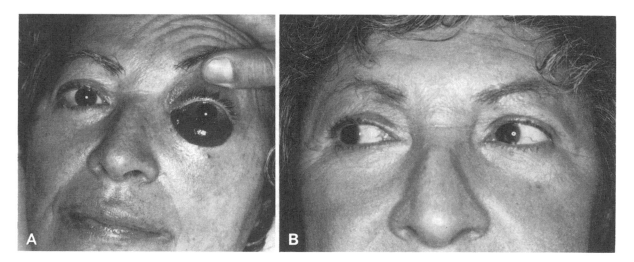

Fig. 6.1 A, B. TCCF following motor vehicle accident. **A** Clinical picture 3 weeks after the accident. The patient complained of hearing a noise and double vision. Note, the proptosis, conjunctival and lid engorgement. Associated secondary glaucoma ptosis and muscle entrapment were also present. **B** 10 days after balloon repair of the fistula. All signs and symptoms resolved

Table 6.2. Neuro-ophthalmic abnormalities before and after embolization (Kupersmith, 1986)

Pre-embolization	Postembolization improvement	Postembolization[a] normal
Ptosis 62%	85%	52%
Third nerve 68% (1b)	69%	35%
Fourth nerve 50%	76%	41%
Sixth nerve 85% (1b)	76%	55%
Pupillary defects III 35% sympathetic-3 9%	(III) 8% sympathetic 67%	8% 67%
Iris dilated vessels 9% (1b)	33%	33%
Proptosis 88% (1b)	100%	80%
Chemosis 59% (1b)	67%	63%
Dilated conjunctival vessels 100% (4b)	100%	88%
Bruit 85%	100%	100%
Thrill/pulsation of globe 15%	100%	100%
Lid engorgement 47%	100%	94%
Venous retinopathy 38% (2b)	85%	85%
Disc edema 15% (1b)	80%	80%
Visual loss 50% (1b)	35%	24%
Increased intraocular pressure 79% (3b)	96%	96%
Pain[b]	100%	100%

[a] 2 weeks to 5 years follow up

[b] Pain may start ort aggravate following treatment, when the cavernous sinus collapses. It will resolve in 3–5 weeks.

b=bilateral

a) Type of Venous Drainage

α) Anterior (Fig. 6.2). Drainage to the ophthalmic venous system produces proptosis, chemosis, dilated conjunctiva, lid engorgement, venous retinopathy, disc edema, increased intraocular pressure with secondary glaucoma, and visual loss. The reversed blood flow in the ophthalmic system will then drain toward the facial venous system and external jugular vein. Similar symptoms may be present in the absence of anterior drainage if sufficient venous hypertension exists (see DAVMs, Fig. 6.26).

Associated symptoms related to anterior venous hyperpressure may be congestion of the extraocular muscles and anterior displacement of the eyeball (exophtalmos). Mechanical restrictions to movement of the eye secondary to venous hypertension and orbital congestion (Fig. 6.1A) will occur, but this will resolve after repair of the fistula (Fig. 6.1B) and should be differentiated from cranial nerve impairment (see below).

β) Posterior (Fig. 6.3). The fistula may drain directly into the inferior petrosal sinus, the superior petrosal sinus, or the occipital transverse sinus.

Patients usually present with complaints of a noise and/or some dysfunction of the VI, IV, III or V_1 cranial nerves.

γ) Superior (Fig. 6.4). Drainage to the sphenoparietal sinus (superficial sylvian vein) or deep sylvian veins involves cortical venous routes.

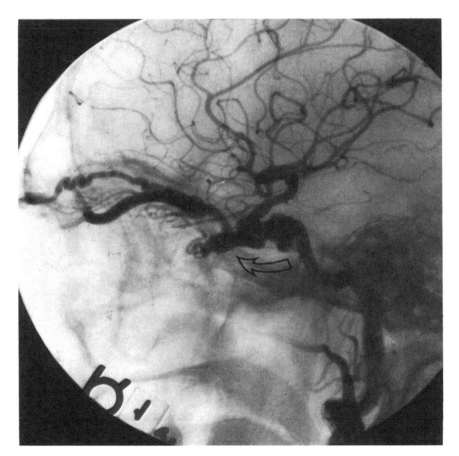

Fig. 6.2. Lateral substraction angiogram of the right internal carotid artery, in midarterial phase. Carotid cavernous fistula with purely anterior drainage is seen (same patient as Fig. 6.15) *(open curved arrow)*. Relatively small fistula, but with significant ocular findings

Fig. 6.3. Posterior drainage. Lateral subtraction angiogram of the left internal carotid artery. Post traumatic fistula with purely posterior drainage is noted *(arrow)*. Inferior petrosal jugular confluence *(open curved arrow)*. (By permission of Manelfe and Berenstein 1980)

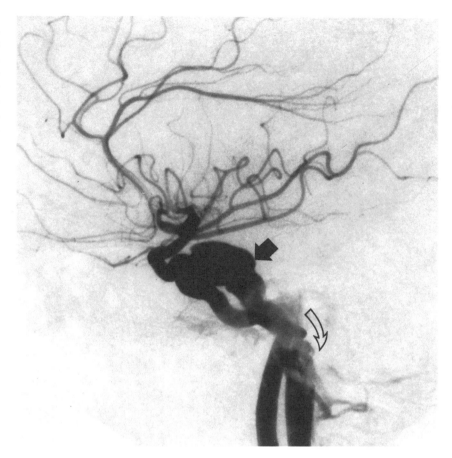

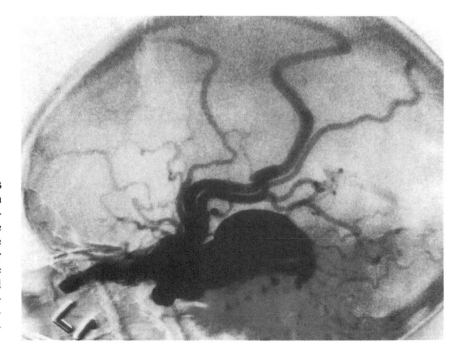

Fig. 6.4. Superior venous drainage. Lateral subtraction angiogram of a chronic post-traumatic fistula. Note the aneurysmal dilatation of the cavernous sinus and superior cortical venous drainage through the sphenoparietal sinus. Note the complete angiographic "steal" on the cerebral arterial system (same patient as Figs. 6.19 and 6.36)

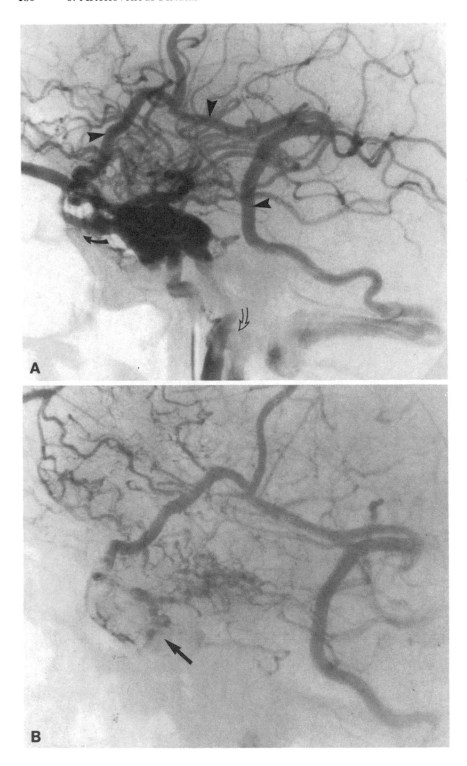

Fig. 6.5 A-C. TCCF with mixed venous drainage. **A** Lateral subtraction angiogram of the left internal carotid artery demonstrates a CCF with drainage anteriorly towards the ophthalmic venous system *(curved arrow)*, posteriorly towards the inferior petrosal sinus, jugular vein *(open curved arrow)* and superiorly towards cortical veins *(arrowhead)*. **B** Lateral subtraction angiogram immediatly after balloon *(arrow)* repair of the fistula. Note the dilated, ectatic looking cortical veins, filling antigrade and in normal sequential time

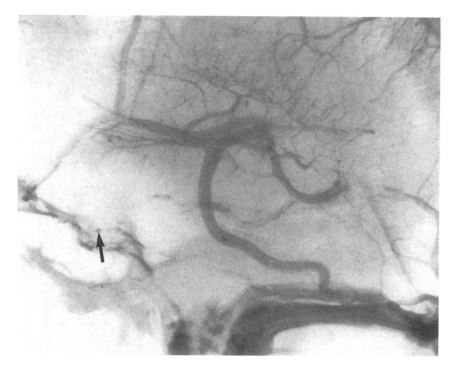

Fig. 6.5. C Follow up angiogram three months later in venous phase. Note, the return to a normal appearance of the veins. The balloon has deflated *(arrow)*. The cavernous sinus is not opacified

One may see an aneurysmally dilated cavernous sinus that may even act as a large extradural mass (Fig. 6.4) which, although impressive, does not seem to have a high risk of rupturing. This is usually seen in chronic fistulas.

Tortuous and ectatic cortical veins can be seen (Fig. 6.5A), but even if arterialized, intracranial hemorrhage is very rare (Dohrmann, 1985). After repair of the fistula these venous changes are seen in the immediate postembolization study but are now filling in the normal sequential time (Fig. 6.5B) and will regress to normal on a follow-up angiogram some months later (even if a balloon is in the cavernous sinus) (Fig. 6.5C).

δ) Contralateral (Figs. 6.6, 8.1A). Both cavernous sinus plexuses anastomose anteriorly and posteriorly. A given CCF drainage, therefore, can produce all the signs of the lesion on the contralateral side. In general, the more severe symptoms, are on the side of the fistula, however, if ipsilateral ophthalmic venous thrombosis is present, the opposite eye will be the more symptomatic one.

ε) Inferiorly. Usually of minor importance, flow can be to the vein of the foramen rotundum or laterally through the vein of the foramen ovale (Fig. 6.8). This inferior drainage then drains into the pterygoid plexus. It is usually associated with other drainage (ophthalmic vein or mixed).

ζ) Mixed Drainage (Fig. 6.4, 6.5). This is actually the most frequent situation. The symptomatology is usually mixed. Predominance of one type of drainage will then correspond to the main clinical manifestations.

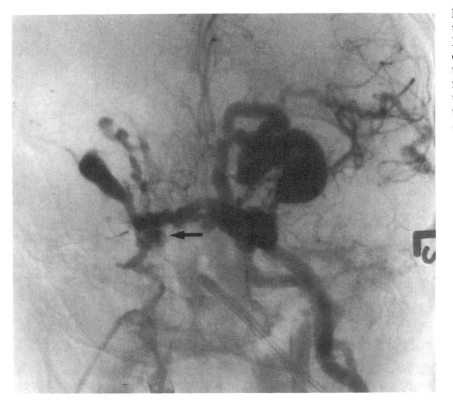

Fig. 6.6. Left TCCF with bilateral ophthalmic drainage. Frontal subtraction angiogram of the left internal carotid artery in late arterial phase. Note filling of both cavernous sinuses and ophthalmic veins, through the coronary sinuses *(arrow)*

Prominent mixed venous drainage can be associated with complete or nearly complete hemodynamic "steal" (Fig. 6.4).

η) Altered and/or Aberrant Drainage. On occasions, previous procedures such as surgical ligations or partial occlusion of the venous drainage may alter the pattern of drainage. This may cause aggravation of the symptoms in the remaining venous return, and the patient may present with prominent facial vein(s) which have prominent pulsations and thrills (Fig. 6.7A) which will reverse following successful embolization (Fig. 6.7B).

b) Bruit

This is the most constant finding (in association with a hyperhemic conjunctiva) in traumatic fistulas and is due to the high flow of the lesions. It is usually maximal over the ipsilateral eye.

The bruit can radiate to the frontal, temporal, jugular, or other areas depending on the venous outflow of the fistula. Subjective bruits are related to posterior drainage and bone conduction.

Thrills and/or pulsations of the globe are infrequent and related to a dominant anterior drainage.

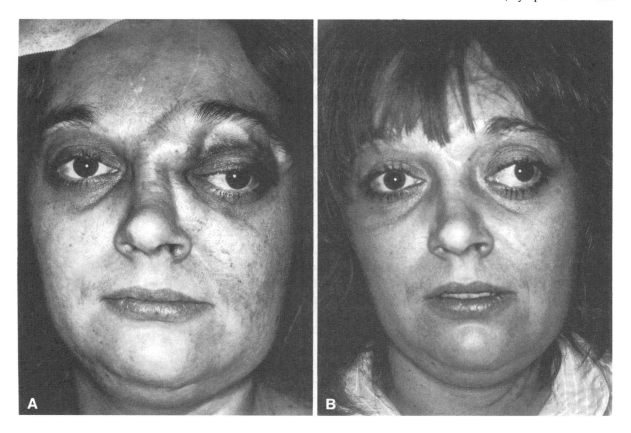

Fig. 6.7 A, B. TCCF with ligation of the internal carotid artery, external carotid artery and internal jugular vein. **A** Clinical picture of a patient with prominent collateral venous dilatation, following surgical ligation of the internal jugular vein. Note the prominent angular and upper eyelid veins. **B** Complete regression following successful embolization of the fistula, after surgical exposure of the previously ligated internal carotid artery

c) Arterial "Steal"

This may affect the ophthalmic artery territory, and produce impaired vision. However, in our experience this is infrequently present, unless compression of the ophthalmic artery and nerve in the optic canal (hematoma, contusion, edema, etc.) are associated. The hypoxia of the anterior segment of the eye is manifested by changes in corneal epithelium and the presence of cells in the anterior chamber; occular dysfunction is further aggravated by the increased intraocular pressure, that if severe enough, will further contribute to visual loss. It may even result in occlusion of the central retinal artery (Kupersmith, 1986). The hypoxic venous retinopathy is an added or aggravating factor that further affects visual function.

d) Hemispheric Arterial Insufficiency

When the fistula is large and a complete hemodynamic "steal" (Fig. 6.4) is superimposed on a congenitally and/or acquired underdevelopment of cerebral collateral circulation, usually at the level of the circle of Willis, an acute neurological deficit may be the presenting symptom or may accompany the development of the fistula (Day, 1982). It is important to emphasize that this insufficiency, though rare, may represent a true emergency necessitating immediate treatment (see section on emergency treatment). It may also be a contributing factor in patients with a depressed level of consciousness secondary to "steal". Occlusion of the fistula will improve cerebral perfusion.

e) Associated Traumatic Lesions

Traumatic fistulas represent part of a more complex clinical problem where other structures have been injured; these may be associated with epidural and/or subdural hematomas, intracerebral hematomas, contusions, depressed fractures, CSF leaks, and traumatic pseudo-aneurysms in other segments of the internal carotid artery (Fig. 6.8), or other brachiocephalic vessels (Fig. 6.9, Table 6.3).

Some of the eye findings in traumatic carotid fistulas may be related to the trauma itself and not the high flow fistula, such as rupture of the globe or laceration of the extraocular motor nerves and/or the optic nerve (Fig. 6.10). Demonstration of a fracture in the optic canal (Fig. 6.10A) and/or angiographic evidence of ophthalmic artery damage (Fig. 6.10) carry a poor prognosis of visual recovery. Other ophthalmic manifestations may actually be secondary to compression from reversed venous flow which produces orbital congestion with mechanical entrapment of the extraocular muscles restricting muscle function (Fig. 6.1A). These mechanical restrictions resolve after repair of the fistula (Fig. 6.1B) and should be differentiated from traumatic neuropathies.

f) Cranial Nerve Involvement in Traumatic Carotid Cavernous Fistulas
(Tables 6.2, 6.4)

The III, IV, VI, and V_1 cranial nerves can be impaired as they course in the wall of the cavernous sinus. As mentioned previously, nerve dysfunction may occur at the time of the trauma (as a direct injury to the nerve) or may present later (as a compression of the nerve by the dilated cavernous sinus or secondary to arterial "steal" of the blood supply to the cranial nerves) or a combination of these factors.

Table 6.3. Associated traumatic lesions in CCFs

Brain	Contusion
	Hematoma
	Subdural hematoma
	Epidural Hematoma
	Contre coup
Bone	Frontal fracture
	Orbit roof fracture
	Orbit floor fracture with muscle entrapment
	Medial wall of orbit fracture
	Petrous bone fracture (± VIIth, VIIIth damage)
	Sphenoid fracture
	Optic canal fracture
	Nasal fracture
	Craniofacial fracture
Sinuses	Fluid level
	Intracranial air
	Contralateral side
Soft tissue	Soft tissue injury
Others	Cervical trauma
	Other fractures

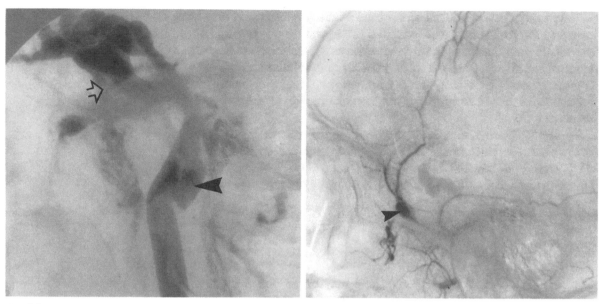

Fig. 6.8   **Fig. 6.9**

Fig. 6.8. Associated vascular injuries. Lateral subtraction angiogram of the right internal carotid artery, early arterial phase. A traumatic pseudoaneurysm of the petrous carotid *(arrowhead)* is associated with a high flow CCF with mixed drainage. Note the vein of foramen ovale *(open arrow)* draining towards the pterygomaxillary plexus. (By permission of Berenstein, 1980)

Fig. 6.9. Lateral subtraction angiogram of the right (contralateral) middle meningeal artery in the same patient as Fig. 6.20, and after balloon trapping of the internal carotid artery, shows a middle meningeal artery false aneurysm *(arrowhead)*

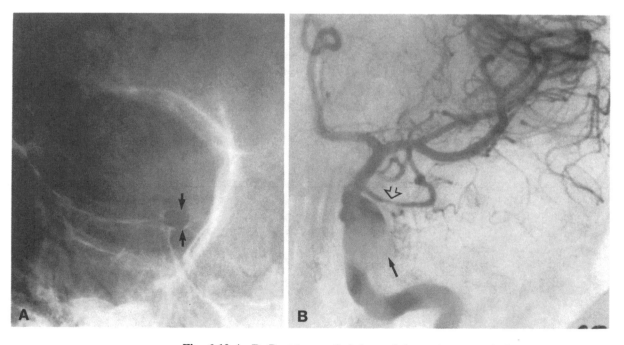

Fig. 6.10 A, B. Post-traumatic injury of the optic nerve. **A** Optic foramen view demonstrates a fracture of the optic canal *(arrows)* that resulted in immediate nonreversible visual loss. **B** AP subtraction angiogram of the same patient after balloon *(arrow)* repair of the fistula. Note the focal narrowing of the ophthalmic artery *(open arrow)* at the level of the optic canal

When the nerve is injured at the time of the trauma, there may be no recovery after treatment of the fistula. When the dysfunction is delayed, there is higher chance of improvement or complete recovery after treatment of the fistula (Fig. 6.11), although it may take several months for complete normalization. When the limitation in ocular motion is due to mechanical factors, resolution will uniformly follow soon after repair of the fistula (Fig. 6.1B).

Paralysis of cranial nerves other than those that course through the wall of the cavernous sinus is more likely due to direct injury such as fracture of the petrous bone with damage of the VII cranial nerve. Deafness in general is usually secondary to traumatic impairment of the inner and/or middle ear.

2. Etiology and Epidemiology

CCFs by far are traumatic in origin and may be produced by direct or indirect trauma during head injury, with or without skull base fracture (Hamby, 1966). Blunt trauma, usually frontal and on the same side of the lesion (Pool, 1965), penetrating orbital injuries associated with optic globe injury, gunshot wounds with laceration of the carotid artery and/or cranial nerves can be encountered. In the latter (Fig. 6.12), the CCF is usually of large size.

Iatrogenic fistulas have been described secondary to transphenoidal surgery (Takahaski, 1969), internal carotid artery thromboendarteriectomy (Baker, 1968) (Fig. 6.13), and thermocoagulation or rhizolysis of the gasserian ganglion or vidian nerves. In some patients no history of trauma or only minor trauma can be elicited; there may be some mechanical precipitating factor such as vomiting, sneezing, or acute hypertension. The angiographic findings are those of a typical TCCF. In some of these cases can one suspect a traumatic rupture of a pre-existing aneurysm and may actually see it during angiography (Fig. 6.14). One must also be aware that in some cases no or minor trauma may produce a fistula in a vessel involved with an angiodysplasia such as Ehler Danlos syndroma (Graf, 1965) or pseudoxanthoma elasticum (Koo and Newton, 1972). When no history of

Fig. 6.11 A, B. 31 year old male with left side ophthalmoplegia that developed some weeks after trauma. **A** Clinical picture showing the inability to medial gaze of the left eye. **B** 2 weeks after treatment, there has been complete recovery

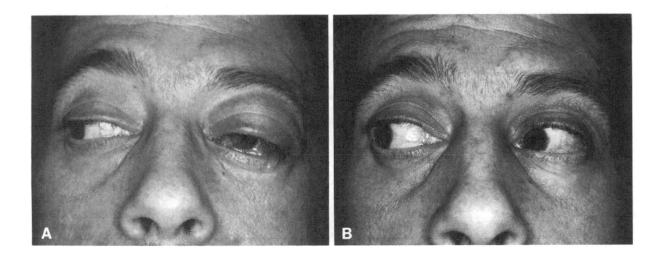

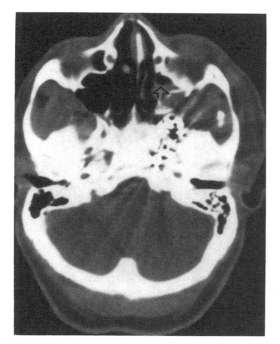

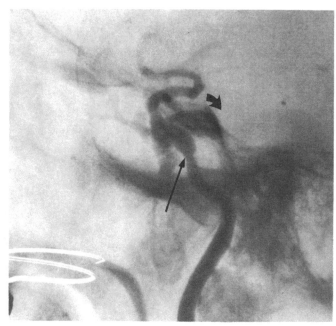

Fig. 6.12   **Fig. 6.13**

Figs. 6.12. Axial CT after gunshot wound. Prominent soft tissue swelling on the left malar region, in the bullets trajectory. Note the air fluid level in the maxillary sinus *(open arrowhead)* secondary to bony fracture of its lateral wall

Fig. 6.13. Lateral subtraction angiogram of the left internal carotid artery. Iatrogenic CCF following Fogarty (surgical) thrombo-endarterectomy. Note the dilated cavernous carotid artery where the Fogarty balloon was inflated *(arrow)* and filling of the cavernous sinus *(curved arrow)*

trauma is available one should look for the evidence of associated vascular disease (angiodysplasia) during the angiographic exploration (Fig. 6.15).

As expected, traumatic carotid cavernous fistulas most frequently present in young adults, usually males. By far the most frequent trauma is secondary to motor vehicle accident. In children, they are more frequently seen following a penetrating orbital injury. Because of their traumatic nature, these patients have associated injuries at multiple levels and a thorough clinical assessment of the extent and type of injury is mandatory to prevent manipulation of unstable injuries (Table 6.3). Spontaneous direct arteriovenous fistulas are uncommon, but seen more frequently in females, whereas the congenital type prevails in children with a slight female predominance.

3. Natural History

In review of the extensive literature on TCCFs the natural history discussed in most series includes traumatic and spontaneous type fistulas together. The risk of untreated lesions as reported by Hamby (1966) includes loss of vision in 25% of cases and visual impairment in another 20%. Our own series (Kupersmith, 1986) shows visual loss in 54% of cases, of which 23% were blindness and in the other 31%, the visual loss was reversible and returned to normal after treatment (Table 6.4).

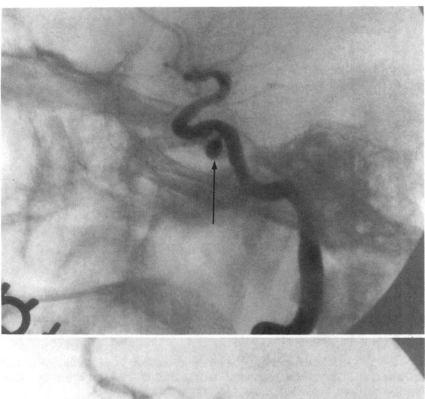

Fig. 6.14. Lateral subtraction angiogram of the right internal carotid artery in early arterial phase. Only minor trauma preceded the onset of symptoms. A narrow neck aneurysm of the cavernous internal carotid artery is noted *(arrow)*

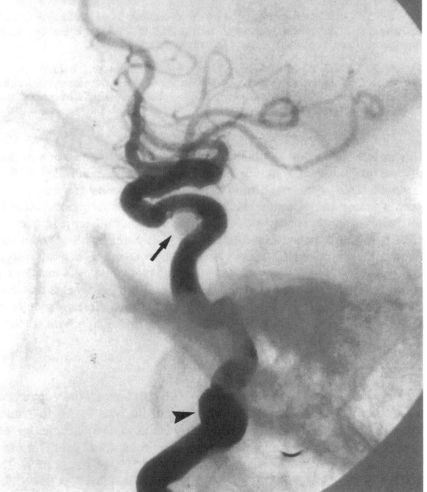

Fig. 6.15. Lateral subtraction angiogram of the left internal carotid artery following repair of a "spontaneous" CC fistula. Note dysplastic aneurysmal dilatation of the cervical internal carotid artery *(arrowhead)*. Similar dysplastic changes were noted in the opposite internal carotid and vertebral arteries. The internal carotid flow was preserved with a balloon *(arrow)* in the venous side

Fig. 6.16. Frontal subtraction angiogram of the left common carotid artery in a 26 year old male. The patient was referred to us because of severe and repeated epistaxis that started 1 year after incomplete repair of a traumatic fistula. Note the large pseudoaneurysm *(arrow)* projecting into the sphenoid sinus. Two silastic balloons are seen in the cavernous sinus *(arrowheads)* from the previous treatment (same patient as Figs. 6.9, 6.20)

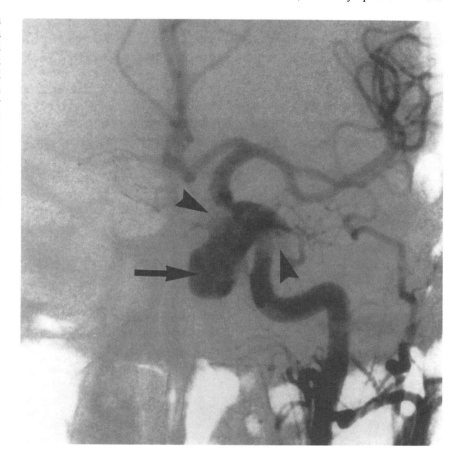

Sattler (1920) reported a 3% mortality as a result of intracranial or nasal hemorrhage. Based on our own material and the more recent reports of TCCFs by Debrun (1981) and Tsai (1983), it has become apparent that patients with nasal hemorrhage most likely are those that have a pseudoaneurysm in the sphenoid sinus (Fig. 6.16), whereas those with intracranial hemorrhage most likely have a direct intracranial vascular injury. The presence of these findings during angiography indicates immediate treatment (see section of emergeny treatment).

Spontaneous regression has been reported in 6% by Hamby (1966) and 10% by Dandy (1928); in both series it is a combined number of TCCFs and DAVMs of the cavernous area. It has been our experience that spontaneous regression of these lesions has been by far more frequent in the DAVMs than in the TCCFs where it is extremely rare.

4. Visual Symptoms

a) Visual Loss (Table 6.4)

Visual loss occurs in approximately 54% of cases (Kupersmith 1986). In a TCCF progressive visual loss represents one of the main indications for emergency treatment.

Henderson (1959) reported the spontaneous progression of the secondary glaucoma to blindness; even when the fistula is surgically treated, it may still progress to blindness or will be associated with the late formation of cataracts. A similar observation by Hamby (1966) prompts his recommendation of rapid aggressive intervention. We believe that progressive visual loss and epistaxis represent the two main instances where endovascular treatment is a true emergency. The significantly better results in recovery of visual loss by the endovascular embolization treatment as compared with Henderson's (1959) or Hamby's (1966) methods, is directly related to the closure of the fistula, preservation of the ophthalmic artery, and restoration of the normal ophthalmic arterial venous oxygen gradient. In Hamby's (1966) method the ophthalmic artery is ligated as part of the trapping procedure and further aggravates the ocular hypoxia.

Table 6.4. Visual loss in TCCFs (Kupersmith, 1986)

Pre-embolization causes of visual loss (54%)	Post-embolization
Traumatic optic neuropathy (15%)	no change
Post surgical optic neuropathy (6%)	no change
Optic globe damage (6%)	no change
Reversible optic neuropathy "steal" (12%)	normalized
Venous hypoxic retinopathy[a] (9%)	2 normalized
Surgical anophthalmous (3%)	no change
Central retinal artery occlusion secondary to elevated intraocular pressure (3%)	no change

[a] 1 Patient with venous hypoxic retinopathy represents our only unsuccessful embolization.

b) Corneal Ulcerations and/or Infections and Secondary Glaucoma

Acute and chronic exposure from proptosis can lead to infectious conjunctivitis, keratitis; Vth nerve involvement diminishes corneal sensitivity leading to noninfectious ulceration of the cornea. These complications were reported as frequent problems in the early series, but are not a problem in modern times, as proper protection of the exposed globe with lubricants and/or temporary tarsorraphy will prevent ulceration.

Glaucoma secondary to poor aqueous outflow and elevated episcleral venous pressure may be difficult to control medically. Visual loss occurs despite Pilocarpine, Timoptol, Epinephrine drops, and/or carbonic inhibitors (Diamox, Reptozaine). Rarely intraocular pressure is high enough to cause a central retinal artery occlusion requiring glycerol or intravenous mannitol. The intraocular pressure normalizes in all cases where the shunt is successfully occluded (Table 6.1). In those cases where embolization is not curative, laser trabeculopathy has been effective in preventing further glaucomatous visual loss. As long as the fistula remains patent the patient is not a candidate for any intra-ocular surgery, therefore, embolization should be done first.

c) Diplopia

The frequent involvement of cranial nerves in the cavernous sinus often produces diplopia; although cranial nerve function improves in the great majority of cases, complete normalization of extra-ocular muscle function is observed in 32% of cases. Extra-ocular eye muscle palsies which remain may cause diplopia. Prism therapy (temporary fresnel) may help in giving binocular vision during the recovery phase. Some cases with permanent cranial neuropathy may benefit from ptosis repair and/or strabism surgery if no improvement is made within six months of the fistula closure.

5. Pretherapeutic Evaluation

Based on the clinical picture one will have a high degree of certainty that one is dealing with a TCCF. However, for planning the best therapeutic regimen we must consider all of the clinical problems caused by the precipitating trauma and not only the vascular injury. As mentioned previously, emergency treatment of cerebral injuries or unstable fractures may precede repair of the fistula.

To evaluate the extent of orbitocranial injury, CT scanning is probably the best imaging modality to assess the degree of trauma and in some instances to predict some of the potential problems (Table 6.3).

a) CT Findings in TCCFs

The CT studies are important for the evaluation of the structures in the orbit, intracranially or in the face.

The findings concern the effects rather than the fistula itself and include: exophthalmus, evidence of prominent ophthalmic vein(s) (Fig. 6.17), extraocular muscle congestion (Fig. 6.17), a markedly enhancing cavernous sinus, that is convexed outwards producing dilatation of its tributaries (Fig. 6.18) or may even compress the 3rd ventricle (Fig. 6.19) producing hydrocephalus. Associated injuries include: bony fractures at the same side of the fistula or at a distance with soft tissue injuries or intracranial

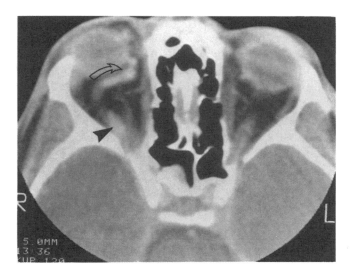

Fig. 6.17. Axial enhanced CT shows the characteristic prominence of the ophthalmic vein *(open curved arrow)* and the engorgement of the superior rectus muscle *(arrowhead)*

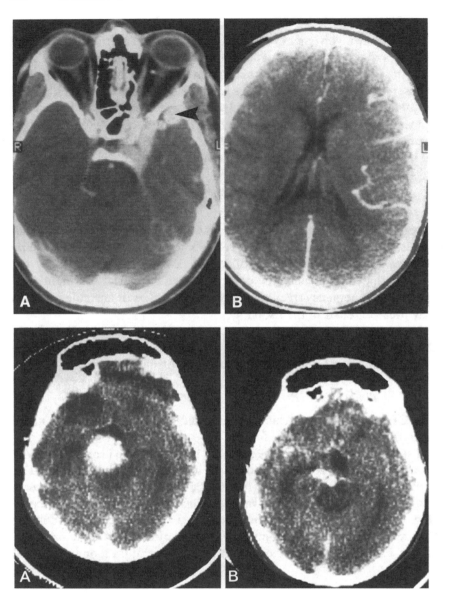

Fig. 6.18. Axial enhanced CT. **A** Multiple aneurysmal dilatations of the left cavernous sinus including the sphenoparietal sinus *(arrowhead)* and mild exophthalmus. **B** Axial CT at the level of the lateral ventricle. Note the prominent cortical veins in the left cerebral hemisphere

Fig. 6.19 A, B. Same patient as Figs. 6.4, 6.36. **A** Pre-embolization enhanced axial CT demonstrates the aneurysmally dilated cavernous sinus compressing the 3rd ventricle. **B** Enhanced CT after embolization. Note collapse of the cavernous sinus. Two balloons are seen (see Fig. 6.37). (By permission of Berenstein, 1980)

blood collections (Fig. 6.20), paranasal opacification and/or air fluid levels, usually the result of additional trauma can also be seen (Fig. 6.12).

Although the more precise topographical diagnosis of the fistulas supply and drainage is done by angiography, associated lesions are best demonstrated by CT scan and may modify the overall patient management.

The importance of this pretherapeutic evaluation will give the physicians preliminary information that can influence the urgency and/or proper importance of the treatment of the TCCF in the total management of the patient.

b) Angiography of TCCFs

Topographical Assessment of TCCFs. It is important to establish the vascular anatomy in an orderly and a systematic manner with the aim of answering the following questions:

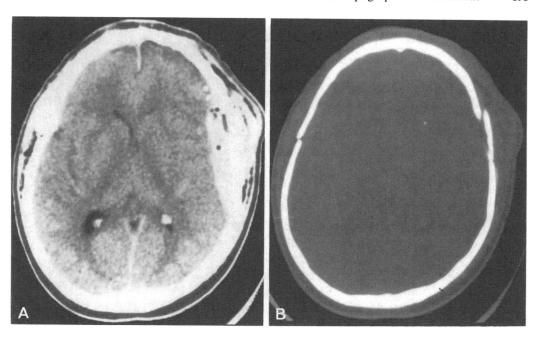

Fig. 6.20 A, B. Same patient as Figs. 6.9 and 6.16. **A** enhanced axial CT demonstrates bilateral epidural hematomas and soft tissues injuries. **B** Bony windows, demonstrate bilateral skull fractures

Location of the Fistula

A. Is the fistula in the internal carotid wall? And if so, what is its location?

B. Is it rupture of a branch of the C4 or C5 segments of the internal carotid artery, and if so, can it be reached from the external carotid side (Fig. 6.21)?

C. Is there a complete arterial "steal" from the fistula (Fig. 6.4) and what is the circulation to the normal brain?

D. Status of the collateral circulation: anterior and posterior portions of the circle of Willis, leptomeningeal collaterals of the brain.

E. Internal maxillary to ophthalmic circulation, and ascending pharyngeal contribution.

F. Associated vascular lesions:

1. Associated pseudo-aneurysms, proximal and/or distal to the fistula in the internal carotid artery (Fig. 6.8).

2. Other arteriovenous fistulas (Fig. 6.22).

3. Aneurysms (pseudo or bony) in other brachiocephalic arteries (Fig. 6.9).

4. Evidence of arterial disease (atheroma, stenosis, angiodysplasias, etc.) (Figs. 6.14, 6.15).

G. Venous drainage of the fistula:

1. Is it compatible with the clinical symptoms?

2. Is it purely sinus drainage or is there cortical venous rerouting?

3. Is there evidence of venous thrombosis?

4. Is there evidence of venous ectasias?

5. Is there crossfilling to the opposite cavernous sinus and its tributaries (Fig. 6.6).

In an attempt to answer these questions, we suggest the following angiographic protocol to be used.

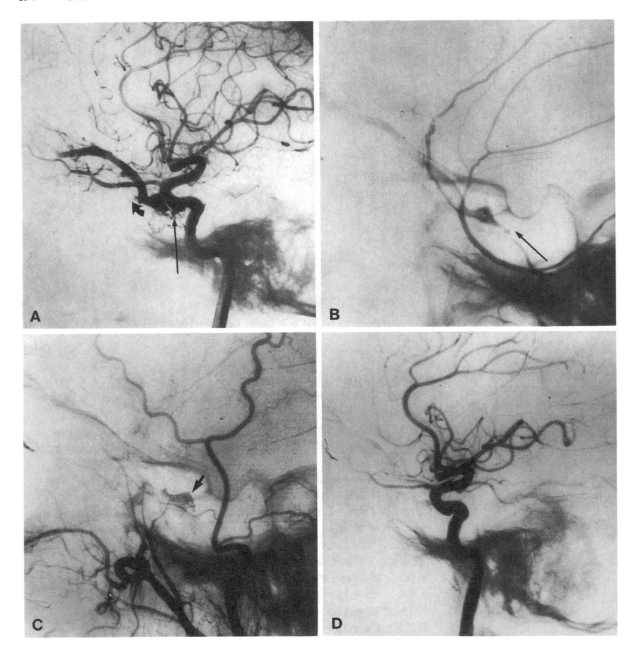

Fig. 6.21. A Lateral subtraction angiogram of the left internal carotid artery (arterial phase). There is early filling of the cavernous sinus and ophthalmic venous system *(curved arrow)* with a prominent ILT *(arrow)*. **B** Lateral subtraction angiogram of the ipsilateral middle meningeal artery. The cavernous sinus is also opacified without filling the internal carotid artery; representing laceration of the ILT. **C** Lateral subtraction angiogram of the left external carotid artery after IBCA embolization of the middle meningeal artery. Note the subtracted IBCA cast in the cavernous sinus *(arrow)* and no filling of the fistula. **D** Left internal carotid artery control after MMA embolization. There is no filling of the ILT fistula (the internal carotid artery was not embolized but used to control the result of embolization)

Fig. 6.22. Lateral subtraction angiogram after repair of the internal carotid to cavernous fistula *(arrow* points to the subtracted balloon). The orbital bruit persisted, control angiogram demonstrates a traumatic fistula of the ophthalmic artery to the superior ophthalmic vein *(curved arrow)*. This fistula was not treated, and disappeared spontaneously on a 3 months follow-up

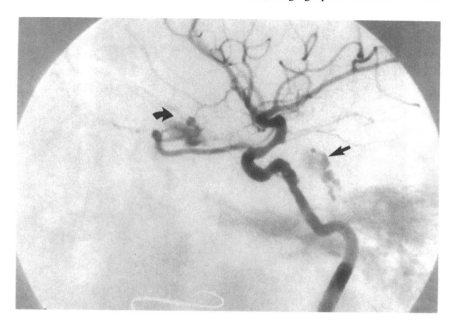

c) Angiographic Protocol

First Injection. Ipsilateral internal carotid artery. Although rapid sequential angiography has been said to be best for high flow lesions, and although very useful, it is not mandatory. The correct information can be obtained with slower rates and an equal total volume of contrast injection. The ipsilateral internal carotid injection confirms the fistula and its venous drainage. It also document the degree of distal hemodynamic "steal", and assesses other vascular injuries. The origin of the ophthalmic artery must be sought; if it originates in the C4 segment (Vol. 1, Fig. 15.4) and does not fill from the internal maxillary injection, the internal carotid artery flow must be preserved. Frontal filming in Caldwell projection may demonstrate contralateral venous drainage (Fig. 6.6). During internal carotid exploration special attention should be paid to the venous phase of the cerebral circulation. Opacification of the cavernous sinuses, both prior and after treatment should be noted (Fig. 6.5). Some special (unusual) vascular arrangements can occur if the fistula(s) remains patent after multiple proximal ligations or incomplete embolizations (Vol. 1, Figs. 9.19, 10.4, 15.13).

Second Injection. Lateral view of the ipsilateral internal maxillary artery. This injection may directly opacify the lesion if the ruptured vessel is part of the inferior lateral trunk (ILT) (Fig. 6.21), indirectly when the rupture is in the internal carotid wall by opacifying the internal carotid artery via the ILT (Fig. 6.23); the ophthalmic artery may be better studied through the internal maxillary artery as there is less superimposition of venous structures, retrograde filling of the siphon and the fistula can also be seen.

Third Injection. Ipsilateral ascending pharyngeal artery in the lateral projection. If the fistula is in the posterior and/or medial portion of the internal carotid artery at the C5 level, one may opacify the fistula via its carotid branch or from the clival branches (medial and/or lateral). When

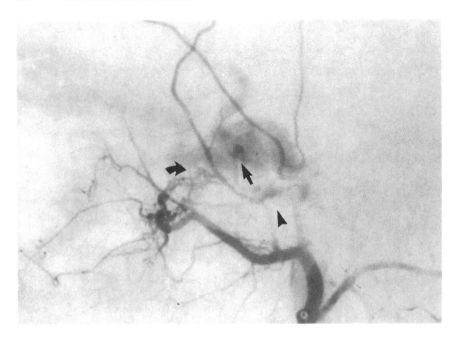

Fig. 6.23. Lateral subtraction angiogram of the distal external carotid artery. Middle meningeal artery *(arrowhead)* and artery of the foramen rotondum *(curved arrow)* fills the ILT, the internal carotid artery and then the fistula. The lesion is therefore located on the internal carotid wall and not on the ILT

the fistula is in the posteromedial wall of the internal carotid artery (C5), one will examine the contralateral ascending pharyngeal artery in frontal Caldwell projection, as both ascending pharyngeal arteries anastomose via the medial clival arcade (see Vol. 1, Figs. 10.4B, 15.13B).

Fourth Injection. Dominant vertebral artery in the lateral projection. This injection evaluates the posterior portion of the circle of Willis and the degree of spontaneous "steal". It may show the exact level of the fistula. If not, a fifth injection will be needed (vide infra). During the vertebral artery study, as in all others, other vascular injuries and embryonic vessels may be encountered (3.5% of our fistulas) (Vol. 1, Fig. 15.11).

Fifth Injection. Dominant vertebral artery in the lateral projection with manual compression of the symptomatic internal carotid artery.

This permit a downward flow of contrast material to the fistula and precise localization of the abnormal communication (Hubner, 1982) (Fig. 6.24). Vertebral angiography is of value in complex lesions where there has been ligation of the external carotid artery branches and/or the internal carotid artery (Fig. 6.26).

If the posterior circle of Willis is incompetent during the fourth injection, retrograde filling of the lesion will not be accomplished. In this instance, or when the flow is too rapid, the fistula site can be determined by the use of a double lumen balloon catheter in the involved internal carotid artery (Berenstein, 1979) (Fig. 6.25). By inflating the balloon the carotid flow is stopped and contrast material is slowly injected until it becomes diluted. A jet effect can be appreciated as the contrast material comes in contact with nonpacified blood flowing retrograde from above, demonstrating the exact fistula site.

In addition, one can, at the same time test for tolerance of internal carotid occlusion (see section on tolerance test and Chapter 7). An important point of caution: when the balloon is occluding the internal carotid artery proximal to the fistula, the development of a neurological deficit during the tolerance test may be

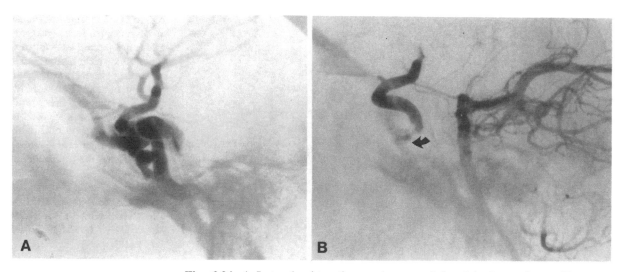

Fig. 6.24. A Lateral subtraction angiogram of the right internal carotid artery, demonstrating a CCF. **B** Lateral subtraction angiogram of the left vertebral artery with manual compression of the right internal carotid artery. Note filling of the internal carotid artery via the posterior communicating artery and downwards filling of the fistula *(curved arrow)*

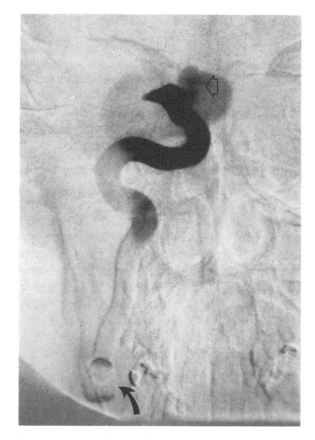

Fig. 6.25. Frontal subtraction angiogram of the right internal carotid artery. A double lumen occlusive balloon catheter *(curved arrow)* is occluding the internal carotid artery. The fistula site is clearly demonstrated *(open arrowhead)*. (By permission from Berenstein, Radiology 132:762–764, 1979)

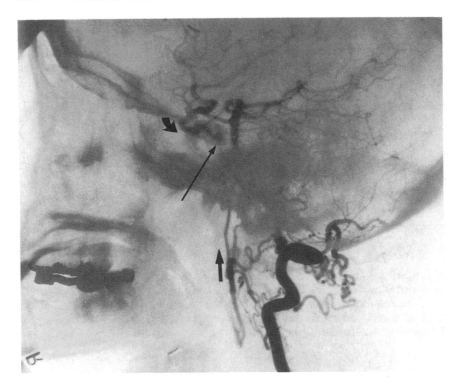

Fig. 6.26. Lateral subtraction angiogram of the left vertebral artery in a patient with multiple previous surgical ligations. The ascending pharyngeal artery *(arrow)* opacified via C3, fills the C5 segment of the internal carotid artery via its carotid branch. A surgical clip in the supraclinoid internal carotid artery above the ophthalmic is incompetent and permits downwards filling of the internal carotid artery *(curved arrow)* and then filling of the fistula *(long arrow)* (same patient as Fig. 6.28)

created by the added demand to the collateral circulation [by the downwards (retrograde) "steal" created by this maneuver] and this does not necessarily mean intolerance to internal carotid artery occlusion with fistula closure.

One additional maneuver for fistula site localization can be accomplished by placing the detachable balloon distal to the fistula site and injecting contrast material proximally while bringing the balloon to a more proximal position until the position of the balloon is actually at the level of the fistula.

Sixth Injection. Contralateral internal artery in the frontal view with a Caldwell projection.

This study will be important to demonstrate the presence or absence of transellar (medial capsular artery) or retroclival (medial clival artery) supply between the two internal carotid arteries (see Vol. 1, Fig. 15.3). If there is a clinical suspicion of bilateral involvement and/or the pretherapeutic evaluation demonstrates a basal skull fracture that crosses the midline, a lateral projection may be valuable to document or exclude bilateral fistulas (3% of cases in our own series). Contralateral internal carotid artery injection is also used to assess the status of the anterior segment of the circle of Willis. When cross filling to the contralateral side is poor or only the contralateral anterior cerebral artery is seen, a 7th injection may be advisable.

Seventh Injection. Contralateral internal carotid injection with manual or balloon occlusion of the diseased (ipsilateral) internal carotid artery. This injection appreciate the degree of cross filling and, may demonstrate the fistula site by retrograde filling.

Eighth Injection. Contralateral ascending pharyngeal injection in the lateral projection.

As stated previously, if the fistula is in the C5 segment (posteromedially) the lesion could be demonstrated by supply from the medial clival arcade. Although rarely important in traumatic CC fistulas, this route may become the only access to the lesion in complex cases where previous occlusions (ligation, proximal embolizations) have been done without satisfactory occlusion of the fistula. One other indication for contralateral ascending pharyngeal exploration is when the pretherapeutic screening demonstrates a contralateral posterior extension of the fracture. If the ascending pharyngeal on either or both sides has been ligated, one may use the anastomosis to demonstrate the fistula (see Vol. 1, Figs. 10.4B, 15.13B).

Ninth Injection. Contralateral internal maxillary injection. For the most part, this is not necessary, except in bilateral fistulas when the preliminary studies demonstrate traumatic changes such as fractures, soft tissue injuries, or fluid levels in the contralateral orbit, sphenoid sinus or maxillary antrum, or when looking for additional vascular injuries (Fig. 6.9). One additional instance for contralateral internal maxillary artery exploration would be in complex lesions where multiple procedures or occlusions have been done and an alternate route to reach the lesion is sought.

6. Therapeutic Objectives and Strategy

After a thorough analysis of the patients problem from clinical, anatomical, and hemodynamic points is understood, a therapeutic goal or objective is planned.

As stated in each specific instance of traumatic fistulas, there are situations in which therapy should be done immediately or even on an emergency basis. In some instance, treatment should be done to improve cosmesis. When the risks outweigh benefits, treatment may be deferred.

a) Embolization

From Brooks (1930) original conceptualization and successful management of a carotid cavernous fistula using an endovascular approach with muscle, it became apparent that this approach permits closure of the fistula itself and not at a distance. Various reports of the successful treatment of carotid cavernous fistulas by the Brooks method or a variation of it (Lang, 1964) confirmed its efficacy. This included balloon catheters of various designs that permit reaching the fistula and occluding it by balloon inflation (Caras 1978; Prolo 1971; Picard 1974). However, all these techniques would occlude the internal carotid artery flow. Isamat in 1970 reported the first case of successful endovascular occlusion in a TCCF with preservation of the carotid flow. He used a 1 × 0.5 cm piece of omohyoid muscle with a radiopaque clip attached to it that was carried to the fistula by the carotid blood flow. No other reports of this technique appeared. The authors failed to mention the risk of not occluding the fistula, retrieving the muscle, prevention of the cerebral embolization and the need for an operation. Serbinenko's (1974) introduction of a controllable flow guided balloon that could enter the fistula and then be detached, has made this technique the treatment of choice not only for TCCF, but probably for all AVFs throughout the body.

The endovascular approach to CCFs is by far the treatment of choice (Tables 6.2, 6.4). Various reported series confirmed the effectiveness and safety of this technique (Serbinenko, 1974; Debrun, 1981; Berenstein, 1980; Scialfa, 1983; Kendall, 1983; Kupersmith, 1984; Hieshima, 1983, 1985). At present the most frequently used endovascular approach is via the femoral artery. However, direct cervical carotid puncture can be used, when tortuosity at the arch or common carotid ligation prevents femoral catheterization of the internal carotid artery.

In the traumatic laceration of the internal carotid artery the use of detachable balloons is the best available method of treatment. The balloon can enter the cavernous sinus and with progressive inflation permit occlusion of the pathological arteriovenous communication with preservation of the carotid flow (Fig. 6.15).

In the largest reported series, the lesions have been cured from 85% to 98% of cases with a recurrence rate from 1.3 to 9% which usually responds to a second transvascular treatment.

The permanent complication of cerebral infarctions secondary to a stray balloon or thromboemboli has been reported in less than 2%. Permanent cranial nerve deficit that was not present prior to balloon treatment has been reported from 0–5%. Death related to the embolization occurred in 1 (1.8%) in Kendall's patients and 1 (3%) of Scialfa's patients.

Premature balloon detachment (Kendall, 1983; Scialfa, 1983; Flashner, 1984), dislodgment of previously detached balloons (Chalif, 1983), or intracranial migration secondary to delayed balloon deflation (Tsai, 1983) has been reported to be from 1 to 2.7% of which 3 cerebral dysfunctions occurred. One of our own patient, resolved after expeditious surgical removal of the balloon intracranially (Chalif, 1984). Immediate measures to increase the blood pressure can resolve some of this neurological ischemia and gain time to permit surgical extraction of the dislodged balloon. One patient in Kendall's series, an 83 year old, died from a stray balloon.

Although preservation of the carotid blood flow is one of the main advantages of the technique, in most reported series successful preservation of carotid flow has occurred in 50–100% of cases. Most authors in the largest series have reported a preservation of carotid flow between 60 and 70%. If the carotid flow cannot be preserved, a higher success rate may be obtained if the procedure is stopped and a new attempt is made at a later time (Scialfa, 1983).

Even in those instances where the internal carotid artery was intentionally occluded (Berenstein, 1981) or when it is technically impossible to preserve carotid flow, the transvascular approach is still preferred, as it has the advantage of closing the carotid artery at the fistula site and therefore, preventing collateral filling or recanalization of the pathological arteriovenous communication (see Chapter 1., XIII, XIV and Chapter 7, II 5c).

The exception for the use of balloon catheters in the management of these fistulas would be in cases of traumatic lacerations of the C4 or C5 branches of the internal carotid artery, where the lesion can be reached from the external carotid system (Fig. 6.21). In these instances, balloons may not enter the small cavernous branches, or occlusion of the internal carotid artery will not solve the problem. In these instances, the venous side can usually be reached with a fast polymerization tissue adhesive such as

IBCA introduced superselectively from the external carotid side, and the internal carotid artery can be used to control the effectiveness of the treatment (Fig. 6.21).

b) Emergency Treatment

1. Progressive visual loss: We have analyzed the course of visual loss previously, and divided it into permanent and irreversible, and progressive and reversible (Table 6.4). This latter type is the one in which treatment is most effective and rewarding. In some instances, the visual loss is slow and progressive, but in others it can be very rapid and measured in hours and days. If visual loss has already been established, without traumatic injury to the globe and/or optic nerve, immediate treatment should also be carried out. Although the yield may be low, it represents the only chance for improvement or recovery.

2. Epistaxis: Nasal bleeding in this disease is probably the most urgent problem to solve as it represents a true threat to life and should take precedence to any other treatment (Fig. 6.16).

Epistaxis in the acute phase of the traumatic incident is most often related to maxillofacial trauma and can be managed by internal maxillary artery and/or facial embolization (Fig. 6.16).

3. Sphenoid sinus aneurysm: If during pretherapeutic evaluation a soft tissue mass is noted in the sphenoid sinus which during angiographic evaluation proves to represent a (pseudo) aneurysm of the internal carotid artery (Fig. 6.16), treatment should be immediately undertaken as this lesion has a significant potential of rupture with its potential lethal implications.

4. Comatose patients: In patients with a depressed level of consciousness where intracranial lesions have been excluded, treatment should be instituted. This probably also applies to the unconscious and/or stuporous patient that has increased intracranial pressure, even if no cortical venous rerouting is noted.

5. During the course of treatment if a balloon is placed in such manner that the posterior venous drainage is blocked, or if in the immediate postembolization period the balloon migrates to block the posterior venous drainage following partial balloon deflation or vomiting (Fig. 6.27), a rapid aggravation of ophthalmic symptoms may occur; it requires immediate treatment. Every attempt to preserve the internal carotid flow should be done; if not possible, and depending upon the severity of symptoms the internal carotid artery should be sacrificed, if the patient can tolerate it.

c) Surgical Approach to Carotid Cavernous Fistulas

At present we strongly believe that there is no indication for any type of nonendovascular surgical attack on carotid cavernous sinus fistulas as the primary treatment. In Isamat's (1970) review of 545 reported cases of surgically treated carotid cavernous fistulas, cervical ligation of the internal carotid or common carotid arteries or both had a cure rate of 31–40%. "Trapping" the carotid cavernous fistula in a combined intracranial internal carotid clipping and internal carotid ligation in the neck resulted in good results in 56.7%. A "complete trapping" approach would include intracranial occlusion of the internal carotid and ophthalmic arteries followed by

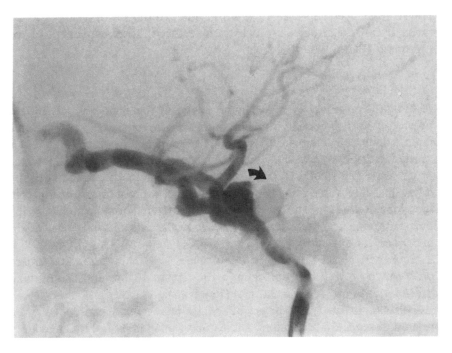

Fig. 6.27. Lateral subtraction angiogram of the internal carotid artery 8 h. following "satisfactory" repair of a TCCF with preservation of the internal carotid flow (not shown). The balloon *(curved arrow)* has migrated posteriorly after severe vomiting and has blocked the posterior drainage; aggravation of ocular signs and symptoms including rapid deterioration of visual acuity developed which responded readily to immediate secondary embolization. The internal carotid artery had to be sacrificed (not shown)

cervical ligation of the internal carotid and external carotid arteries. This technique achieved satisfactory results in 78.8% of 76 patients. Morley (1976) showed that the operative mortality and cerebral morbidity in the surgical approach to CCF has been distressingly high. Parkinson (1973) shows that it is surgically possible to repair these fistulas and preserve the carotid flow, however, this is a complex and major surgical endeavor. Hosobuchi, in 1975 reported a venous approach to cavernous sinus electrothrombosis, and although successful, it was apparent that significant technical skill was needed for operation. Mullan (1979) reported 33 fistulas treated by a variety of ingenious approaches to the venous side using thrombogenic technique with good results. Probably the only indication for surgical embolization is where previous procedures (surgical ligations or proximal embolization) have taken away the percutaneous accesses (Fig. 6.28).

d) Conservative Treatment of Traumatic CC Fistulas

When the symptoms are mild, and there is no immediate risk for vision, or when the patient refuses or is reluctant to take the risks of treatment, conservative follow-up should concentrate on intra-ocular pressure, visual acuity, and cranial neuropathies (see section on medical treatment of CCF).

7. Technical Aspects of Embolization

a) Balloon Selection

At present various detachable balloon systems are available. These are discussed in detail in Chapter 1. For the treatment of CCFs the involved physician has to familiarize himself with one or more types of detachable balloons so that he can have reliable and reproducible results.

Fig. 6.28. Plain film of the skull in the lateral projection, after surgical exposure of the supra-clinoid carotid artery below the lower surgical clip (see Fig. 6.26) and after the injection of IBCA. A second clip *(arrow)* was placed in the posterior communicating artery *(arrow)*. Note the radiopaque cast of the cavernous carotid artery, the fistula and the ILT *(open curved arrow)*

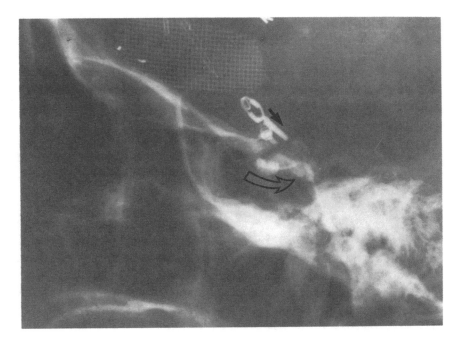

In this chapter we will consider the specific aspects of balloons as they relate to CCFs, such as balloon deflation, development of stenosis, aneurysmal pouches, etc.

A latex balloon filled with contrast material will eventually deflate in weeks to months, even silastic balloons filled with iso-osmolar contrast material can or will eventually deflate. This deflation produces venous pouches in a significant number of patients, usually without symptoms (Fig. 6.29).

We have seen one case of a large post-traumatic pseudoaneurysm after an incomplete occlusion of a TCCF with 2 silicone balloons of the Hieshima type (Fig. 6.16). This aneurysm pointed to the sphenoid sinus

Fig. 6.29. Lateral subtraction angiogram, 6 months after balloon repair of a TCCF. The patient is asymptomatic. The contrast filled balloon has deflated. An aneurysmal pouch *(arrow)* has formed at the site of the original balloon repair (same patient than Fig. 6.5)

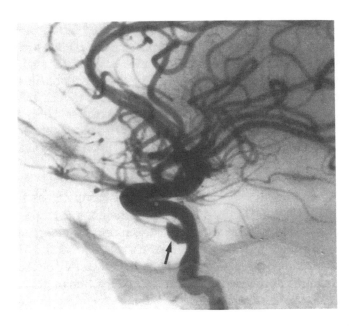

and the patient presented with severe repeated epistaxis. It is interesting to note that in Kendall's series of his 2 fistulas that still had persistance of some shunt, 1 resolved clinically and the other was his only symptomatic aneurysm (untractable V_1 pain). In most reports on traumatic fistulas when only minimal filling of the fistula persists the lesion thromboses spontaneously. Debrun makes no mention of the relationship between his symptomatic pouches and persistent minimal shunting.

Although theoretically balloon deflation could be a problem in the management of aneurysms, it may actually be of some advantage in the management of fistulas (see below). One considers that the main object of balloon deflation is the avoidance of a venous pouch at the site of the repair. However, one should remember that venous pouches have been observed to occur in 28.5% of cases even after filling the balloon with silicone (Debrun, 1981). Tsai (1983) reports a 19% presence of venous pouches; however, he did not have to retreat any of his cases. Debrun (1981) found 44% cases developed pouches and had to retreat 15% of his cases. In our experience, small pouches are not infrequent, although we have not had to treat any patient for a symptomatic pouch. Kendall had to retreat only one of his 49 treated patients and Scialfa reported that 75% of pseudoaneurysms at the site of the repair related to the pouch, did not need re-embolization. There are multiple examples of shrinkage and/or stabilization of the pouches rather than the relatively rare symptomatic pouches (which respond to a secondary embolization); no other adverse effects of these pouches have been reported. To our knowledge, there have been no reports of cerebral embolization from these pouches in up to 11 years follow-up. In Debrun's report there was a 21% incidence of carotid stenosis when he inflated the balloons with silicone, whereas there was none with iodinated contrast material. In our experience, we had one carotid stenosis out of four instances where we filled the balloon with silicone. Our only other instance of carotid stenosis in a patient with a carotid cavernous fistula was secondary to a gunshot wound. In one instance, a delayed occlusion of the ICA occurred in a patient with an iatrogenic CCF (following endarteryectomy). A similar experience was reported by Tsai and Hieshima (1983). The development of oculomotor palsies after the repair in Debrun's series was 36% when the balloon was filled with silicone and 17% when inflated with iodinated contrast material. Debrun makes no mention of the material used to fill the balloon in his patient with a permanent oculomotor palsy. Peeters and De Werf (1980) filled their latex balloons in 6 (out of 7) patients with silicone, and only 1 of 3 patients with oculomotor palsy had recovery of the IIIrd nerve but not the VI nerve. Tsai who uses nondeflating silicone balloons has reported at 5.4% of permanent ophthalmoplegia after treatment.

Although we do not have a full explanation of this variable evolution of the postdeflation pouches, one must realize that these lesions which in the internal carotid artery usually follow trauma could represent either rupture of a developmental arterial aneurysm or a secondary one (traumatic) not appreciated previously. The overwhelming carotid flow supplying the artiovenous fistula following repair is then exerted on the weakened or false wall of the pre-existing aneurysm. Observation of the venous phase of the postembolization angiogram, paying attention to the patency of the ipsilateral cavernous sinus, in the presence of a "venous" pouch, may

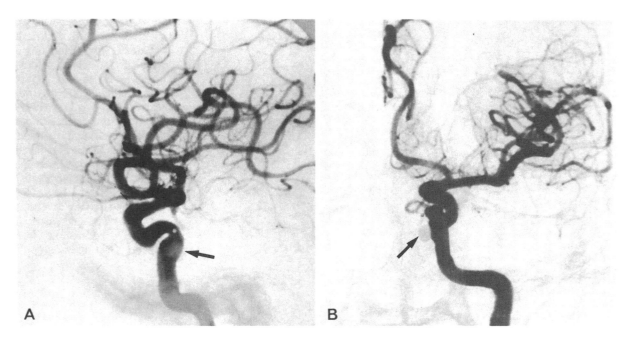

Fig. 6.30. A Lateral subtraction angiogram of the left internal carotid artery after balloon occlusion of the traumatic CCF. Note the substracted balloon and silver clip project into the carotid lumen *(arrow)*. **B** Frontal projection, same patient. The balloon is clearly outside of the carotid artery *(arrow),* and can be safely detached

suggest the evolution of (small) pre-existing traumatic or developmental arterial aneurysm; it may be an indication for prophylactic treatment or at least sequential follow-up angiograms. As seen during the dicussion of traumatic aneurysms, they carry a potential for growth, rupture and life threatening hemorrhage.

Therefore, we believe that the balloon deflation may be advantageous if an oculomotor palsy occurs after treatment. In dealing with fistulas of the internal carotid artery and vertebral artery in specific, prior to detaching a balloon, one must be certain that the balloon (or most of it) is in the venous side and not in the carotid lumen. The balloon may project onto the carotid lumen in one or two views, therefore, if needed oblique projections should be obtained until one can be certain that the balloon clears the lumen of the carotid (Fig. 6.30).

b) Venous Approach (Fig. 6.31)

1. Inferior petrosal approach (Mullan 1979; Manelfe 1980; Debrun 1981; Kendall 1983).

If the anatomy of the fistula and its venous drainage are favorable, with the fistula being in the posterior superior compartment and draining exclusively into the inferior petrosal sinus occlusion of the fistula can be accomplished by the retrograde transjugular approach using a Fogarty or a detachable balloon catheter system. The technique is difficult with an approximately 50% success rate in the various reports. This route, although elegant and safe, is not easy and should be reserved for special occasions as described earlier. Transient neuropathies are more frequent by the inferior petrosal approach. A point of caution when using this approach is to convert the posterior drainage into a purely anterior one. This would actually aggravate the ocular signs and symptoms.

2. Retrograde ophthalmic vein catheterization:

Although a logical and tempting route, it carries potential dangers for control of bleeding and orbital damage. There may be difficulty in

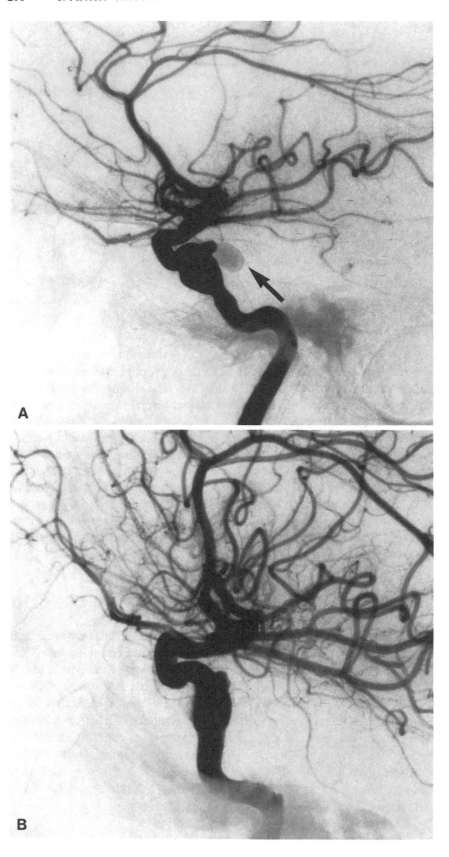

Fig. 6.31 A, B. Same patient as Fig. 6.3, venous approach. A Lateral subtraction angiogram of the right internal carotid artery after a Fogarty balloon catheter *(arrow)* was introduced retrograde via the jugular inferior petrosal route. Note preservation of the internal carotid artery. A small cavernous aneurysm remains. B Lateral subtraction angiogram 3 month later. The balloon has deflated and the cavernous aneurysm has decreased in size. (By permission from Manelfe, Neuroradiology 7: 13–19, 1980)

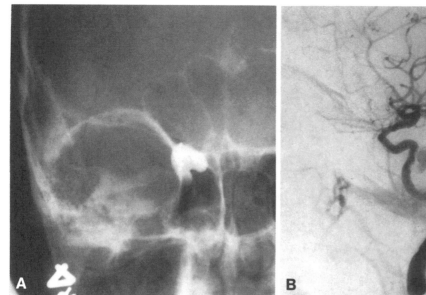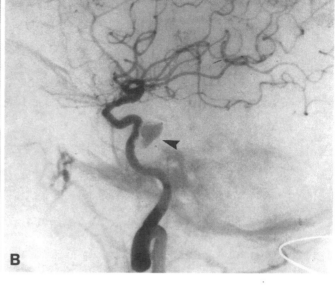

Fig. 6.32. A Frontal plain skull film after balloon repair of a TCCF. Note the lobulated configuration of the balloon as it conforms to the septations of the cavernous sinus. **B** Lateral subtraction angiogram same patient. The lobulated balloon *(arrowhead)* is in the posterior cavernous sinus. The internal carotid artery flow is preserved

advancing a balloon or nonballoon catheter, as it is being negotiated against the blood flow and significant tortuosities of the ophthalmic veins are frequent. Three cases have been reported using detachable balloons or coils (Santos de Lima, 1984). This approach can be considered in cases of previous ligations of the internal carotid artery where there is no access via the arterial or posterior venous side to avoid the need for open surgical embolization. In Santos de Lima's (1984) experience, the procedure is done after cutting down on the frontal division of the vein and not percutaneously. Furthermore, the safety of the technique is directly related to the age of the fistula. In the chronic group the thickened wall of the ophthalmic vein permits easy control; whereas in acute fistulas the venous wall is thinned and fragile.

c) Balloon Configuration in the Cavernous Sinus

Balloons of any type when entering the cavernous sinus may take a lobulated configuration as they mold to the septations in the cavernous sinus (Fig. 6.32). They may also have large oval shapes, as they fill an aneurysmally dilated sinus or a pre-existing developmental or post-traumatic pseudoaneurysm. When (latex) balloons are filled with tantalum (or Bismuth) opacified silicone a variable interface may be seen as the radiopaque metal will precipitate depending on the patient position (Fig. 6.33). In Debrun's (1975) model balloons (Fig. 1.9) the main body of the balloon should inflate first. If the distal tip that harbors the radiopaque silver clip is seen to inflate first there is a high chance of rupture with distal embolization of the silver clip. If this occurs when testing the balloon in vitro, or at any point in vivo, the balloon should be changed. For the most part 1 balloon is usually needed to close most fistulas, but on occasions, however, multiple balloons may be needed (Fig. 6.36). When one cannot preserve the carotid artery the second best treatment is to trap the fistula by putting a balloon distal to or at the fistula site and a second balloon proximal to the fistula (Fig. 6.34) as close as possible to insure occlusion of the

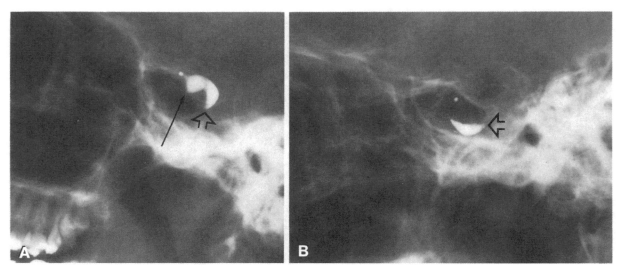

Fig. 6.33. A Lateral skull X-ray. Approximately 20 min after balloon detachment (patient is lying supine). The ballon is filled with silicone fluid mixture and tantalum powder. Note how the heavier tantalum powder has settled in the posterior part of the balloon *(open arrow)*, whereas some contrast material from the dead space of the catheter is in the superior (anterior) portion of the balloon *(arrow)* with nonopaque vulcanized silicone in between. **B** Same patient 24 hours later after being ambulatory. Note the radiopaque tantalum in the dependent (inferior) portion of the balloon *(open arrow)*

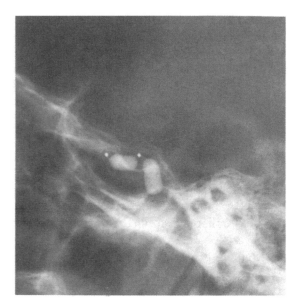

Fig. 6.34. Lateral skull film shows 2 balloons in the C4 and C5 segment of the internal carotid artery trapping a large TCCF

communication. On occasions the fistula track is too small or the venous side may not permit entry of an inflated balloon in it (Fig. 6.35A, B), the balloon itself (uninflated) may then plug the fistula (Fig. 6.35C, D).

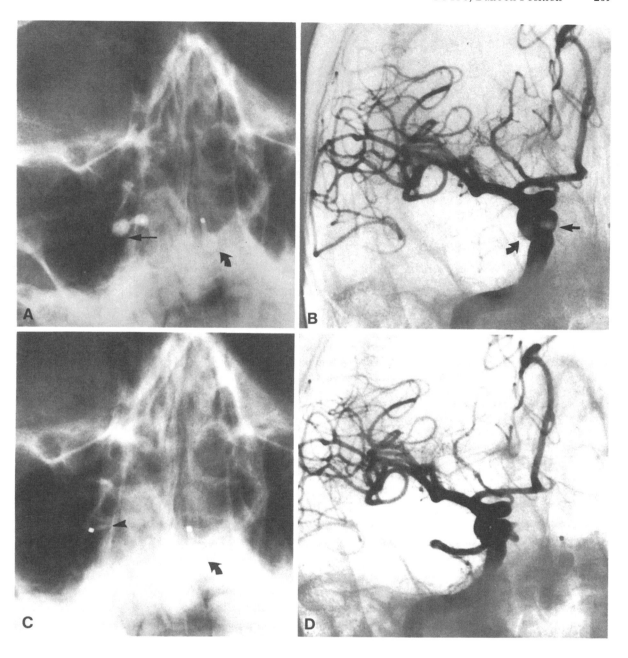

Fig. 6.35. A Frontal skull film in waters projection. A balloon has been detached in the left cavernous sinus for a left CCF *(curved arrow)*. On the right side, an hour glass balloon (Debrun # 15) is partially in the cavernous sinus and partially in the internal carotid artery *(arrow)*. The narrow portion of the balloon demonstrates the fistula site. The balloon is not detached. **B** Frontal subtraction angiogram same projection. Note the subracted balloon with a portion into the internal carotid artery lumen *(arrow);* the portion into the cavernous sinus *(curved arrow)* occludes the fistula. **C** Plain film, waters projection. The right side balloon has been detached uninflated *(arrowhead)* and was sufficient to occlude the fistula. **D** Control post embolization angiogram. The fistula is closed and the carotid arteries were preserved bilaterally

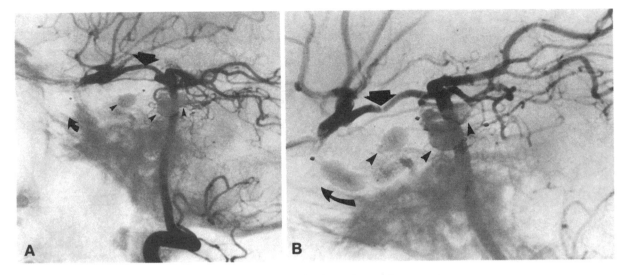

Fig. 6.36 A, B. Same patient as Figs. 6.4, 6.19. **A** Lateral subtraction angiogram of the left vertebral artery after 3 balloons were placed in the aneurysmally dilated cavernous sinus *(small arrowheads)*, and a 4th balloon *(curved arrow)* in the internal carotid artery trapping the fistula. Note elevation of the posterior communicating artery by the distended cavernous sinus *(solid arrow)* (compare with Fig. 6.4). **B** 24 hours after embolization, while the patient was ambulant, a severe headache developed, associated with the development of a VIth nerve palsy, which resolved spontaneously in 4 weeks. Note collapse of the dilated cavernous sinus with the corresponding downwards displacement of the left posterior communicating artery *(broad arrow)*. (By permission of Berenstein, 1980)

d) The Use of IBCA in the Management of CCF

IBCA has limited indications in the management of CCF. Kerber (1979) reported the successful occlusion of 3 patients with traumatic CCF using flow guided catheters and IBCA. All 3 patients developed IBCA cerebral embolization and although in all patients the symptoms reversed, the chances of retrograde IBCA embolization into the cerebral circulation make this technique more hazardous.

In our experience, IBCA is the agent of choice for lesions of the ILT (Fig. 6.21) where balloons cannot enter the small ruptured vessel or when there is no percutaneous access and a surgical repair of a traumatic fistula is the only alternative (Fig. 6.28). Prior to IBCA injection one must insure reliable protection of the cerebral and ophthalmic circulation.

e) Trigeminal Participation in Cavernous Fistulas

The participation of the trigeminal artery persistance in the supply of the fistula, mainly if the trigeminal artery enters the fistula directly (both of our cases, Vol. 1, Fig. 15.11) must be assessed. An attempt to enter the cavernous sinus via the carotid route is probably the first choice (Kerber, 1984). If this fails, one may attempt entering the fistula via the vertebrobasilar route; to facilitate this maneuver ipsilateral manual compression of the carotid artery will be of assistance. In one of our 2 cases these maneuvers failed for which the internal carotid artery was occluded above the fistula and large particles (PVA) were flow guided to occlude the cavernous sinus fistula primarily to resolve the symptomatic ophthalmic vein filling.

f) Cavernous Origin of the Ophthalmic Artery (Vol. 1, Fig. 15.4)

When the ophthalmic artery originates at C4, if the cavernous sinus cannot be entered, analysis of the collateral circulation to the orbit is imperative prior to trapping. Or the retrograde venous approach (posterior or anterior) may be attempted.

g) Internal Carotid Artery Occlusion

Sacrificing the internal carotid artery for the management of a CCF is an aggressive measure that should be thoroughly weighed as to risks vs. benefits. As stated in the aneurysm and techniques chapters (Chapter 1, XIII, XIV, and Chapter 7, II 5c) a tolerance test should be done first. The procedure should probably be stopped and an additional attempt to preserve the internal carotid artery should be done at a later date.

8. Postembolization Care

This is primarily related to the early postembolization period and refers to bed rest, control of nausea and vomitting or other maneuvers to prevent balloon migration (Fig. 6.27); 24–36 hours appears sufficient. Analgesics are needed to control the pain that may occur in the first weeks as the cavernous sinus and/or the fistula is thrombosing. On occasions, a delayed cranial nerve dysfunction may occur as the distented cavernous sinus collapses (Fig. 6.36), it usually resolve in 2–5 weeks (a more frequent event following treatment of cavernous aneurysms).

A frontal and lateral skull X-ray to document the position and size of the balloon(s) should be obtained immediatly after detachment as a baseline. If any clinical problem occurs a repeat plain skull film will be of assistance to explain the clinical change or deterioration.

If the internal carotid artery had to be sacrificed the postoperative care reviewed in the postoperative care (Chapter 1) should be followed.

III. Vertebral Arteriovenous Fistulas (VAFs)

1. General

Arteriovenous fistulas of the vertebral artery are uncommon lesions and they are usually of traumatic origin. They may occur spontaneously with no history of trauma. In rare cases the fistula may be congenital.

In the past surgical excision of the fistula has been the preferred method of management in these lesions; however, this may not be possible. The enlarged feeding vessels and arterialized veins that drain through the fistula may cause excessive blood loss at surgery. Ligation of the feeding vessels proximal to the fistula may be the only surgical option; however, this results only in temporary control due to the vast collateral network in the head and neck (Shumacker, 1966; Wage, 1974; Stapleford, 1981).

With the advent of transcatheter endovascular techniques and new embolic agents, embolization has become the treatment of choice for these lesions. Several reports have appeared in the literature describing embolization of these lesions using a variety of embolic agents (Goodman, 1975; Debrun, 1979; Berenstein, 1980; Miller, 1984).

Fistulous connections of the vertebral artery occur frequently after trauma (Markham, 1969). They can present without a previous history of trauma; these are usually present at birth and manifest at a more advanced age. As a separate group there are reports of "spontaneous" vertebral arteriovenous fistulas associated with fibromuscular dysplasia (FMD) (Bahar, 1984) and neurofibromatosis (Deans, 1981).

In Markham's (1969) review of 41 cases of vertebral artery fistulas, 37 were of traumatic origin.

2. Clinical Findings

The clinical manifestation of VAFs, as other fistulas, is related to arterial depravation in the territory distal to the fistula which can result in vertebrobasilary insufficiency (Reivich, 1961) or spinal cord ischemia (Nagashima, 1977). Venous hyperpressure and/or congestion is the second mechanism by which VAFs produce signs and symptoms of spinal cord ischemia and/or nerve root compression (Deans, 1982). These symptoms include spasticity, spastic quadraparesis, painful torticolis, blurring of vision, and facial pain. The high AV shunting manifest itself by a prominent paraspinal bruit that usually does not change with manual compression of the carotid arteries, but may be associated with decrease in distal pulses in the ipsilateral upper extremity. In our personal experience hemisensory deficits are more frequent than motor dysfunction; a bruit was present in all cases and in 70%, was the only symptom.

3. Natural History and Indications for Treatment

The natural history of the fistulas is still not completely understood. However if symptomatic (neural compression and/or distal insufficiency), they are usually progressive (Markham, 1969).

The discussion of treatment concern the asymptomatic fistulas only presenting with a bruit; Chou (1967) suggested that untreated VAFs will increase in size and become unmanagable by conventional surgical techniques. Contrary to other fistulas there is seldom spontaneous thrombosis; cardiac decompensation is an indication for treatment.

All previous discussions as to the advisability for or against treatment have been based on the difficulty of surgery where complete irradication is needed and not merely ligation of some feeders. At present, there is a high degree of success (95–100%) in the percutaneous endovascular management of VAFs by experienced hands (Moret, 1979; Debrun, 1979; Berenstein 1980; Heishima, 1985; Miller, 1984); there were no serious complications and this makes endovascular treatment of relatively asymptomatic fistulas more attractive. In case of doubt, one can follow the patient; even if the fistula increases in size, endovascular management is not necessarily more difficult.

a) Traumatic VAFs

The anatomical location and relationship of the vertebral artery and surrounding veins, as well as the mechanism of formation in traumatic

Fig. 6.37. A Clinical picture of a 19 year old male demonstrating an old scar from the original injury as well as the pulsatile soft tissue mass in the retroauricular region. **B** Lateral subtraction angiogram of the left vertebral artery demonstrates a fistula at C1 with an aneurysmally dilated venous outflow *(open curved arrow)*. **C** Lateral subtraction angiogram in mid arterial phase of the left occipital artery *(arrow)*. Additional fistulas are demonstrated *(arrowheads)*. **D** Clinical picture of the same patient three weeks following embolization, with complete disappearance of the abnormal pulsations and mass

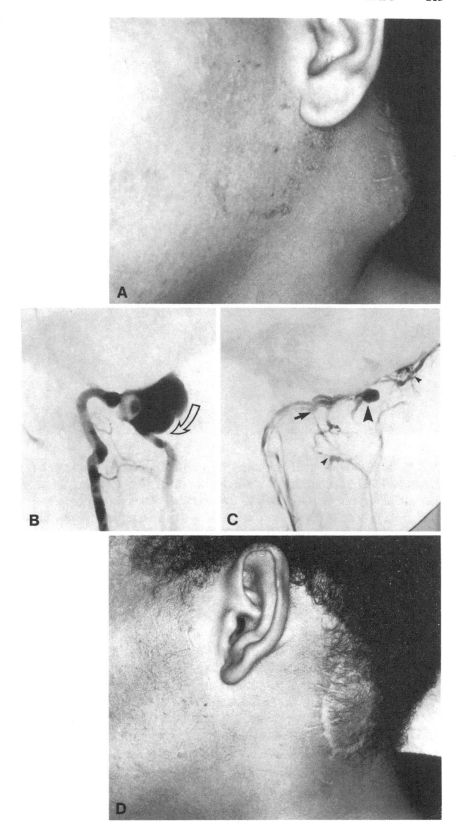

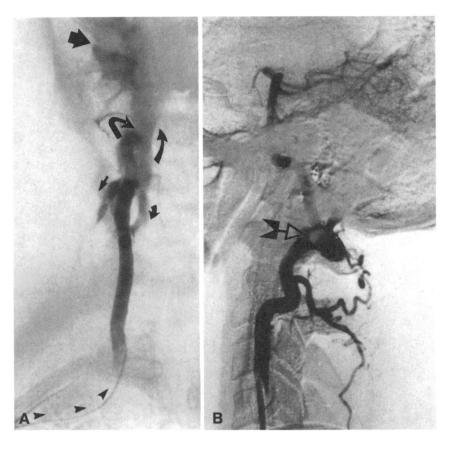

Fig. 6.38. A Vertebral angiogram by axillary approach *(arrowheads)* in case of TVAF following gunshot wound injury. The fistula *(broken arrow)* is at the C2 level. The venous outflow is rostral towards the epidural venous plexus *(curved arrow)* and to the paravertebral venous plexus *(solid arrow)* and caudal to the epidural plexus *(small curved arrow)*. Note a vein following the C3 nerve *(arrow)*. **B** Lateral subtraction angiogram after balloon embolization. The subtracted balloon *(arrow)* is in the venous side. Note the patent vertebral artery without filling of the fistula

VAFs, is similar to that reviewed on traumatic pseudoaneurysms (see Chapter 7). It appears that AV fistulas are more frequent than traumatic pseudoaneurysms in the vertebral distribution; this is probably related to the proximity of the vertebral artery and its surrounding venous plexus (Davis, 1983) (see Chapter 7).

Traumatic lesions can occur at any level of the vertebral artery. They may be associated with a large expanding false aneurysm (Fig. 6.37) and/or multiple AV fistulas on other vessels (Fig. 6.37C) as well as other traumatic vascular injuries such as thrombosis.

They may follow gunshot wound injuries (Fig. 6.38). The most frequent location is high at the C1, C2, or C3 level (Figs. 6.37, 6.38) (Goodman, 1975). Those that follow percutaneous vertebral angiography (Bergquist, 1971) are usually in the proximal 1/3 of the vertebral artery (Fig. 6.39).

Hematomas in the neck may follow the acute injury with tamponade or delayed presentation of the fistula days, weeks or even years later. They may be secondary to direct injury of the vertebral artery by a fractured bone and therefore careful analysis of associated bony injuries is important (see Pretherapeutic Evaluation).

b) Nontraumatic VAFs

These can be divided into congenital and spontaneous fistulas. Congenital fistulas are those that are present at birth without preceding trauma; they usually are asymptomatic and found incidentally by the parents and/or during a routine examination by the pediatrician they may occasionally

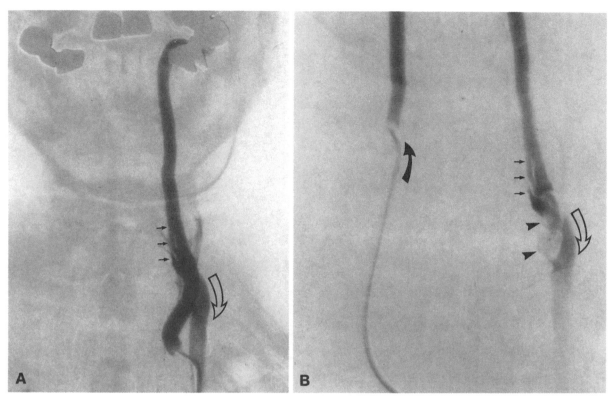

Fig. 6.39. A Frontal subtraction angiogram early arterial phase demonstrates a iatrogenic fistula following accidental puncturing of the vertebral artery during angiography. A fistula in the proximal 1/3 of the vertebral artery associated with subintimal dissection *(small arrows)* is seen to drain primarily downwards the innominate vein *(open curved arrow)*. **B** Opposite right vertebral injection *(curved arrow)* for control before balloon detachment the fistula fills in a retrograde manner. The dissection *(small arrows)* is best seen, as well as downwards filling of the innominate vein *(open curved arrow)*. Two balloons are seen in the proximal left vertebral artery *(arrowheads)*. Complete obliteration of the fistula could be obtained by further inflation of the second balloon

present with signs and symptoms of cardiac overload (Bartal, 1972) or cardiac failure (Norman, 1950). The diagnosis of congenital fistula may be assisted by the presence of other congenital vascular anomalies. In some of these lesions the fistula is associated with a large venous structure with the proximal vertebral artery entering at one point and the distal vertebral artery entering at another point (Fig. 6.40) (vide infra).

The second category is considered "spontaneous". These fistulas occur without a history of trauma and are encountered at a later age, usually in young males. They present as a bruit or swishing noise of acute onset (Goody, 1960) that follows sudden neck movement, straining or sneezing (Bartal, 1972). These fistulas may follow a previous thrombosis or rupture of a pre-existing aneurysm, although it is difficult to prove.

Some spontaneously occurring fistulas can occur with other vascular dysplasias such as fibromuscular dysplasia (Bahar, 1984) (Fig. 6.41, see also Chapter 7), or neurofibromatosis (Fig. 6.42) (Deans, 1982). Since Reubi's (1945) report there has been increased awareness of the vascular lesions in neurofibromatosis which include stenosis, aneurysms (Itzchak,

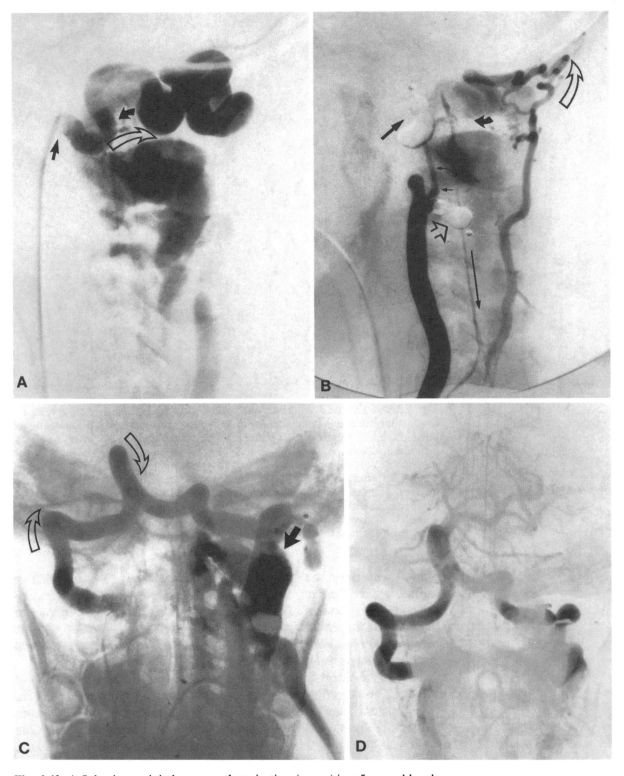

Fig. 6.40. A Selective occipital artery catheterization *(arrow)* in a 5 year old male
with clinical and radiographic evidence of cardiac overload and a congcuital VAF.
The occipital artery is markedly hypertrophied and tortuous. The fistula fills via the
artery of the first space *(curved arrow)* and enters into a large venous structure
(open curved arrow) **B** Left vertebral injection following occlusion of the occipital
artery with a detachable balloon *(arrow)*. The vertebral contribution to the fistula

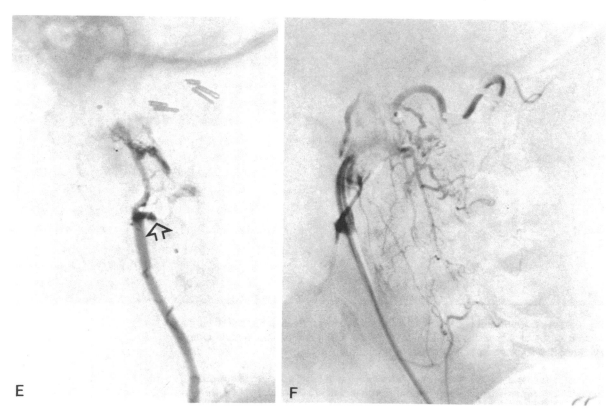

E

F

Fig. 6.40 (continued)
has been occluded with a second balloon *(open arrowhead)*. Note the congenitally abnormal proximal VA, ending in an aneurysmal pouch *(arrowheads)*. The lateral spinal artery *(small arrows)* fills the anterior spinal artery *(long arrow)*. There is reflux into the dorsocervical artery which reconstitutes the distal occipital artery *(open curved arrow)* with the artery of the first space *(small curved arrow)* still filling the upper portion of the fistula with opacification of the large venous structure. **C** Control into the right vertebral demonstrates complete "steal" *(open curved arrow)* and filling of the fistula from above *(solid arrow)*. The superior portion of the fistula could not be successfully catheterized. **D** Right vertebral angiogram after surgical ligation of the dorsocervical and left vertebral artery by exposing it a C1–2. Note filling of the posterior fossa circulation, without filling of the fistula. **E** Left vertebral injection after the surgery. Note the significant decrease in the caliber of the right vertebral artery following treatment. An aneurysmal pouch at the site of the original repair *(open arrow)* is noted after balloon deflation. **E** Control occipital injection. Note the decrease in caliber of the occipital artery without filling of the fistula and its patency from the external carotid trunk although it had been occluded

1974) and AV fistulas. Deans (1982) reported 2 cases of such fistulas in patients with neurofibromatosis and one had a spontaneous fistula of the left internal maxillary artery that presented with spontaneous hemorrhage. All of Deans' patients and one of the 2 patients we have seen presented between the 4th and 5th decade of life (Fig. 6.42).

The histological analysis of some of these patients with neurofibromatosis shows proliferation of Schwann cells in the adventitia of the arterial wall, as well as intimal fibrosis and fragmentation of the elastica and thinning of the smooth muscle with aneurysm formation, nodular masses of spindleshaped cells are also seen between the media and adventitia in the involved artery (Deans, 1982). Saylor in 1974 actually found such lesions in

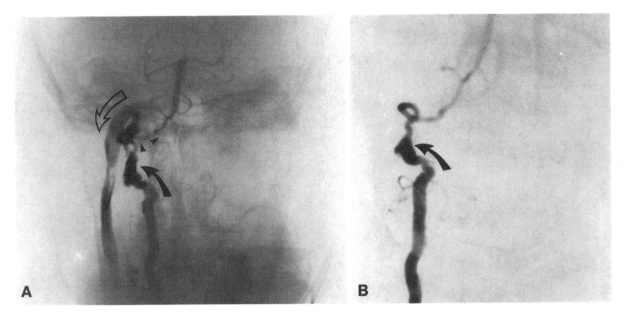

Fig. 6.41 A, B. Spontaneous fistula in a 48 year old female which presented with a sudden onset of a "swishing" noise on the right side. The patient demonstrated evidence of fibromuscular dysplasia at multiple brachiocephalic vessels *(not shown)*. **A** Frontal subtraction angiogram of the right vertebral artery. Note the dysplastic segment of the vertebral artery *(curved arrow)* filling of the internal jugular vein *(open curved arrow)* and a dysplastic distal vertebral artery *(arrowheads)*. **B** Frontal subtraction angiogram of the right vertebral artery following "spontaneous" closure of the fistula while attempting balloon embolization. The dysplastic vertebral artery involved by fibromuscular dysplasia is better seen *(curved arrow)*

almost 50% of neurofibromatosis patients studied at autopsy even if they did not have fistulas. Green (1974) in his study of aneurysmal and nodular lesions in patients with neurofibromatosis found no evidence of Schwann cell proliferation, and the EM characteristics of the spindle cells in these lesions were those of smooth muscle. They suggested that some of the vascular changes in these patients are due to a primary dysplasia of the arterial wall. Either dysplasia of the arterial wall or neurofibromatosis proliferation in the arterial wall, or a combination of both, can lead to aneurysm formation and eventual rupture into an adjacent vein which produces a pathologic AVF.

Alternatively, a VAF could arise congenitally as a manifestation of mesodermal dysplasia (Deans, 1982). Angiographically the feeding vessels to the fistula are markedly abnormal with multiple irregular dilatations and constrictions and ectasias pointing to the dysplastic abnormal vessels (Fig. 6.42). Even after the fistula is occluded the feeding vessels shows dysplasia and stasis and a relative inability to react (Fig. 6.42); the vessel probably should be occluded completely to prevent delayed embolization. The prominent and chronic venous drainage can produce widening of bony foramen that should not be confused with the frequent presence of tumors in the nerve roots in patients with neurofibromatosis. "Spontaneous" fistulas may be present simultaneously at multiple levels, may not be appreciated on the initial study (Fig. 6.43). They will be demonstrated in oblique projections (Fig. 6.43) or become apparent after occluding the

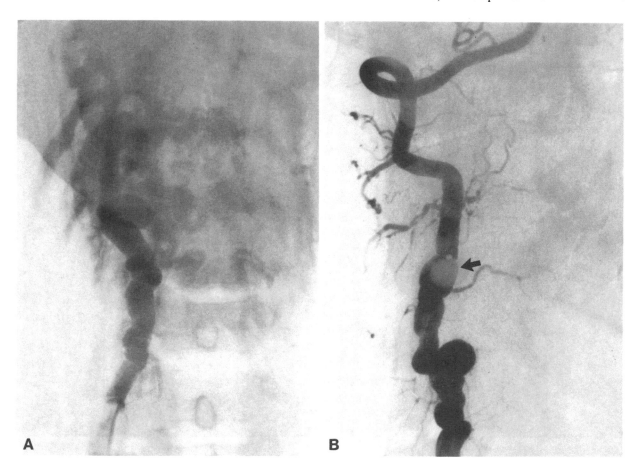

A   **B**

Fig. 6.42 A, B. Spontaneous fistula in a 52 year old female which presented with a sudden onset of "swishing" noise on the right side. The patient was presenting cutaneous signs and a family history of neurofibromatosis. **A** Right vertebral injection demonstrates the C3–4 AVF. **B** After balloon occlusion of the fistula *(arrow)* the proximal dysplastic segment demonstrated significant stagnation for which the vertebral artery was completely obliered. Note the dysplastic appearance of the VA, proximal to the fistula

most distal one. Multiple balloons will be needed to trap all the fistulas. In the case illustrated in Fig. 6.44 an associated blood dyscrasia (Willebrand's disease) with deficiency of factor VIII at 12.5% (normal is more than 40%) and low procoagulant assay was found. Liquid embolic agents or particles should probably not be used as they may enter vessels supplying the spinal cord.

4. Pretherapeutic Evaluation

In general, VAFs are of the high flow type, and their exact localization may be difficult. Proper assessment of the circle of Willis is important when considering a trapping procedure. The normal blood supply to the spinal cord must be established, particulary in patients with congenital variants (Fig. 6.40). Differentiation must be made between a true VAF and a fistula of the anterior spinal artery that may present with subarachnoid hemorrhage (Fig. 6.44).

5. Angiographic Protocol

The pretherapeutic evaluation is similar to that discussed for other fistulas. Here we will review the angiographic evaluation:

First Injection. Ipsilateral vertebral artery. Biplane studies of the vertebral artery harboring the fistula will help determine the presence of a fistula, its

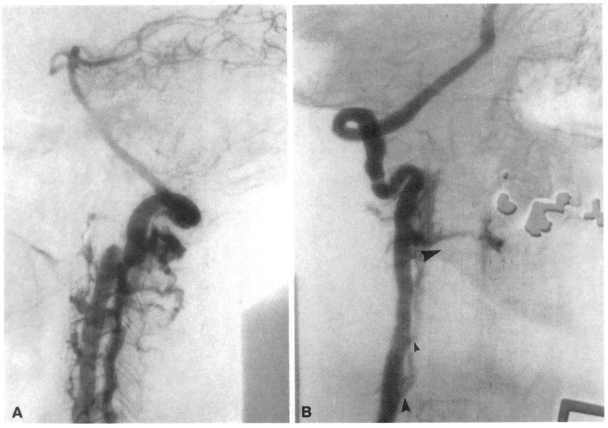

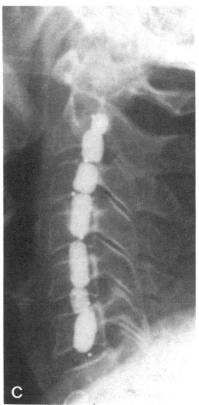

Fig. 6.43. A Lateral subtraction angiogram in a patient with von Willebrand disease and deficiency of factor VIII. The multiplicity of fistulas or exact fistula site could not be accuratly demonstrated. **B** Oblique subtraction angiogram demonstrates seperate AVFs. *(arrowheads)*. The largest fistula at C3 drains anteriorly towards the contralateral epidural venous plexus. **C** Lateral plain film of the cervical region demonstrates multiple balloons in tandem from C2–C5. As balloons were placed in the most superior portion of the vertebral artery, additional fistulas were seen. All signs and symptoms were relieved after the embolization

Fig. 6.44. Oblique subtraction angiogram in early arterial phase demonstrates a congenital arteriovenous fistula of the anterior spinal axis. The right vertebral artery is markedly hypertrophied. The artery of the cervical enlargement *(open curved arrow)* is markedly enlarged, and joins a hypertrophied anterior spinal artery *(arrow)*

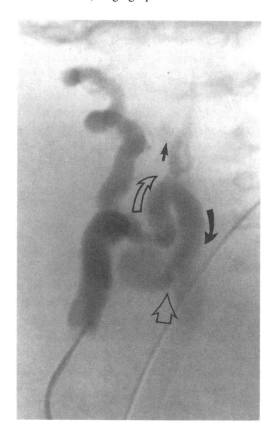

location (vide infra), and its venous drainage towards the paravertebral jugular, epidural or medullary venous system. The presence of "partial" or complete angiographic "steal" and the presence of associated dysplasia in the involved vessel (primarily in the "spontaneous" type) can be evaluated.

Second Injection. Contralateral vertebral artery. Frontal subtraction angiography of the opposite vertebral artery will rule out associated dysplasias or vascular lesions and will demonstrate the importance of each vertebral artery in the perfusion of the vertebrobasilar circulation, and the retrograde "steal" towards the fistula (Fig. 6.40).

Third Injection. Ipsilateral occipital injection. Due to the proximity of the occipital artery, its frequent involvement in FMD (see FMD, Aneurysm chapter) and its relationship in the collateral circulation to the vertebral artery, the ipsilateral occipital artery should be routinely studied, as it may be the site of associated vascular injuries (Fig. 6.37). It may show the exact site of fistula via the C1 or C2 collaterals. Furthermore, in fistulas that are proximal to C1 or C2, the occipital artery may be a main source of collateral circulation towards the brain, and may even be an avenue to reach the lesion (Moret, 1979).

Fourth Injection. Ipsilateral dorsal and ascending cervical arteries. As in the ipsilateral occipital injection, these natural collaterals to the vertebral artery may be best to demonstrate the fistula (Fig. 6.40); they may also offer an alternative route to reach the fistula. Of outmost importance is the assessment of these vessels in the supply to the normal spinal cord.

Fifth Injection. Ipsilateral and contralateral internal carotid artery. The main purpose of internal carotid angiography is in the presence of angiodysplasia, where one should rule out associated vascular lesions, such as aneurysms (Chapter 7, FMD) and evaluate the circle of Willis.

Sixth Injection. Ipsilateral vertebral artery injection with flow arrest. When the fistula site cannot be ascertained during the previous injections (contralateral vertebral artery, ipsilateral occipital, dorso or ascending cervical arteries), one can use a double lumen balloon catheter to produce flow arrest and pinpoint the fistula(s) as done in other high flow AVFs (Figs. 6.25 and 6.50).

6. Embolization

The technique and principles are similar to those reviewed in techniques (see Chapter 1, IV and XII). Of specific importance in VAFs is the need for larger balloons, as the venous structures draining the fistula are usually of large caliber. Preservation of the VA flow (Fig. 6.38) although ideal, is less critical than in the internal carotid artery, with the exception of particular anatomical dispositions, such as a small or absent contralateral vertebral artery on an incompetent posterior circle of Willis.

Even in cases where the vertebral artery cannot be preserved, balloon trapping is adequate to cure the lesion. In the rare instance where the fistula cannot be trapped due to a complete tear or a congenital variant (Fig. 6.40), balloon occlusion of the vertebral artery proximal to the fistula may be the first stage of a combined embolization-surgical trapping (Fig. 6.40).

In general, the femoral approach is best; however, if not possible, one may use a retrograde brachial-axillary approach (Fig. 6.38). Finally, if possible, one may use the occipital route via C1 or C2 (Moret, 1979). It may be advisable to have 2 separate catheters if fistula trapping is needed (Fig. 6.39).

In comparison to fistulas in the internal carotid artery, preservation of flow in the VAF is less frequent, and in our experience of 19 patients, it was possible in 65% of cases (Berenstein, 1980). Spontaneous thrombosis is rather unusual in these fistulas; however, we heve seen thrombosis in one case following attempted balloon occlusion of the fistula (Fig. 6.41). Multiple balloons were once needed (Fig. 6.43).

Other agents such as coils or IBCA may close the fistulas; however, they are less reliable than detachable balloons (see Chapter 1, VI) in this type of lesions.

a) Post-Embolization Control

Due to the multiple anastomosis of the vertebral artery and their presence at multiple levels, collateral circulation can be used to trap a VAF. The vertebral segment distal to the fistula must be visualized prior to final balloon detachment (Figs. 6.30, 6.40).

b) Pediatric (Congenital Fistulas)

Cardiac manifestations of AVFs are unusual, and except for those infrequent debilitated patients with pre-existing cardiac history, cardiac failure is almost exclusively seen in the pediatric population. In these children staged embolization should be considered if multiple fistulas are present (Fig. 6.40) and one must be prepared to deal with acute cardiac overload (see Chapter 1).

c) Post-Operative Care

In general, bed rest for 36 hours is recommended, and if one wishes to decrease neck motion during the immediate post-embolization period neck immobilization with a soft collar may be a good precaution.

In patients presenting with VAFs after trauma (mainly blunt), thorough assessment of associated cervical injuries should precede the management of the fistula.

d) Balloon Deflation

If balloon deflation occurs early, within hours of the embolization, the fistula may recur. However, for the most part, if the balloon remains inflated for more than 24 hours the fistula does not recur. The formation of an aneurysmal pouch at the site of repair following balloon deflation (Fig. 6.40) has not produced any clinical symptoms to our knowledge. If balloon deflation is to be avoided the balloon(s) can be filled with HEMA (see Chapter 1).

IV. Common Carotid Fistulas

The incidence, natural history, and clinical presentation of these lesions is difficult to assess in view of their infrequency. They usually follow trauma, generally penetrating injuries. It was the least frequent type of fistula in our experience; we had only 1 case and it occurred after percutaneous placement of a Swan-Ganz catheter (Fig. 6.45) in an 80 year old female with congestive heart failure (CHF). The fistula further aggravated a pre-existing cardiac failure and required immediate treatment.

The pretherapeutic evaluation, principles, and techniques of treatment are similar as in other fistulas; detachable balloons are the agents of choice (Fig. 6.45C).

V. External Carotid Fistulas (ECFs)

1. General

Arteriovenous fistulas of the external carotid artery are uncommon lesions. As reviewed in other fistulas the most frequent cause is trauma. However, a certain group of patients may present without a history of trauma and therefore are called "spontaneous". Some of which may be present from birth and therefore may be considered congenital (Stucker, 1974; Berenstein, 1985).

Excision of the fistula has been the preferred method in these lesions; however, this may not be possible in all cases. The enlarged feeding vessels and arterialized draining veins may cause excessive blood loss at surgery

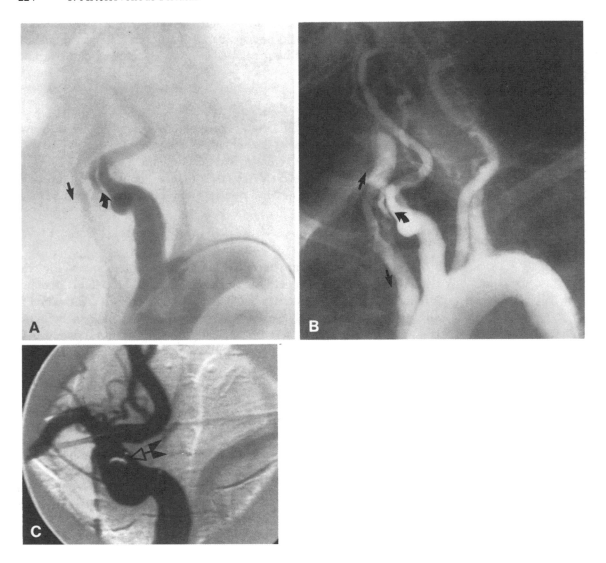

Fig. 6.45 A-C. Iatrogenic common carotid fistula following percutaneous placement of a Swan Ganz catheter in an 80 year old female with congestive heart failure
CHF. The fistula further aggravated the cardiac insufficiency. **A** Right anterior
oblique subtraction angiogram in early arterial phase of an arch study demonstrates
a small fistula at the proximal segment of the right common carotid artery *(curved
arrow)*, draining into the jugular vein *(arrow)*. **B** Later phase demonstrates the
fistula *(curved arrow)* as well as filling of the jugular vein *(arrow)*. **C** Digital
subtraction angiogram of the innominate artery after balloon repair of the fistula.
Note preservation of the common carotid artery with no filling of the fistula. The
CHF resolved after occlusion of the fistula

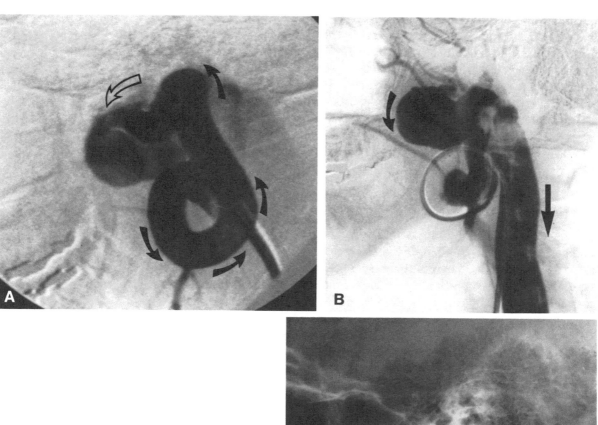

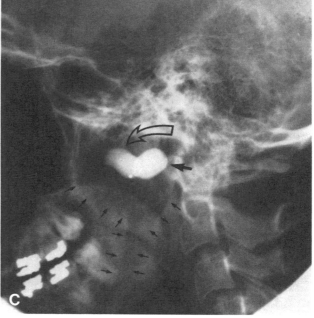

Fig. 6.46 A-C. 23 year old female with left facial asymmetry and a pulsatile tumefaction on the left side of the face. No previous history of trauma was found. **A** Lateral DSA of the distal external carotid artery on the left side. Note marked tortuosity of the distal external carotid artery and internal maxillary artery *(curved arrow)* as well as the abrupt transitional caliber at the site of the fistula *(open curved arrow)*. **B** Later phase, demonstrates the large venous dilatation *(curved arrow)* and drainage into the jugular venous system *(arrow)*. **C** Plain film following balloon embolization. The most distal balloon shows an hour glass appearance as part of the balloon is at the fistula site *(open curved arrow)*. A second balloon is placed in tandem as a safety to prevent distal displacement of the balloon. Note the well circumscribed bony expansion in the pterygoid region and inferior alveolar canal *(small arrows)*

(Holt, 1980). Ligation of the feeding vessel may be the only surgical option; however, this results only in temporary control due to the vast collateral network in the head and neck (Stucker, 1974; Reizine, 1985).

These lesions are infrequent, but will occur where external carotid artery branches are close to venous structures. Therefore, ECFs are most frequently seen where branches of the ECA pass through the basilar osseous foramena, as they are near emissary veins and the basilar venous plexus. Fracture through these bony structures can therefore result in a ECFs, even congenital fistulas are frequently at or near bony passages (Fig. 6.46).

2. Incidence

The incidence of ECFs of any kind is very low. In our own experience, ECFs represents 7% of all AVFs in the head and neck, and 11% of all carotid artery fistulas. There is slight male predominance in the traumatic type, whereas there appears to be a higher incidence of females with the congenital type (Callbucci, 1974; Berenstein, 1985). The middle meningeal artery (Figs. 6.47, 6.48) is most frequently involved in traumatic fistulas, followed by the occipital (Fig. 6.37) and superficial temporal arteries (Fig. 6.49). Extracranial fistulas are most frequently of the "spontaneous" or congenital type (Fig. 6.46). Reizine (1985) found 3 congenital facial AVFs in over 200 cases of vascular lesions of the face (a distinction has to be made between direct AVFs and the AV fistulas seen as part of a facial AVM or DAVM which are not considered here and are discussed in their respective chapters). The history of trauma although suggestive of a traumatic AVF, should be taken with caution, as trauma may be the triggering factor in AVMs.

3. Natural History

As to their natural history, one can separate them best by location and venous drainage than by etiological cause into: 1. intracranial, 2. extracranial, a) with intracranial venous drainage or b) purely extracranial.

a) Intracranial ECFs

These fistulas originate intracranially from dural branches of the external carotid artery. Because of their intracranial location they may present with intracranial hemorrhage that may be an extra-axial collection, either acute or chronic (Fig. 6.48), or they may also present with intracerebral hemorrhages if they have a cortical venous drainage.

In Treil's (1977) review of 30 patients with trauma to the middle meningeal artery, 16 patients had an AVF and 80% had a skull fracture. Although most of the fistulas were seen at the site of the fracture, some may be seen at a distance or even on the opposite side. In Roski's (1982) review from the literature of 38 patients with middle meningeal fistulas, 26 were associated with intracranial hematomas. In both series there was a poor prognoses; however, most AVFs were associated with significant head trauma, probably accounting for the poor outcome of these patients. In traumatic middle meningeal fistulas there was a frequent association with AVFs and pseudoaneurysms.

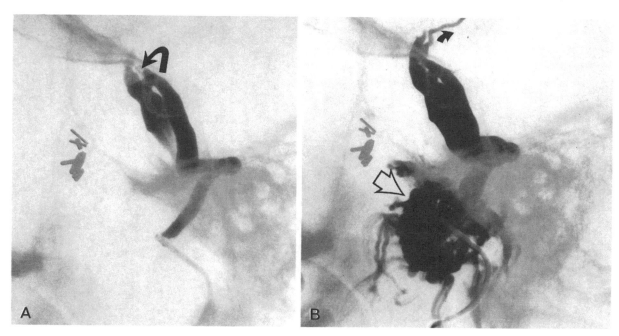

Fig. 6.47 A, B. Traumatic intracranial fistula of the peritoneal portion of the middle meningeal artery secondary to blunt trauma. **A** Lateral subtraction angiogram of the middle meningeal artery shows a direct AV fistula draining into a dural vein *(broken arrow)* **B** Later phase the lesion is secondarily draining into the pterygoid venous plexus via the vein of the foramen ovale. Note the normal caliber of the middle meningeal artery *(small curved arrow)* distal to the fistula

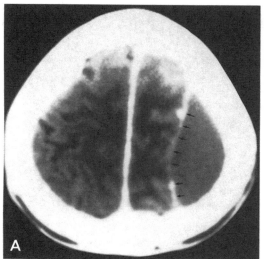

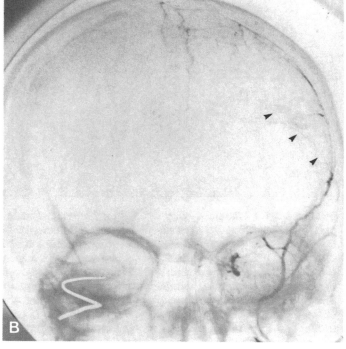

Fig. 6.48. A Axial CT following intravenous administration of contrast material, demonstrates a typical chronic subdural hematoma with enhancing membrane *(small arrows)*. **B** Frontal subtraction angiogram of the selective middle meningeal artery with demonstrates some "extravasation" *(arrowheads)* suggesting either small leakage of contrast material or blushing of the subdural membrane. After embolization of the middle meningeal artery with medium sized particles to prevent ophthalmic embolization and surgical evacuation of the chronic recurrent subdural hematoma via a burrhole there is no evidence of recurrence of the extra-axial collection with 2 years follow-up

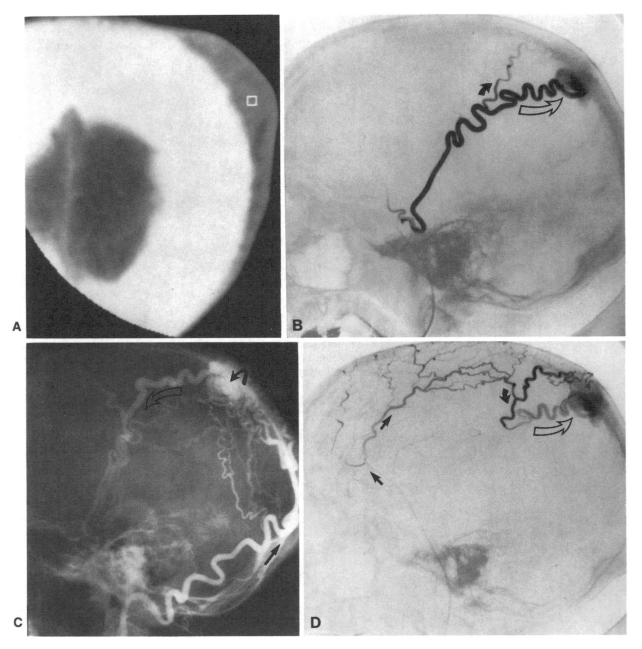

Fig. 6.49 A-G. Traumatic scalp fistula in a 13 year old male presenting with a pulsatile tumefaction of the left side of the scalp. **A** Enhanced CT scan demonstrates the soft tissue tumefaction. **B** Superselective catheterization of the parietal branch of the superficial temporal artery *(open curved arrow)* demonstrates the fistula *(broken arrow)*. Note the smaller branch *(curved arrow)* to be compared with **D** and **F**. **C** Lateral angiographic examination of the occipital artery *(arrow)* demonstrates the region of the fistula *(broken arrow)* and retrograde filling of the parietal branch of the superficial temporal artery *(open curved arrow)*. **D** Catheterization of the frontal branch of the superficial temporal artery *(arrow)* fills the same collateral pathway demonstrated in **B***(small curved arrow)* and the parietal branch of the superficial temporal artery *(open curved arrow)*. **E** Tangential view following IBCA embolization in this distal fistula and using a "push" technique. Note the radiopaque IBCA. **F** Post-embolization control angiogram of the external carotid artery in late phase. Note filling of the frontal branch of the superficial temporal artery, the same collateral anastomotic pathway *(small curved arrow)* with no filling of the fistula.

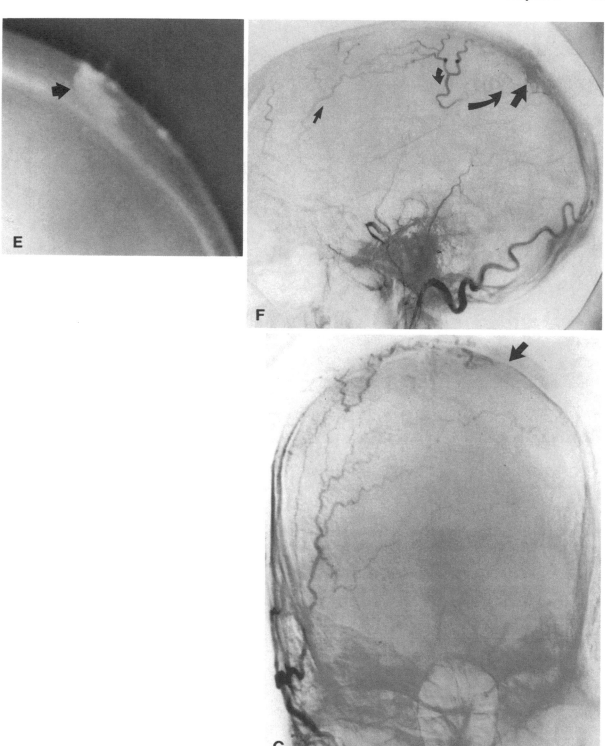

Fig. 6.49 (continued)
The IBCA cast of the main parietal branch of the superficial temporal is subtracted
(curved arrow). The IBCA in the fistula is also subtracted *(solid arrow)*. The
occipital artery does not reach the lesion although this vessel was not embolized
(compare to **C**). **G** Contralateral superficial temporal control angiogram demonstrates cross circulation without filling of the fistula

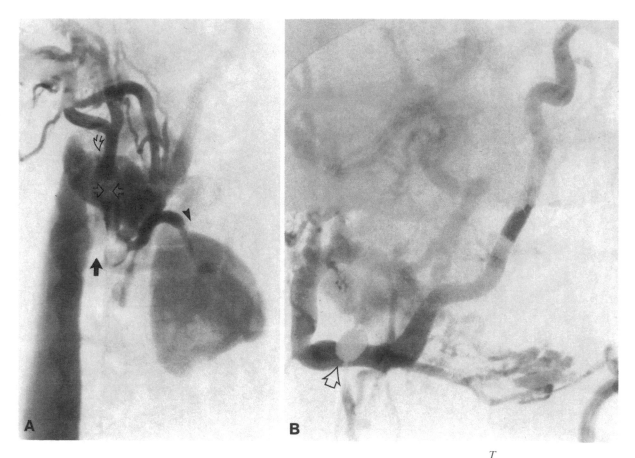

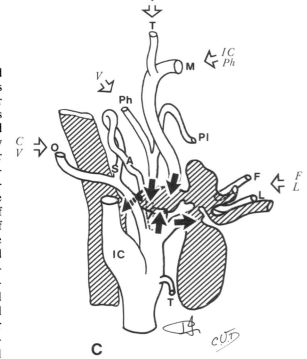

Fig. 6.50 A-C. Complete laceration of the external carotid main trunk following penetrating trauma. Same patient as Volume 1, Figs. 4.6, 9.9, 9.15, 9.25, 10.8, 11.3. The upper segment of the fistula could be demonstrated in those injections via collateral circulation. However, the proximal transsected segment was difficult to assess; in addition, due to the high flow hemodynamic "steal" towards the fistula associated vascular injuries could be missed. **A** Proximal external carotid angiogram under flow control with a double lumen Berenstein occlusive balloon catheter *(arrow)*. Note the transsection of the external carotid artery *(double arrowhead)*, the distal portion of the fistula *(open curved arrowhead)* and the pseudoaneursym of the facial artery *(arrowhead)*. **B** Late phases of the same injection demonstrating the venous anatomy with marked dilatation of the facial veins and some venous changes throughout the face compatible with venous hyperpressure. **C** Diagrammatic representation of this complex lesion. *IC* Internal carotid, *T* Superior thyroidal artery, *F* Facial artery, *L* Lingual artery, *O* Occipital artery, *S* Stylo mastoid artery, *A* Posterior auricular artery, *Ph* Ascending pharyngeal artery, *Pl* Ascending palatine artery, *M* Internal maxillary artery, *T* Superficial temporal artery, Legends in *italic* correspond to contralateral opacification of the arteries listed above. *C* Cervical arteries, *V* vertebral artery

When reviewing pure AVFs as compared with pseudoaneurysms, the course is far more benign (Roski, 1982) and spontaneous thrombosis can occur (Sato, 1983).

In review of the literature on middle meningeal fistulas, no distinction was made between the type of venous drainage and intracranial hemorrhage; but we believe that if a middle meningeal fistula or orther intracranial fistula has a purely dural or diploic drainage, chances of hemorrhage are probably low, whereas with cortical venous drainage it carries a higher risk of hemorrhage and they can present with convulsions or neurological deficits (Bitoh, 1980) (see DAVMs).

In patients with purely dural drainage, if the drainage is towards the cavernous sinus they will present with neuroophthalmologic findings similar to those of CCFs.

b) Extracranial ECFs

Those with extracranial venous drainage may have similar presentation than intracranial ones. In general, in patients with extracranial AVFs of the external carotid artery the clinical manifestations will be primarily those of a pulsatile tumefaction (Figs. 6.49, 6.50) associated with a thrill and bruit. Cardiac manifestations are even more rare than in other type of AVFs. Two of our cases presented with a transient facial palsy related to the development of a "swishing" noise. Both fistulas involved the extracranial segment of the middle meningeal artery and presumably were related to a hemodynamic "steal".

In both the palsy resolved spontaneously while the fistula was still patent. One patient underwent embolization without problems and the second refused treatment of the fistula. To our knowledge no AVF in the distribution of the neuromeningeal branch of the ascending pharyngeal artery producing dysfunction of the lower cranial nerves has been reported. Fistulas that drain into the cavernous sinus can present with ophthalmoplegia as discussed above and in Chapter 8.

Pretherapeutic evaluation and indications for treatment are similar as those of the area where the fistula is located. Similarly the principles elucidated in other fistulas and aneurysms apply. Proper analysis of the collateral circulation to localize the fistula and to assess the effectiveness of treatment is essential (Figs. 6.49, 6.50).

c) Embolization

Based on our experience (Berenstein, 1985) and that of others (Scialfa, 1979; Reizine, 1981) endovascular embolization is the treatment of choice with a cure rate of over 95%, with very little risk and significantly less morbidity and hospitalization than any other form of treatment.

The choice of embolic agents depends upon the location of the fistula and its flow characteristics. In most cases a permanent agent should be used with the possible exception of those traumatic fistulas where there is no intrinsic vascular pathology. Although we have personally seen recurrence in one such fistula. In general, particulate agents are usually not suitable since they tend to pass through the large arteriovenous connections of these lesions. The goal of embolization is the occlusion of the fistula itself rather than occlusion of the feeding pedicles. Due to the vast collateral network in the head and neck the fistula will recur if only proximal embolization is performed as has been the surgical experience.

Whenever possible, detachable balloons are the preferred embolic agent and are usually best in large arteriovenous fistulas in the proximal portion of external carotid artery branches. The high flow aids in guiding the balloon to the site of fistula. Balloons, available in multiple sizes (see Chapter 1), can be placed directly at the site of the abnormal arteriovenous communication.

When using detachable balloons in these high flow conditions, precise placement of the balloon at the fistula site may be difficult, as the high flow may push the balloon into the venous side with significant force. Therefore, the balloon should be well attached to the catheter when using the Serbinenko (1974) or Debrun (1979) techniques. The arteriovenous fistula is usually at the site of an abrupt change in caliber between the artery and the vein.

The exact site of fistula communication can be easily demonstrated with a double lumen balloon catheter with flow arrest (Fig. 6.25). A stenotic area can be seen at the acute transition point, it usually represents the best place to wedge the balloon and close the fistula (Fig. 6.46). Therefore, to prevent distal migration of the balloon (primarily after detachment) we recommended to rapidly inflate the balloon several centimeters proximal to the fistula; the fast flow will then push the inflated balloon which will stop at the stenotic transition between the artery and vein. Not infrequently an hour glass appearance of the ballon may be noted. It is our feeling that 2 balloons in tandem are usually best to insure good closure and prevent distal migration of the balloon (Fig. 6.48C).

For those fistulae that are more distal in location and are unreachable with detachable balloons (Fig. 6.49), a liquid embolic agent such as IBCA, whose polymerization time can be controlled (see Chapter 1) is injected through very small superselectively placed catheters or open end guidrewires, and occludes the distal fistula. In general, detachable balloons are preferred whenever possible.

Gianturco coils are usually less desirable as they are less efficient and difficult to retrieve if extruded in the wrong location (see Chapter 1).

d) Post-Embolization Care

No specific post-embolization care is usually necessary except for a precautionary period of rest.

VI. Other Types of AVFs

1. Fistulas of the External Carotid Main Trunk

AVFs of the main trunk of the external carotid artery can occur secondary to trauma, including complete transsection of the external carotid artery, they may be difficult to demonstrate. Collateral circulation analysis may be useful to localize the fistula (see Vol. 1, Figs. 4.6, 9.9, 9.15, 9.25, 10.8 and 11.3). However if complete transection of the main trunk occurs the proximal segment may be difficult to visualize. In addition, they may be part of a complex vascular hemodynamic "steal" will fail to opacify other branches. In these instances the use of flow arrest with a double lumen balloon catheter can be useful to see the fistula and other vascular injuries such as pseudoaneurysms (Fig. 6.50).

2. Malignant Fistulas

Vessel erosion by malignant infiltration or following radiation of a malignant lesion may result in a fistula between an eroded artery(s) and the tumor. These lesions can even communicate with other vessels through the same fistula (see Figs. 2.2, 5.12) which may be a major unexpected danger during embolization. For the most part malignant invasion of a major artery will manifest itself as a pseudoaneurysm with massive bleeding, requiring immediate management (Fig. 5.11).

During treatment a point of caution is the fragility of the involved vessels. The principles of management discussed in pseudoaneurysms should be followed (Fig. 7.22).

CHAPTER 7
Aneurysms

I. Introduction

Aneurysms of the extradural carotid and vertebral arteries are significantly less common than intracranial aneurysms, but their precise incidence is not known, they are not as rare as once believed (Margolis 1972). They are usually described in relation to the vessel involved, or etiological origin. They occur most frequently in the internal carotid artery, followed by the vertebral artery; and least frequently in the extenal carotid artery and its branches.

The most common etiological factors vary depending on the location of the aneurysms, the age of the patients, and the type of population analyzed. In general, lesions may be secondary to atherosclerosis, congenital or developmental defects, trauma, infection, radiation or connective tissue disorders. In some cases no pre-existing or associated abnormality can be found.

II. Extradural Carotid Artery Aneurysms

1. General

Extradural aneurysms in the craniofacial area most frequently involve the internal carotid artery; the most common area affected is the cavernous segment (Table 7.1).

Symptomatic cavernous aneurysms are usually greater than 2.5 cm (and therefore are referred to as "giant"). In the literature, they are usually discussed with "giant" intradural aneurysms; they represent 5% of those reported by Drake (1979) and 39% of those reported by Morley (1968). However, their incidence in relation to other extradural carotid aneurysms is unknown. In our experience of 53 internal carotid artery aneurysms (Table 7.1) 83% were in the carvernous segment, 7.5% were in the petrous segment and 9.5% were located in the cervical internal carotid artery. In this selected population some cervical and bifurcation aneurysms

Table 7.1. Extradural internal carotid aneurysms, etiology and location

Location			Congenital Developmental	Traumatic	Mycotic	Atherosclerotic
Cervical	6	(91.5%)	2 (33%)	3 (50%)	–	1 (16%)
Petrous	5	(8.7%)	–	5	–	–
Cavernous	46	(80%)	40 (87%)	6 (13%)	–	–
Total	57	(100%)	42 (73.6%)	14 (24.5%)	–	1 (1.7%)

may not come to the attention of the surgical neuroradiologist as they are usually operated upon.

The etiological classification of extradural internal carotid aneurysms includes: congenital or developmental (including angiodysplasias), traumatic, mycotic and atherosclerotic disease (Table 7.1).

2. Aneurysms of the Common Carotid Artery

They are very rare. We have personally seen one false aneurysm (Fig. 7.1) and one CCA to jugular vein fistula (Fig. 6.45) following attempted placement of a central line.

The most frequent type of aneurysm involving the cervical internal carotid artery, is congenital or developmental, followed by traumatic, atherosclerosis, and mycotic pseudoaneurysms (Margolis 1972). In our series the most frequently encountered were traumatic. In the past infectious aneurysms were more frequently seen, but these are now relatively uncommon (Houser 1968; Resenberg 1964).

In the petrous segment of the internal carotid artery, our 4 cases were all of traumatic origin (either secondary to blunt trauma or iatrogenic following biopsies of aberrant courses of the internal carotid artery).

In the cavernous carotid artery, 86% of aneurysms are congenital or developmental. It is difficult to exclude the possibility that some of these

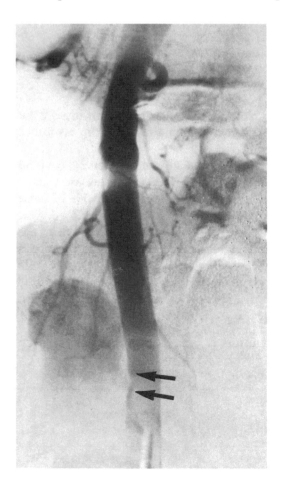

Fig. 7.1. Iatrogenic pseudoaneurysm of the right CCA. Oblique subtracted angiogram of the right CCA in a patient with a large pulsatile neck mass following placement of a central venous line. Note a small dissection at the mouth of the large pseudoaneurysm *(double arrow)*. The false aneurysm was surgically resected

lesions have an atherosclerotic origin. In the older symptomatic patients the presence of associated atherosclerotic lesions in other locations, or other segments of the carotid arteries, does not prove or exclude an atherosclerotic origin to the aneurysms. The presence of atherosclerosis, hypertension, diabetes or other systemic diseases influence the assessments of the need, safety, and risks of treatment. On the other hand, once the symptomatic side has been studied and the diagnosis of aneurysm is confirmed, a complete cerebral angiographic study is mandatory to assess collateral circulation, and to exclude other associated aneurysms. Subarachnoid aneurysms pose a greater threat to the patient's life and should be treated first. If the subarachnoid aneurysm is on the contralateral side or in the posterior circulation, increased compensatory flow and other altered hemodynamics following occlusion of the carotid artery or vertebral artery may increased the risk of rupture.

In our discussion of extracranial aneurysms we will consider first those of the internal carotid artery below the cavernous segment; those involving the cavernous segment of the internal carotid artery, the external carotid artery and the extracranial vertebral arteries will be analyzed separately.

3. Cervical Internal Carotid Aneurysms

a) Epidemiology

Developmental. Margolis (1972), in his review of 20 aneurysms in the cervical portion of the internal carotid artery, found that developmental aneurysms were the most frequent affecting 7 of their patients (35%); in our smaller series of 11 patients, 2 (33%) had a developmental aneurysm. One of our patients had associated dysplastic aneurysms of both vertebral arteries. He presented with symptoms due to embolism from the carotid artery (Fig. 7.2) and had spontaneous thrombosis of the internal carotid artery seven days later. In our patient, the dysplastic aneurysm was associated with a carotid cavernous fistula that followed minimal trauma (Fig. 6.15). The contralateral internal carotid artery and both vertebrals were dysplastic without evidence of atherosclerosis.

The diagnosis of a congenital or developmental aneurysm is made by exclusion, when no previous history of trauma, infection or sign of atherosclerosis exists (Alexander 1966; Melot 1966). The presence of other aneurysms (primarily intracranial aneurysms) is suggestive of congenital aneurysms (Duplay 1957; Houser 1968; Kramer 1969; Manelfe 1974), polyarteritis nodosa (Rob 1954) or pseudoxanthoma elasticum (Dixon 1956). On occasions, congenital aneurysms may be found incidentally in the investigation of a neck mass (Fig. 4.7).

Traumatic pseudoaneurysms were next in frequency in Margolis's series (1972) with 30% of their cases and were the most frequent type of aneurysms involving the cervical ICA (50%) in our cases (Table 7.1); as well as in the series of 7 patients reported by Beall (1962).

Penetrating Trauma. Traumatic aneurysms may result from penetrating injuries such as a stable wound, a high velocity gunshot wound (Fig. 7.3), or from iatrogenic trauma (Teal 1972). These injuries most often result in a false sac or pseudoaneurysm, which is produced by disruption of the continuity of the arterial wall. A periarterial hemorrhage forms and is

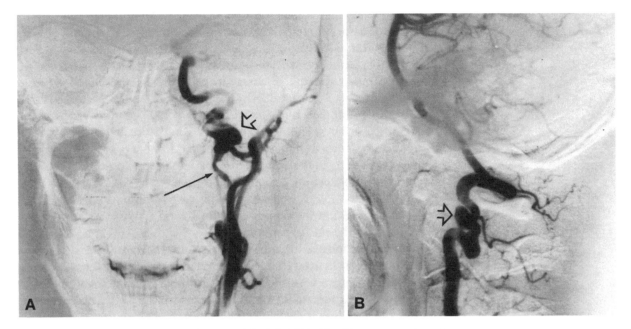

Fig. 7.2. A Frontal subtraction angiogram of the left CCA. Significant narrowing of the proximal carotid artery suggesting a dissection is noted, although there was no history of pain *(arrow)*. An irregular aneurysm *(open arrow)* is present in the distal cervical ICA. The patient presented with transient hemiparesis and aphasia with no previous history of trauma or infection. One week later the ICA thrombosed spontaneously (not shown). **B** Lateral subtraction angiogram of the right vertebral artery in the same patient. Note a dysplastic aneurysm at the C2 level *(open arrow)*. A third dysplastic aneurysm of the left VA at the C1 level was also present (not shown)

contained by the vascular sheath. During systole, arterial blood pressure forces blood into the periarterial region. Blood accumulates at the site of leak until the extraarterial pressure equals the mean arterial pressure (Deysine 1969). During diastole, blood tends to return into the vessel lumen. This "to" and "from" motion produces a turbulant blood flow which generates a typical murmur. The periarterial blood clots and then retracts; the center of the hematoma becomes cavitied and thus communicates with the arterial lumen. The fibrotic reaction produced in the surrounding tissues forms the wall of the false aneurysm (Figs. 7.3B, 7.4A, B).

Lesions due to penetrating trauma have been more prevelant in military situations, where the majority are produced by fragments of explosive devices. Rich (1970) and coworkers, in their analysis of acute arterial injuries in 1000 patients during the Vietnam war, found that 88% of carotid injuries resulted from shrapnel. However, carotid injuries were relatively infrequent; only 5% of all arterial injuries occurred in the carotid arteries. In Perry's (1971) review of penetrating arterial injuries in the civilian population, only 7.5% occurred in the carotid arteries; of these 4.7% involved the common carotid artery, 1.6% the internal carotid artery, and 1.2% the external carotid artery. Beall in 1962 reported an equal number (17%) of carotid injuries due to stab wounds as compared to gunshot wounds.

Changes in the epidemiology of traumatic lesions of the carotid arteries have shown interesting shifts associated with the significant mortality of

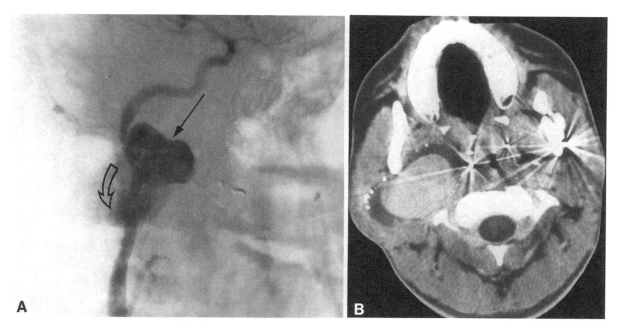

Fig. 7.3. A False aneurysm of the cervical ICA following a gunshot wound. Oblique subtraction angiogram of the right CCA. Two pouches are evident; filling of the pseudoaneurysm *(arrow)* is followed by laminar flow into a second pouch *(open curved arrow)*. Note the posterior displacement of the ICA distal to the injury, and the filling defects within the pseudoaneurysm, representing a significant quantity of clot. Although the level of the arterial tear is well documented by angiography, the true size of the lesion cannot be fully assessed by the angiographic picture. **B** Same patient: axial CT Image after IV administration of contrast material. Best shows the true size of the false aneurysm. Note the enhancement of the patent lumen which is surrounded by an area of low attenuation, representing the thrombosed portion of the false aneurysm. Metallic artifacts from fragments of the gunshot can be seen in the bullet trajectory

neck wounds due to modern weapons (Davis 1983). In 1926, Winslow was able to find 26 pseudoaneurysms of the carotid arteries secondary to penetrating injuries. These are rarely seen today, as most carotid injuries at present are due to fatal gunshot wounds.

False carotid aneurysms may also occur following carotid endarterectomy, infections complicating carotid surgery or following deterioration of silk sutures (Ehrenfeld 1972) and may progress to vessel thrombosis (Madison 1970). Lord reported carotid injury after tracheostomy and following radical surgery, and Barrett (1960) reported it as a complication of mastoidectomy. The formation of pseudoaneurysms of the carotid arteries following direct carotid puncture for cerebral angiography has also been reported (Miller 1977; Huckman 1979) or after radiationtherapy (Fig. 5.11).

In the pediatric population an additional type of carotid injury follow intraoral trauma. After a fall onto an object that enters the mouth or a fall with an object in the mouth, an injury is produced in the tonsillar region. Bickerstaff reported that these "pencil injuries" have a mortality of about 30% (1964). Subsequent neurological complications have been felt to be secondary to distal embolization on intracranial arteries, although in the absence of embolization the lesion may be asymptomatic because children can tolerate unilateral carotid occlusion in many instances.

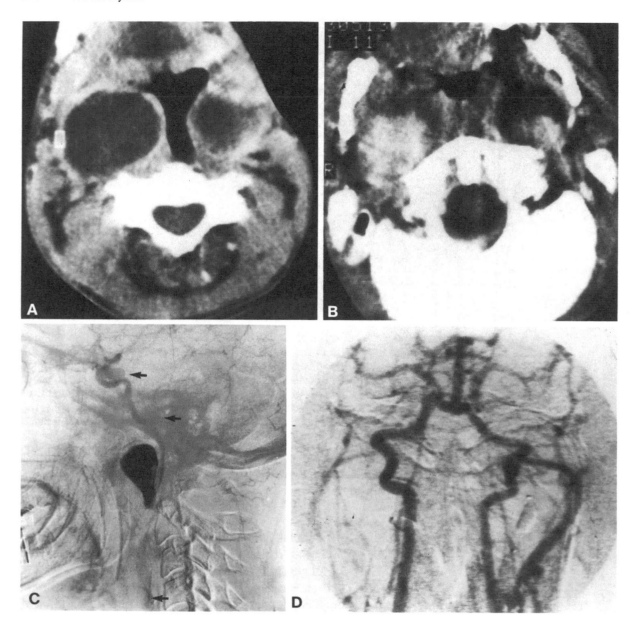

Fig. 7.4 A-D. Bilateral pseudoaneurysms following blunt (MVA) trauma. **A** Axial CT scan at the level of C4 demonstrated bilateral large (right more than the left) areas of low attennation coefficient representing old lobulated thrombosed portions of both false aneurysms with encroachment of the airway (at oral examination this nonpulsatile portion of aneurysm could be mistaken for a peritonsillar abcess. **B** At the odontoid level, there is eccentric contrast enhancement of the intraluminal portions of both aneurysms. Note the inhomogeneous enhancement due to the thrombi. **C** Late phase of a lateral subtraction angiogram of the left CCA shows the recanalized lumen of the aneurysm. Only a very small portion of the pseudoaneurysm is opacified during angiography (compare to **A** and **B**). Subtracted balloons *(arrows)* in the contralateral right cavernous, petrous and cervical ICA are seen, following trapping of the right sided pseudoaneurysm. Prior to bilateral carotid trapping, bilateral EC-IC bypass were done (not shown). **D** Digital intravenous angiogram (DIVA) 2 weeks later, confirms complete thrombosis of both aneurysms. DIVAs can be useful as a noninvasive imaging modality for the easy follow up of these patients

Fig. 7.5. Lateral view of the right CCA in a patient after motor vehicle accident with acute thrombosis of the proximal internal carotid artery. Note the filling defects produced by the thrombi *(arrows)*. (Same patient than in Figs. 1.6 and 7.10)

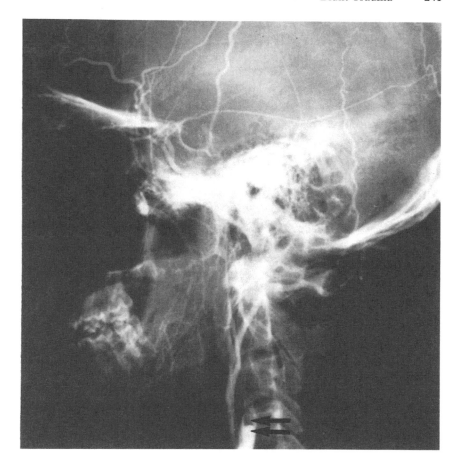

Blunt Trauma. Other mechanisms of vessel injury following blunt trauma (Beall, 1962) affect the vessel wall in the same manner as penetrating injuries and may occur following the application of force to the angle of the mandible which is then transmitted to the carotid wall; if the mandible is fractured, a bony spickle may lacerate the internal carotid artery producing a pseudoaneurysm (Beall, 1962). Ingested foreign bodies have also been reported to cause pseudoaneurysms of the internal carotid artery (Morris, 1969).

Blunt injuries of the cervical internal carotid artery are relatively uncommon (Davis, 1983). They may follow motor vehicle accidents (Fig. 7.4), altercations, falls, direct blows (Beatty, 1977), strangulation, or digital carotid compression (Nelson, 1963). The most frequent lesion resulting from blunt trauma is spasm or thrombosis (Fig. 7.5). Followed in frequency by pseudoaneurysms, dissections, extraluminal and/or intramural hematomas (Fig. 7.6) which may then become dissecting aneurysms. Rarely complete transsection and AV fistulas may occur (see also Vol. 1, Fig. 10.8B), (Jiminez 1969). One form of blunt trauma involves combined rotatory hyperextension of the neck which stretches and compresses the internal carotid artery over the lateral mass of the atlas and axis, resulting in damage of the arterial wall. This type of injury occurs more frequently in young patients, as in the elderly tortuosities of the carotid arteries tend to straighten so that they are not stretched during sudden hyperextension and rotation movements. The internal carotid artery is usually damaged at the level of the atlas (Boldrey, 1957; New, 1969). A similar injury may occur at the side of fixation of the internal carotid artery at its point of entrance into the petrous bone, at the level of the carotid canal (Davis, 1983).

The most frequent lesion resulting from blunt trauma is an intimal tear with subsequent intimal dissection and thrombosis. The intimal tear forms a nidus for thrombosis and clot propagation occurs over a variable distance distally and/or proximally (Yamada, 1967). This clot propagation is at least partially responsible for the high incidence of neurological complications in this type of patient. Soft tissue swelling may displace and compress the carotid arteries, further aggraving the compromised lumen. Yamada in 1967 reported the clinical significance of this thrombosis which was associated with a high mortality and neurological morbidity. The initial symptoms characteristically appear hours or even days after the initial trauma. In addition to the neurological symptoms of carotid occlusion and/ or progressive thrombosis, the presence of Horner's syndrome secondary to disruption of the sympathetic fibers in the carotid wall (Yamada, 1967) may be an important clinical sign of carotid injury, especially when external signs of trauma are absent, as is not infrequently the case following blunt trauma (Davis, 1983).

Frequently, false aneurysms of the cervical internal carotid artery protruding into the posterior pharyngeal wall are misdiagnosed as peritonsillar abscesses (Fig. 7.4A). Anatomically, the carotid is separated medially from the lateral pharyngeal constrictor muscles, whereas laterally it is better protected by the muscles attached to the styloid and by the cervical fascia.

Additional signs and symptoms include those related to cerebral embolization from the aneurysmal sac, subjective and objective murmurs, cervical pain, headaches, tinnitus and vertigo, and/or Horner's syndrome which results from disruption of the carotid sympathetic fibers. As with carotid dissection, the symptoms may be delayed from hours to several years (Batzdorf, 1979). On occasion massive hemorrhage is the presenting symptom.

Dissecting Aneurysms. These may occur when an intimal tear permits the penetration of blood into the vessel wall with or without the formation of a pseudoaneurysm. In both traumatic (Fig. 7.5) and spontaneous (Fig. 7.2) types, the dissection usually extends cranially and frequently terminates where the internal carotid artery enters the petrous carotid canal. The internal carotid lumen is narrowed, frequently with intimal irregularities. If the blood dissects in a subadvential rather than a subintimal plane, a pseudoaneurysm can be formed (Davis, 1983). In contrast to aortic dissecting aneurysms extending in the carotid arteries, opacification of the false and true lumens is usually not identified (Fig. 7.6).

Atherosclerotic aneurysms of the extradural internal carotid arteries are usually seen in older patient (Margolis, 1972) and typically occur just distal to the common carotid bifurcation in areas of severe atherosclerotic involvement.

The mechanism of formation of these aneurysms has been the subject of much discussions. Although lipid metabolism may play a role, local factors play the initial and perhaps predominant role i.e. deposition of fibrin and

Fig. 7.6. Post-traumatic dissection of the cervical internal carotid artery *(small arrows)* with a smooth extraluminal, subendothelial compression *(curved arrows)* due to mural hematoma

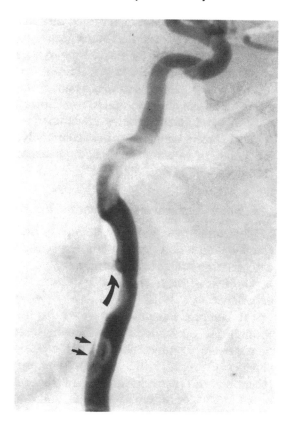

other blood substances in the intima, accumulation of ground substances, disruption of elastic lamellae, and perhaps disturbance of circulation of the vasa vasorum. Formation of atheroma may weaken the wall and atheromatous ulcers, in particular may be the basis for aneurysm formation in some cases (Gore 1966, Rob 1954, Wood 1969). Associated stenotic lesions or other atherosclerotic lesions were seen in most cases reported by Margolis (1972). Not infrequently, however, it may be difficult to asign a specific etiology as a congenital weakness may predispose to atherosclerotic changes or cause the artery to be less resistant to adjacent infections, severe atheromatous changes may predispose to arterial weakness. For the most part, aneurysms of the lower cervical carotid or internal carotid artery are amenable to surgery and not to embolization.

Mycotic Aneurysms. Infections of pyogenic or syphilitic origins are a less common cause of carotid aneurysms than in the past. The mechanisms include septic microemboli to the vaso vasorum, septic emboli within the vessel lumen with thrombosis, and perivascular infections (Baker 1954; Lansky 1975; Sunwanwela 1972). Pathological findings in the blood vessel wall include infiltration of polymorphonuclear leukocytes in the adventitia and media, and marked intimal proliferation which is responsible for spasm or vessel occlusion. The inflammatory changes can progress to frank disintegration of the vessel wall resulting in a myotic pseudoaneurysm.

Sequential angiography may demonstrate rapid changes in the size and shape of the aneurysm (Johnston 1979; Lansky 1975). At present, staphylococci are the most frequent organisms.

In the cervical region the internal carotid artery courses cranially within its sheath, which also contains the internal jugular vein and the vagus nerve. It lies posterior to the lateral pharyngeal space and lateral to the retropharyngeal space with the internal aspect of the vertebral bodies (Finney 1964). Aneurysm may result from the focal extension into the arterial wall of contiguous pharyngeal infections.

At present, postoperative infections are the most frequent cause of cervical carotid aneurysms. Less commonly, aneurysms may follow ionizing radiation or vascular erosion secondary to advanced malignancies (Margolis 1972) (Figs. 5.10, 5.11).

b) Clinical Presentation and Natural History

In addition to specific manifestations of the different etiologies, the most frequent and serious manifestations of carotid aneurysms are secondary to embolization, which occurred in over 50% of cases reported by Margolis, in up to 78% of those reported by Gross (1970) and in over 60% in our experience.

The cerebral ischemic symptoms can be aggraved by the narrowing, thrombosis, or embolization seen in these patients; angiography can demonstrate distal cerebral vessel occlusion, in addition to the local changes (Gross 1970; Beall 1962). Other symptoms vary according to the location of the aneurysms. A pulsatile mass in the oropharynx or neck was noted in 35% of Margolis' patients, and was associated with a murmur in 15% of cases. Horner's syndrome may be produced by concomittant alterations in the sympathetic innervation of the carotid wall (15% Margolis' patients) and occurs most frequently with traumatic false aneurysms. The aneurysms may be asymptomatic (Wychulis 1964) or may have a long silent period. Often the symptoms are vague or non specific [e.g. headaches, tinnitus or vertigo (Boatmann 1958; Winslow 1926)], and are therefore neglected; the patient may then present when the aneurysm has ruptured with interstitial or external hemorrhage. Unruptured aneurysms have been misdiagnosed as peritonsillar abscesses or tumors and profuse hemorrhage has been encountered at the time of incision or biopsy. Spontaneous severe epistaxis (Packer 1960) and bleeding from the ear have been reported (Harrison 1954; Young 1941), although these events are significantly more common in higher petrous aneurysms (Barett 1960; Ehni 1960). Acute local mass effect can produce airway obstruction (Fig. 7.4). Local neural compression usually involves the lower cranial nerves producing a retro-pharyngeal syndrome, and pharyngeal abscesses can produce distal facial nerve dysfunction. Fluctuation in size and tenderness to palpation may be present with arterial dissection and the mass may be noted to decrease in size with contralateral manual compression of the carotid artery.

The differential diagnosis should include: peritonsillar abscess, carotid body tumor, tortuous carotid artery, lymphadenopathy and tumors overlying the carotid arteries (Rensberg 1964, Deterling 1952, Rahael 1963).

c) Pretherapeutic Evaluation

In the investigation of patients with carotid aneurysms, angiography of the ipsilateral side is mandatory; complete cerebral angiography with appropriate oblique projections (Fig. 7.3A), including the external carotid artery is needed to assess associated vascular lesions and collateral circulation information necessary in planning treatment. Although angiography very accurately demonstrates the location of the aneurysm and the extend of the dissection, the true size of the aneurysm may be masked by mural or intramural thrombus and is better appreciated on CT (Figs. 7.3, 7.4).

In addition, CT scanning is invaluable to ascertain other soft tissue or bony involvement, the true extent of the lesion, and compression of the airway. Vascular studies are especially important in patients with neurological symptoms and a history of trauma. As mentioned previously, 50% of patients with aneurysms due to blunt trauma have no external signs of injury.

d) Treatment

Due to the high risk of serious complications treatment is probably always indicated. At present, the treatment of choice of cervical aneurysms is surgical resection of the aneurysm with reconstitution of the carotid lumen by venous or dacron grafts, or if possible, by primary anastomosis when significant redundancy of the carotid artery exists (Benvenuto 1961; Buxton 1964; Cifarelli 1971, Halasz 1964; Ohara 1968; Raphael 1963; Shea 1955; Wilson 1961).

Transcatheter treatment is currently less desirable, because of the difficulty in preserving carotid flow and probably should be reserved for those lesions where distal thrombosis of the internal carotid artery has already occurred or when direct surgical intervention may be impaired by associated problems such as soft tissue involvement, infection or significant cephalad extension of a dissection (Figs. 7.2, 7.3).

4. Petrous Carotid Aneurysms

The internal carotid artery courses in the carotid sheath towards the base of the skull. It lies anterior to the longus cervicus muscle and the transverse process of the upper third and fourth cervical vertebrae. A short distance above the lateral mass of the atlas, the carotid enters the petrous bone through the carotid canal, where it is fixed. The anterior surface of the atlas lies directly posterior to the upper most portion of the cervical internal carotid artery. This relationship is variable if the carotid artery deviates laterally or medially.

Extension, and flexion and some lateral flexion of the skull take place at the atlanto-occipital joint. Extension streches the fixed internal carotid artery against the carotid canal and therefore makes this segment prone to traumatic injury.

Due to this anatomical disposition with the protection provided by the bony structures, the lack of significant branches and the rarity of atheromatous changes in the petrous segment of the internal carotid artery, the most common type of aneurysms in this location is the false aneurysm following hyperextension rotation injury as described earlier. Less common causes include penetrating injuries and infection (Davis 1983).

In our own series, all four petrous aneurysms (Table 7.1) were secondary to trauma, primarily blunt trauma. On one occasion, the petrous aneurysm was secondary to a biopsy of the "aberrant" course of the internal carotid

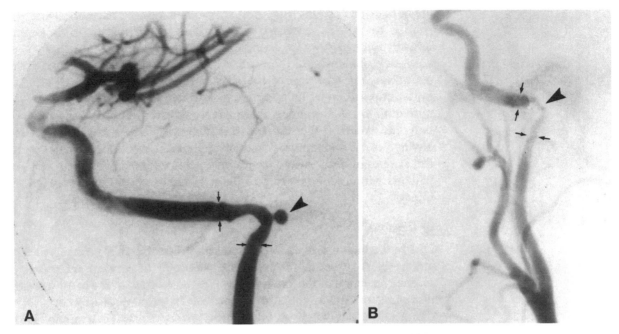

Fig. 7.7 A, B. Iatrogenic (penetrating) pseudoaneurysm following biopsy of middle
"ear" mass. **A** Subtraction angiogram, the left internal carotid artery in Stenvers
view shows a pseudoaneurysm *(arrowhead)* of the "aberrant" intratympanic
(arrows) carotid artery. **B** Same patient as **A**, 2 weeks later. Note the regression of
the false aneurysm and secondary arterial narrowing *(arrowhead)*

artery (Fig. 7.7). Another was associated with a traumatic carotid cavernous fistula (Fig. 6.8).

The clinical symptoms caused by these aneurysms are primarily due to
distal cerebral embolization and hemorrhage, usually manifested as profuse bleeding from the ear (Ehni 1960; Harrison 1954; Young 1941;
Wemple 1966).

They also often directly affect the central nervous system as described
independently by Harrison (1954, 1963) and Wemple (1966), producing
recurrent facial pain, Vth and VIth cranial nerves paresis, deafness, and
less frequently a Horner's syndrome (Fig. 7.8).

The management of these patients is difficult, because of poor surgical
access to the internal carotid artery at the level of the carotid canal. Balloon
occlusion of the aneurysm, if possible is ideal. However, in the presence of
associated dissection, intraluminal thrombi, or a very broad neck, the
internal carotid must be sacrified. Balloon trapping of the aneurysm by an
endovascular technique without surgery, as will be discussed in the section
on cavernous aneurysms, requires proper assessment of intracranial and
extracranial collateral circulation and tolerance to carotid occlusion. On
occasions collateral circulation from the external carotid artery at the C5
and/or C4 portion of the cavernous carotid is important and should be
preserved (Fig. 7.9, see also Vol. 1). Proper assessment of the origin of the
ophthalmic artery is mandatory (Fig. 7.8, see also Vol. 1, Fig. 2.14).

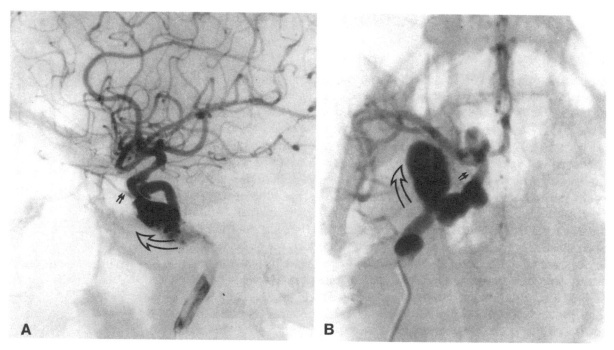

Fig. 7.8. A Dysplastic aneurysm of the intra petrous carotid artery shows on lateral. Subtracted view. **B** Axial subtraction view. The aneurysm *(open curved arrow)* bulges into the foramen lacerum and vidian canal. Note also the C4 origin of the ophthalmic artery *(double arrows)*. This 22 year old patient presented with excrutiating chronic facial pain and a Horner's syndrome which resolved within hours following balloon occlusion of the petrous carotid artery. The vision was preserved

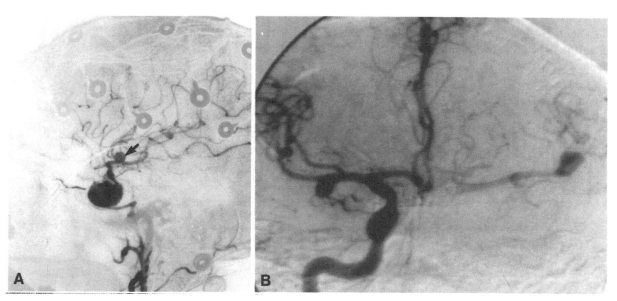

Fig. 7.9 A, B. Associated developmental aneurysm. **A** Lateral subtraction angiogram of the left internal carotid artery shows an aneurysm of the cavernous portion with narrowing of the C4 segment due to compression. An associated left MCA aneurysm *(arrow)* is seen (substracted artifacts represent an EEG helmet). **B** Frontal DSA of the contralateral right internal carotid artery in the same patient. Note the bilateral MCA aneurysms. There is excellent spontaneous cross filling to both ACAs and MCAs from the right. The MCA aneurysm was clipped, prior to balloon occlusion of the left ICA aneurysm

5. Aneurysms of the Cavernous Segment of the Internal Carotid Artery (ACCs)

a) Epidemiology

The most frequent site of extradural internal carotid artery aneurysms is the cavernous segment. They have often been considered to be of atherosclerotic origin. However, the clinical pathological study by Barr (1971) clearly showed that these large saccular aneurysms arise as a result of weakness in the lateral wall of the cavernous segment of the carotid artery at the origin of one of the C4 or C5 branches of the internal carotid artery. Furthermore, similar to the observations of Drake (1979), we have seen these lesions in young patients without evidence of atherosclerosis; we have also seen a relatively high incidence of associated additional berry aneurysms. Among our 44 cavernous aneurysms, we had five patients (11%) with aneurysms at other locations (Fig. 7.9), a statistically significantly higher incidence than in the general population. Mishkin (1965) presented 68 patients with intracavernous aneurysms; three had bilateral aneurysms (4.4%) and nine (13%) had small aneurysms in other locations. Therefore, one can assume that these are true developmental or congenital lesions. Atherosclerotic changes which occur commonly in the cavernous portion of the internal carotid artery may further weaken the arterial wall (Rob 1954) and may be an aggravating factor in the evolution of these lesions. Similarly, the higher incidence of hypertension (Table 7.2) in these patients may be an added factor in their pathogenesis (Barr 1971).

Less frequently, traumatic cavernous pseudoaneurysms may result from motor vehicle accidents (Fig. 7.10), carotid endarterectomy, and trans-sphenoidal surgery.

As with pseudoaneurysms at other levels the clinical presentation may be delayed. Thrombosis (Fig. 7.5), and dissections may also occur in this location primarily following blunt trauma. Only ten cases of mycotic aneurysms of the cavernous carotid artery have been reported in the world literature, seven of which occurred in children (Tomita 1981). In these cases the clinical presentation varied from the typical slow progressive course to an acute onset of ophthalmoplegia with or without fever. WBC count is usually elevated with a shift to the left and CSF glucose levels are decreased (Tomita 1981). Typically, angiography shows an irregular aneurysm with

Table 7.2. Clinical presentation of carotid cavernous aneurysms

	Initial symptoms (%)	Present (%)
Pain (V1)[a]	64.5	82
Diplopia	23.5	82
Ptosis[b]	12	82
Visual loss[c]	–	29
Proptosis	–	6
Additional aneurysms	1	11
HBP or CVD[d]		

[a] Pain in the distribution of the V2 was seen in 12%

[b] Complete absence of levator muscle function was seen in 24% and some degree of ptosis was seen in all patients on careful examination

[c] 1 patient 2.2% had loss of vision secondary to corneal ulceration

[d] HBP high blood pressure, CVD cardiovascular disease

Fig. 7.10. Traumatic cavernous pseudoaneurysm *(arrow)* of the left ICA in the same patient illustrated in Fig. 7.5, with post traumatic thrombosis of the right internal carotid artery. Nonpacified blood from the right PCA *(small arrow)* is seen, and patency of the anterior part of the circle of Willis is confirmed by filling of both ACA and part of the right MCA from the left ICA. This 22 year old male presented with multiple trauma and acute onset of left side ophthalmoplegia. The right ICA thrombosis was asymptomatic (Fig. 7.5). Prior to balloon occlusion of the left ICA, a left EC-IC bypass was performed, and a tolerance test with the bypass was done without problems (see Fig. 1.6)

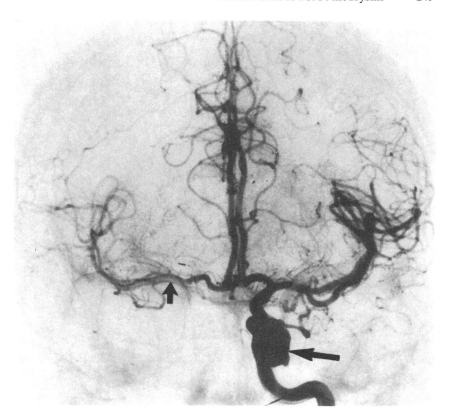

multiple filling defects and mass effect. Sequential angiography may demonstrate rapid changes in the size and shape of the aneurysm and even eventual thrombosis.

Spontaneous dissection or intramural hematoma may occur in patients with blood dyscrasias or coagulopathies such as disseminated intra vascular coagulation (DIC) and often presents with acute ophthalmoplegia. Progressive thrombosis, and the risk of distal embolization (Fig. 7.11) occur as with secondary dissections. Even after the internal carotid artery has thrombosed, embolic episodes to the opthalmic and/or intracerebral circulation may continue from the stump of the internal carotid artery through EC to IC collaterals (Fig. 7.12). To prevent emboli from either the distal carotid or the stump, balloon trapping and stumpectomy is effective (Fig. 7.13).

Rupture may occur when the aneurysm is small, causing a "spontaneous" carotid cavernous fistula (Fig. 7.2), with its typical clinical presentation. If rupture does not occurs early, gradual expansion of the aneurysm brings its wall into contact with the dura covering the cavernous sinus, which in turn provides some protection against rupture.

b) Clinical Presentation

The clinical features and natural history of this condition has been studied by Meadows (1965) who described the sequence of clinical events progressing through cranial nerve palsies, visual impairment, and proptosis, correlating with the way the aneurysm tends to grow laterally and compress the cranial nerves as described by Barr (1971). Compression of cranial

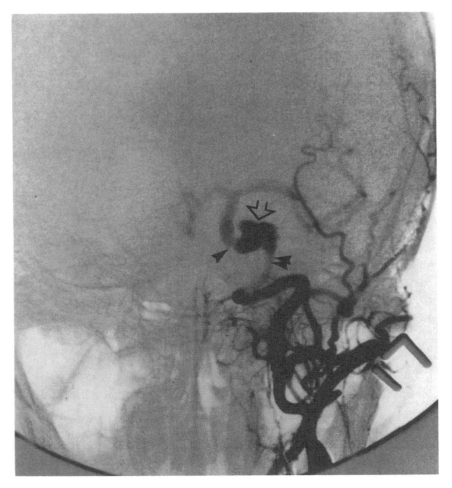

Fig. 7.11. 38 year old female who developed DIC after abdominal surgery and presented with dysarthria, right sided weakness and left sided acute and complete ophthalmoplegia. Frontal subtraction angiogram of the left CCA demonstrates lateral and superior displacement of the cavernous carotid artery with a relatively small irregular aneurysm lumen *(open arrow)*, and significant stenosis distal to the aneurysm. The carotid narrowing due to intramural dissection is seen proximally *(double arrowheads)*. Three days later, she developed a transient episode of amaurosis fugax. The ICA had thrombosed spontaneously and turbulent flow of the IC stump was noted. A balloon stumpectomy was performed (not shown, see Fig. 7.12) to prevent further embolic episodes

nerves III, IV, V, VI and the pericarotid sympathetic and parasympathetic fibers of the IIIrd cranial nerve is frequent. In sequential order dysfunction of the VI nerve occurs first, followed by the IIIrd and then the Vth cranial nerves (Meadows 1965). Further expansion of the aneurysm will eventually strip the dura from the floor of the middle cranial fossa. Anterior extension is usually a late event; this results in erosion of the anterior clinoid process (Fig. 7.14), and eventually inferolateral extension into the optic foramen and superior orbital fissure. Nonpulsatile exopthalmus with compression of the optic nerve result, leading to progressive visual loss and optic atrophy. Conjunctival congestion is rare. Posterior expansion, also a late event, can lead to ipsilateral facial palsy and deafness, sometimes followed by rupture and massive hemorrhage (Barr 1971). Medial expansion may erode the lateral aspect of the sella. Severe epistaxis may occur with aneurysms which erod into the sphenoid sinus (Fig. 6.16).

In Barr's (1971) clinical pathological study, the displacement of cranial nerves due to aneurysm expansion correlated with the clinical manifestations. The motor fibers of the trigeminal nerve ganglion and all divisions of the sensory Vth nerve lie on the posterior and inferior lateral aspects of the aneurysmal sac. Degeneration of some or part of the nerves with demyelination and decrease of Schwann cell nuclei is noted pathologically. All

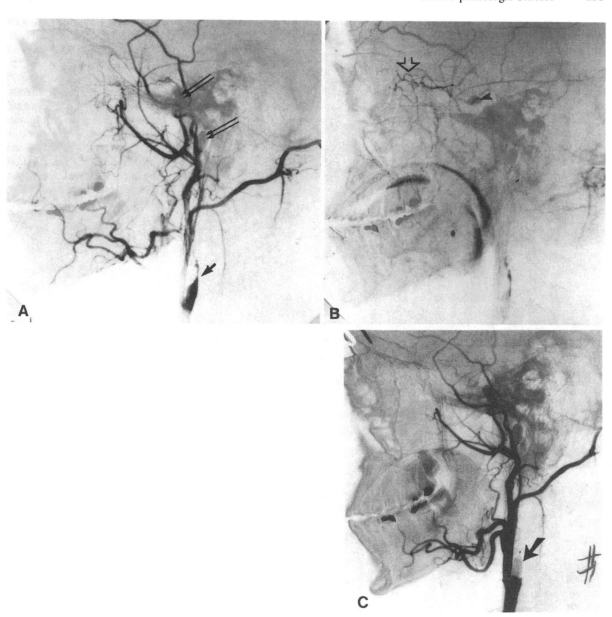

Fig. 7.12 A-C. 39 year old male who developed amaurosis fugax, one week after balloon occlusion of the left ICA for an aneurysm of the cavernous carotid artery. Trapping was not done because of intraluminal thrombi in the aneurysm (not shown). **A** Lateral subtraction angiogram of the CCA. The stump of the left ICA with thrombi *(arrow)* and two partially subtracted balloons in the precavernous and high cervical carotid arteries *(double arrows)* are seen. **B** Late phase of the same injection. Note, stasis of contrast in the ophthalmic artery *(open arrow)* and in the cavernous carotid artery *(arrowhead)* suggesting an embolic event from the turbulent flow of the ICA stump. **C** Lateral subtraction angiogram after a detached balloon was used for stumpectomy *(arrow)*. No further embolic episodes occurred

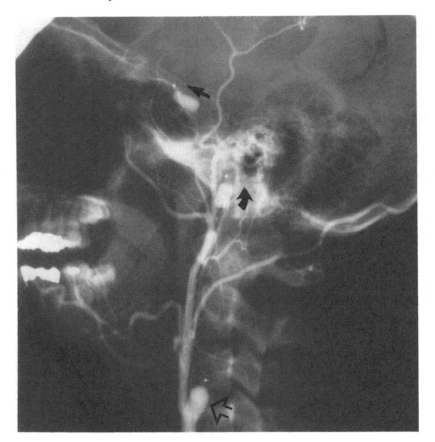

Fig. 7.13. Balloon trapping of the internal carotid artery. Lateral angiogram after trapping with one balloon *(arrow)* in the cavernous carotid artery distal to the aneurysm but proximal to the ophthalmic artery and a second balloon proximal to the aneurysm in the petrous carotid *(curved arrow)* and a third balloon in the origin of the internal carotid artery to prevent turbulence within the stump when sacrificing a major artery

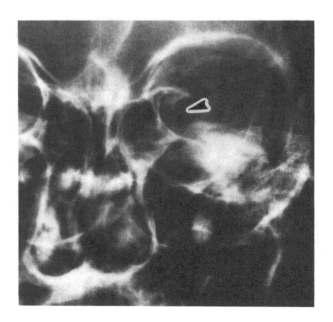

Fig. 7.14. Frontal plain film of the skull in a patient with a cavernous carotid aneurysm. Bone erosion is seen in the left parasellar area with medial and superior erosion of the anterolateral wall of the sella and anterior clinoid process *(arrowhead)*

Table 7.3. Neuro-ophthalmological findings in cavernous carotid aneurysms

	Isolated (%)	Impaired (%)
III[a] (14)	12	82
IV	–	47
VI	12	71
All muscles involved	–	35
Complete ophthalmoplegia	–	18
VI Sensory loss[b]	–	24
Parasympathetic	–	53
Sympathetic abnormality	–	35

[a] 29% of patients with oculomotor nerve palsy had no internal ophthalmoplegia
[b] A profoundly anesthetic cornea in 1 patient (2.2%) resulted in a corneal ulceration and visual loss

patients with autopsy examination had long standing changes. A second saccular aneurysm was frequently encountered.

In our series (Kupersmith 1984), the clinical presentation (Table 7.2) and neuro-ophthalmologic findings were carefully analyzed (Table 7.3). Pain in the distribution of the first division of the Vth nerve was the most frequent initial symptom and was eventually present in most cases. Severe debilitating pain occurred in a third of our patients and was the primary reason for consultation. In the remaining, the pain was either progressive or stable, but in no patient was it explosive. Partial sensory loss in the distribution of the Vth nerve caused diminishing corneal reflex and decreased light touch perception, in the distribution of the first division of the trigeminal nerve. When severe, the sensory loss can lead to corneal anesthesia and ulceration with resulting blindness. Diplopia was the initial complaint in less than a third of the patients, but eventually was present in most. Absence of levator function alone, without internal opthalmoplegia and with normal pupillary function, was seen in a third of patients with ptosis and represented partial third nerve dysfunction. This did not improve in any of our patients following treatment (Berenstein 1984). Progressive unilateral loss of vision occurred relatively late in the course and was usually due to compression of the optic nerve secondary to anterior expansion of the aneurysm. IInd nerve sensory involvement was a less frequent cause of visual loss.

Proptosis occurred rarely in our patients and was mild when present, probably because of our present ability to make an early diagnosis on CT scans, as compared with a higher incidence and degree of proptosis in older series (Jefferson 1938).

Additional aneurysms were seen in 11% and bilateral cavernous lesions were seen in 3% comparable to the experience of Drake (19%) and Mishkin (1965), but less than that reported by Barr (1971). There was a high incidence of associated high blood pressure and cerebrovascular disease, and these are probably significant aggravating factors.

It is interesting to note that our series as well as all other reports showed a significantly higher incidence in females (13:1); of our three males, two had traumatic pseudoaneurysms. If one excludes the younger males with traumatic lesions, the mean age was 58 years. The youngest patient was a 24 year old female in whom symptoms followed pregnancy.

Varying degress of ipsilateral ophthalmoplegia were present in 94% of patients but presented as the initial symptoms in less than a third of patients, probably reflecting compensation of mild ocular motor changes (Morley 1968). Isolated extraocular nerve compression was unusual and involved only the VIth and IIIrd cranial nerves; isolated IVth cranial nerve involvement was not seen. All muscles were involved in 30% and a complete ophthalmoplegia was present in 18%. Contrary to other series (Jefferson 1938; Morley 1968), we found that the IIIrd nerve was involved more frequently than the VIth nerve.

Parasympathetic or sympathetic pupillary abnormalities ipsilateral to the aneurysms were observed in most patients.

c) Pretherapeutic Evaluation

α) **Plain Films.** Bone erosion can be seen on plain films of the skull (Fig. 7.14) (Mishkin 1965), in 8% of cases (Newton and Potts) but could be seen on CT Scans in all of our patients with symptomatic aneurysms.

β) **CT Findings.** In our experience CT scans always show bone erosion which varies depending on the growth characteristics of the lesion. Changes include erosion of the lateral portion of the sella turcica and in larger aneurysms, undercutting of the ipsilateral anterior clinoid process (Figs. 7.15, 7.18A, B). Additional bony changes include erosion of the lesser wing of the sphenoid bone with widening to the superior orbital fissure (Fig. 7.15B).

CT scans prior to and after the intravenous administration of contrast material are excellent for the diagnosis of parasellar lesions and have a high degree of accuracy in differentiating aneurysms from parasellar tumors.

A negative non contrast CT is insufficient to rule out pathology. Following the intravenous administration of contrast material there is a uniformly enhancing lesion with well-circumscribed borders and no edema (Fig. 7.15A). In a small number of cases (3 of our 44 cases) the characteristics CT appearance of a partially thrombosed aneurysm (Pinto 1979), i.e. an area of ring enhancement with an eccentric enhancing lumen surrounded by irregular low attenuation (representing the thrombus) was noted, similar to other partially thrombosed aneurysms (Figs. 7.2, 7.3).

CT scans at the level of the carotid canal should be imaged with bony windows to rule out an aberrant course of the internal carotid artery.

γ) **Angiographic and Functional Investigations.** Angiography is the definite diagnostic study to confirm the diagnosis and permit exclusion of a tumor or an aberrant course of the internal carotid artery and to show the level of origin of the ophthalmic artery (Fig. 7.8). Lateral and frontal projections of the ipsilateral internal carotid artery are done first; after the diagnosis is confirmed appropriate oblique projections are made by rotating the head 30° to the side opposite the aneurysms (Fig. 7.16A).

This is followed by four vessel cerebral angiography in search of associated lesions (11–13%). A cross compression study of contralateral carotid artery in frontal projection and a vertebral angiogram in lateral projection with ipsilateral carotid compression are done to assess the competency of the anterior and posterior segment of the circle of Willis. As an alternative, a high pressure, high volume (6 cc per second for a total of 12 cc at 450 PSI) study may be attempted prior to manual carotid compres-

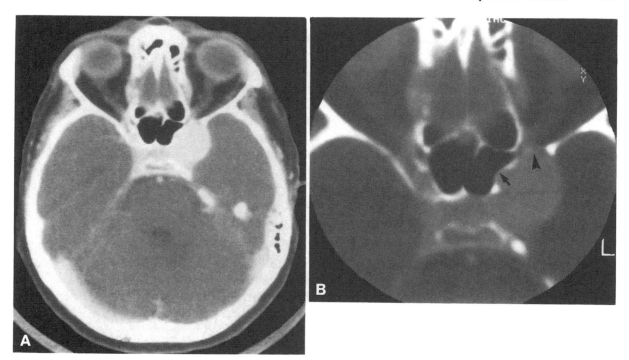

Fig. 7.15 A, B. Aneurysm of the cavernous carotid artery. **A** Axial CT image after IV contrast demonstrates a well circumscribed parasellar mass with homogeneous enhancement and lateral bulging of the cavernous area (compare with right side). There is no edema or bony hyperostosis. **B** Same patient. Bony window demonstrates the bony erosion of the lateral sphenoid bone *(arrow)*, and widening of the superior orbital fissure *(arrowhead)*

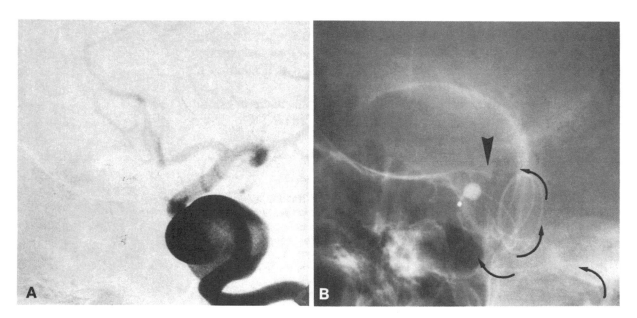

Fig. 7.16. A Oblique projection of the left internal carotid artery shows a giant cavernous aneurysm. A neck could not be shown angiographically on multiple projections. **B** Plain film of the skull in the same obliquity as **A**. The microcatheter is coiled due to the laminar flow within the aneurysmal sac *(curved arrows)*. It would not pass through the exit *(arrowhead)*

sion. In general this type of angiogram will also demonstrate the circle of Willis and prevent the need for manual compression and the concommitant radiation to personel.

Ipsilateral distal external carotid angiography in lateral view allows to assess collateral circulation to the C4 segment of the internal carotid and to the ophthalmic artery. If indicated, a selective injection in the ascending pharyngeal artery in lateral view will demonstrate the collateral circulation to the C5 segment of the internal carotid artery (Vol. 1, Chapter 2). In addition, information is obtained as to the dominant pedicle in the functional anatomy of the superficial temporal, posterior auricular, and occipital arteries to select the best donor in case an extracranial to intracranial bypass is contemplated. In addition, in traumatic, dysplastic or atherosclerotic lesions, associated vascular lesions, even if asymptomatic, must be assessed and treated.

δ) Tolerance to Carotid Occlusion. The carotid and vertebral compression and flow studies will adequately assess the status of the anterior communicating and posterior communicating arteries and are generally reliable. However, if treatment is contemplated during the angiographic work-up prior to embolization, a test of tolerance to acute carotid occlusion is needed. Various tests have been reported, including Xenon cerebral blood flow studies and stump pressures after temporary occlusion (Drake 1979; Gelber 1980; Sharbrough 1973). We have used an intraluminal balloon occlusion test to assess tolerance to acute internal carotid artery occlusion (Berenstein 1984) (see Chapter 1). More recently we have added continuous EEG monitoring as an extra precaution.

If occlusion of the internal carotid and/or vertebral arteries is not tolerated, or if pronounced localized EEG slowing appears with an increase in Delta activity, the balloon should be deflated immediatly. As a point of caution one should assess the function of both hemispheres. On one occasion cerebral dysfunction in the contralateral EEG appeared representing a "steal" across the circle of Willis (Chapter 1). One can determine if the EEG is improved by raising the blood pressure as a measure of collateral reserve (Berenstein 1985).

In those patients with an incompetent circle of Willis bilateral carotid disease, or signs of ischemia during the "tolerance test", an EC-IC bypass is done (Fein 1979), prior to embolization. Even patients that have already an EC-IC bypass receive a tolerance test (Chapter 1, XIII and XIV).

Fig. 7.17 A-E. Bilobed cavernous aneurysm. **A** Lateral subtraction angiogram in patient with a bilobed cavernous aneurysm. The smaller curved arrow points to the anterior inferior lobe and the larger curved arrow to the second lobulation which is larger, more posterior and superior. **B** Plain lateral skull film showing the balloon *(double arrow)* in the anterior inferior lobe. Note the stagnation of contrast material in the posterior lobe *(arrow)*. **C** Control carotid angiogram after the balloon *(arrow)* has been detached in the anterior inferior lobe. Note the preservation of the carotid flow. **D** The same patient 3 months later had recurrence of the retro-orbital pain. The deflated balloon has migrated into the posterior superior compartment *(arrow* points to silver clips). The anterior lobule has recanalized. **E** A silicone filled balloon was placed in the anterior lobe *(double arrow)* with preservation of the ICA. However, the retro-orbital pain did not subside as the pulsatile mass effect has not been removed. The ICA was sacrified at a third procedure with relief of pain. Although the balloon remained, the pulsatile component was removed

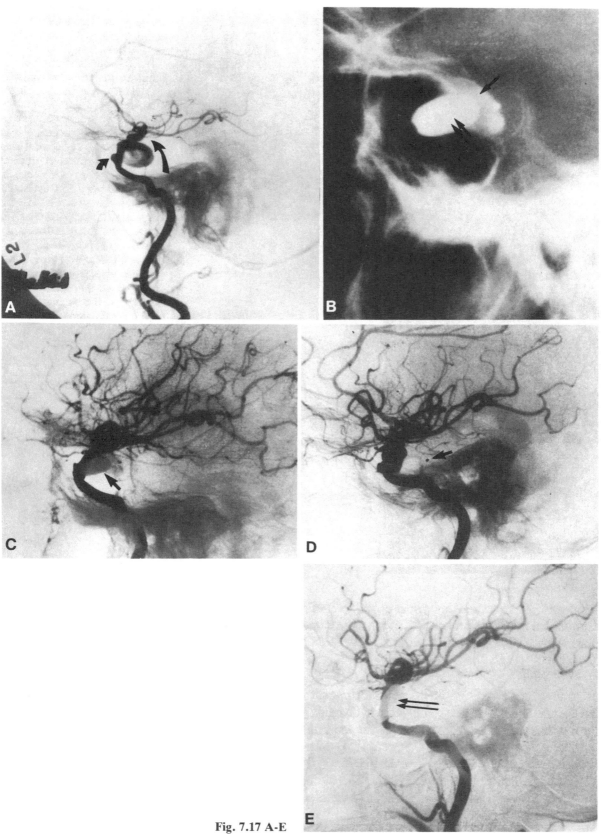

Fig. 7.17 A-E

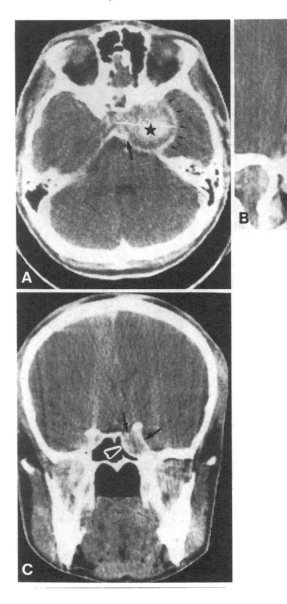

Fig. 7.18 A-C. Thrombosed giant cavernous aneurysm with bony erosion. **A** Axial image. **B** Coronal image on the CT after i. v. administration of the contrast material, two days later after embolization, shows the characteristics CT appearance of a thrombosed aneurysm with the enhancing wall *(small arrows)* and central area of high absorption coefficient *(star)* that does not enhance. Note, the bone destruction involving the posterior clinoid process **(A)** and parasellar **(B)** areas. The foramen ovale *(arrowhead)* is prominent. **C** Coronal CT image made 8 month after embolization. Note the collapse of the aneurysm *(arrows)* and the bulging towards the sphenoid sinus *(arrowhead)*

In patients in whom an associated intracranial aneurysm is found, primarily in another circulation, and in whom carotid occlusion is contemplated, the incidental aneurysm should be treated first (Fig. 7.9).

d) Treatment

α) Embolization. Whenever possible, if the anatomical configuration of the aneurysm permits, an attempt should be made to preserve the internal carotid artery (Fig. 7.17). The balloon should be filled with a vulcanizing or polymerizing substance (see Chapters 1, 6) to prevent deflation. It is important to avoid overinflation of the balloon(s) to permit decompression of the cranial nerves (Berenstein 1984). Therefore, if the internal carotid artery is preserved, the balloon should not completely replace the volume of the aneurysm sac, so that the aneurysm may collapse. Although Hieshima's experience suggests the important role played by pulsations in the production of symptoms in giant aneurysms.

Following internal carotid artery occlusion, primarily at the cervical level, delayed (3–5 days) neurological complications may result from embolization (Oller 1976; Sanoudos 1973) through retrograde filling of the aneurysm via recanalized segments of the cavernous carotid at C4 or C5 (Drake 1983) or from the proximal internal carotid stump (Barnett 1978) (Fig. 7.12). To prevent this complication balloon occlusion of the internal carotid artery has the advantage over cervical (surgical) carotid ligation in that it permits easy percutaneous trapping of the aneurysm in one procedure (Fig. 7.13). Our only two complications in the management of cavernous carotid aneurysms occurred in one of our patients where we were unable to trap the aneurysm. A monocular superior visual field defect without loss of visual acuity occurred ipsilateral to the aneurysm. Over the next six month disc pallor was noted, but the field defect resolved almost completely (Fig. 7.12). The second complication, also involving emboli to the ophthalmic circulation resulted from turbulent flow from the stump of the internal carotid artery (Fig. 7.12). No further episodes occurred after the stump was occluded with a balloon. Since we have used balloon stumpectomy we have seen no episodes of embolism from external carotid to ophthalmic or internal carotid arteries. Delayed ophthalmic artery embolization has three possible origins:

a) Retraction of the thrombus in the occluded segment of the internal carotid artery with retrograde filling of the ophthalmic artery.

b) Antegrade embolization after clot retraction and/or recanalization from C4 or C5 (Kupersmith 1984).

c) Antigrade internal maxillary artery to ophthalmic embolization originating from turbulent flow at the stump of the occluded internal carotid artery (Barnett 1978) (Fig. 7.13C).

The complication can be easily avoided with a balloon stumpectomy (Fig. 7.13C). As an additional precaution the use of inhibitors of platelet aggregation such as aspirin, 650 mgm po q. d. (Fox 1985) has been found to be useful, although Heros (1983) questions the value of antiplatelet drugs in the prevention of embolic complications after internal carotid artery occlusion. One of three patients in Heros' series had an embolic complication during gradual clamp occlusion in spite of antiplatelet therapy.

Minor transient aggravation of ocular symptoms or pain can occur following embolization, and may be due to a traction phenomena of the nerves in the cavernous sinus during collapse of the thrombosing aneurysm sac (Fig. 7.18, and Chapter 6), as discussed by Strenger (1966). Drake has postulated that enlargement of the aneurysm during thrombosis could also be responsible for frequent transient and reversible aggravation of ocular symptoms. On one occasion emergency surgery to decompress the optic chiasm was needed in Drake's experience. Most probably a combination of both phenomena may be responsible for this relatively infrequent transient aggravation.

Aneurysms trapping may not be possible in all cases as the outflow carotid may be at different segments of the aneurysmal sac (Fig. 7.16B). In some instaces the use of an elongated Debrun 16 balloons can be used to reach the distal outflow of the aneurysm. In others, it may be unwise to manipulate a microballoon catheter through an aneurysm if the preliminary angiogram shows obvious intraluminal thrombi or debris (Fig. 7.19C). In the presence of ophthalmic artery origin from the cavernous carotid artery

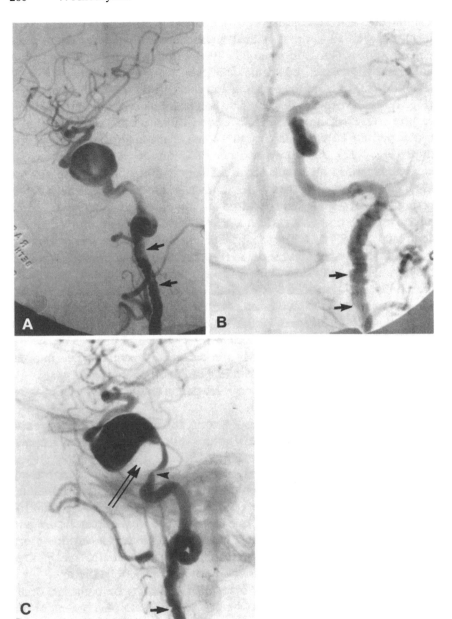

Fig. 7.19 A-C. Cavernous aneurysm associated with FMD of the progressive type. 39 year old female with high blood pressure, chronic headache, fluctuating ophthalmoplegia with rapid onset of diplopia to lateral gaze and delayed onset of Horner's syndrome. **A** Lateral subtraction angiogram of the right CCA. Note the characteristic "string of beads" appearance of type 1 FMD *(arrows)*. The diplopia resolved spontaneously in 3 weeks. She was placed on an antiplatelet aggregation regimen. **B** Frontal subtraction angiogram of the left CCA. The left ICA is also involved with FMD *(arrows)*. **C** Lateral subtraction angiogram of the right ICA, one year later. While still under aspirin therapy, the patient presented with acute onset of a Horner's syndrome. Note the progression of the disease with significant tubular stenosis *(arrowhead)* and partial thrombosis of the aneurysm *(double arrow)*

(Fig. 7.8), this segment must be preserved as its occlusion carries a high risk of blindness. Prior assessment of the quality of the collateral circulation from the maxillary system to the ophthalmic is important.

Before the catheter assembly system is withdrawn, heparinization should be reversed with 1.5 mg of Protamine sulfate per 1000 unit of heparin. Calculation of protamine dose should take into account the total amount of heparin given and the length of the procedure. A simpler way to calculate the protamine dose needed is by ACT determination (see Chapter 1).

β) Postembolization Care. In addition to routine postembolization care (see Chapter 1), special considerations must be taken after occlusion of the internal carotid artery. Frequent and careful neurological and cardiovascular assessment is mandatory. Ischemic deficits may result from fluctuations in blood pressure, position, or cardiac output. These patients have a high incidence of a high blood pressure and periods of relative hypotension may require aggressive management with volume expanders, or vasopressor medication (see Chapter 1). Both cerebral hemispheres must be monitored as a contralateral hemodynamic "steal" may occur when one internal carotid artery is occluded. We have seen this phenomenon twice; each times it readily responded to volume expanders. On occasions when ischemic symptoms develop (early or delayed), artificial increase in cerebral perfusion by medical means may be necessary for up to several days, until the autonomic regulatory system compensates and sufficient collateral flow is established. Theoretically, in precarious situations, and EC-IC bypass could be placed to increase cerebral perfusion. *Strict* bed rest is mandatory during the immediate postoperative period. Patients may start ambulation 36 hours after embolization, but physical activity should be restricted for approximatively 3–4 weeks.

γ) Results of Embolization (Tables 7.4, 7.5) (Kupersmith 1984). All of our patients with cavernous carotid artery aneurysms benefitted from treatment. The most constant improvement was the complete resolution of pain in all patients. Diplopia improved in more than 1/2 of the patients; however, it resolved completely in over 60% of them. Visual loss improved in 20% and stabilized in an additional 40%. Proptosis although infrequent, resolved in all. For our only patient who presented with subarachnoid hemorrhage, we occluded the internal carotid artery and this resulted in thrombosis of the aneurysm (Fig. 7.18). During thrombosis of the aneurysm early after embolization CT will show the typical target appearance

Table 7.4. Clinical results after embolization

	Improved (%)	Resolved (%)	Unchanged (%)	Worsening[a] (%)
Pain	–	100	–	–
Diplopia	62	24	14	14
Ptosis[b]	27	36	36	–
Visual loss	20	–	80[c]	–
Proptosis	–	100	–	–

[a] Transient with eventual improvement as compared to pre-embolization
[b] Including 66% of patients with complete ptosis prior to embolization
[c] Stabilized in 40%

Table 7.5. Neuro-ophthalmological findings after embolization

	Improved (%)	Resolved (%)	Worsened[a] (%)	Unchanged (%)
III	20	60	6	20
IV	17	50	–	33
VI	12.5	50	12.5	37.5
Complete ophthalmoplegia	–	–	–	100
V_1 sensory loss	44	56	6	–
Sympathetic	–	–	–	100
Parasympathetic	–	–	–	100

[a] Transient with eventual improvement as compared to pre-embolization

(Pinto 1979) (Figs. 7.18A, B). We have documented thrombosis and decrease of mass effect with collapse of the sac of the aneurysm (Fig. 7.18C). The results of treatment on cranial nerve dysfunction are seen in Table 7.5. IIIrd, IVth, Vth, and VIth nerve dysfunction resolved in more than 1/2 of the patients, and improved in others. The Vth nerve was the only one which showed either full recovery or some improvement in all patients. No improvement occurred in the sympathetic or parasympathetic dysfunctions.

δ) Other Forms of Treatment: Surgery. Due to the location, anatomical configuration, and the frequent large size of the aneurysm at the time of clinical presentation, primary surgery is usually not possible (Drake 1979, Oller 1976, Pia 1978). Until recently, the recommended treatment of choice has been ligation of the cervical internal carotid arteries either directly or by gradual occlusion with a clamp (Drake 1979, Gianotta 1979, Oller 1976, Pia 1978). We have already discussed the problems of carotid occlusion. Surgical experience seems to favor gradual occlusion with a clamp which presumably allows collateral circulation to develop maximally. This gradual and reversible occlusion theoritically appears safer than acute ligation, as it permits reestablishment of flow if necessary, but ischemic cerebral symptoms can occur as the occlusion nears completion. The hemodynamic basis of this is the fact that significant reduction in the blood flow or pressure does not occur until a cross sectional area of less than 2 mm^2 is reached, regardless of the diameter of the vessel. Although the lumen of the vessel is narrowed gradually, the most significant reduction in flow and pressure actually occurs rapidly during the final adjustment of the clamp (Brice 1974). In addition, the edema of the arterial wall which develops on clamping, further alters the so called "gradual reduction" in pressure and flow (Brice 1974). Distal embolization may occur after reopening the clamp, or prior to complete clamping from residual antegrade flow through the partially thrombosed aneurysm or from partial thrombosis of the carotid artery proximal to the clamp as reported by Heros (1983).

Nishioka (1966) in a cooperative study, reported deficits thought to be ischemic which occurred during gradual occlusion of the internal carotid artery and which reversed when the clamp was reopened in 56% of the patients. However, in some patients the deficit worsened after the clamp was opened, and although the term "ischemic" was used, the worsening of the symptoms after increasing carotid flow must represent an embolic problem. Furthermore, in 62 patients reviewed by Landolt (1970), 38% of patients treated by gradual occlusion developed complications, as opposed to only 24% of those treated by aprupt carotid occlusion. These authors concluded that most of the "ischemic" deficits ecountered during or after therapeutic carotid occlusions are thrombo-embolic in nature. A similar conclusion was reached by Heros (1983) and his coworkers. They recommend the use of detachable balloons or abrupt ligation of the internal carotid artery with the patient awake; following angiographic demonstration of good collateral circulation and proper balloon test occlusion. In the patients who have poor collaterals or those who fail provocative testing, and EC-IC bypass may be advisable. We suggest retesting following this bypass and prior to carotid occlusion (Chapter 1 and Fig. 1.6). Peerless in the comment to Heros' article (1983) concurred with this conclusion and suggested that the balloon occlusion just proximal to the aneurysm will leave a shorter stump in the carotid for thrombi to form. He suggests systemic heparinization with a gradual tapering dose of Heparin for 7 days and then aspirin of one month, a technique and regimen presently used by some authors (Debrun, Peerless). Interestingly, in Peerless group of 15 patients with giant aneurysms so treated, no complication occurred. However, in 3 (20%) after occlusion proximal to the aneurysm, the aneurysms continued to fill and required surgical trapping.

Unfortunately, he failed to mention if any of these aneurysms were beyond the cavernous area.

The technique described by us (Berenstein 1984) has several advantages over those of Debrun, Heros or Peerless. First, we do our tolerance test with a double lumen balloon catheter (see Chapter 1) that permits visualization of the configuration of the aneurysm during flow arrest. Furthermore, the flow arrest permits us to assess retrograde filling of the aneurysm, which if present can easily be handled by balloon trapping. Distal contrast material injection will assess collateral flow from the ophthalmic and will also show contrast washout from the circle of Willis, permitting better assessment or cerebral collateral circulation. The coaxial system permits perfusion of the carotid segment proximal to the balloon occlusion with heparinized saline, so that when the balloon is deflated no thrombi are released. This technique is more effective in preventing thrombosis than systemic heparinization alone.

The other advantage of aneurysms trapping is the inclusion of the C4 and C5 branches of the internal carotid artery which reduces the length of the thrombosed carotid segment even further (Fig. 7.13) [reducing the known risk of delayed (3–4 days) cerebral embolization (see above)].

Finally, we recommend that when a major cerebral vessel is occluded, more than one balloon should be used as a safeguard in case of early deflation. The last balloon should be placed in the cervical internal carotid artery just distal to the bifurcation to obtain an endovascular balloon "stumpectomy" (Fig. 7.13). At present, EC-IC bypass is an excellent adjunct prior to balloon occlusion of the internal carotid artery when one can predict insufficient collateral circulation from the angiographic investigation, or when the patient fails the tolerance test. EC-IC bypass will decrease the potential of ischemic complications, but will not prevent delayed embolic episodes. The value of "prophylactic" EC-IC bypass, however, is still controversial (Heros 1983).

It is important to document exclusion of the aneurysm from the circulation. This can easily be accomplished by a follow-up noncontrast and contrast CT which show the typical appearance of a thrombosed aneurysm described by Pinto; a ring enhancement "bulls-eye" sign and no intraluminal filling after intravenous contrast administration. In addition, it will document the collapse and/or reduction in mass effect (Fig. 7.18C). As an alternative, a digital intravenous study will confirm the exclusion of the aneurysm from the circulation (Kupersmith 1984) (Fig. 7.3D).

e) Indications of Treatment

Preliminary sequential careful neuro-ophthalmological evaluation is mandatory in this group of patients to assess the presence, severity, and progression of symptoms and to choose the adequate timing of intervention. Presently available treatments, including embolization, are not without risks due to the frequent need to sacrifice the internal carotid artery (Oller 1976, Pia 1978, Roski 1980, Kupersmith 1984).

Since subarachnoid hemorrhage is rare in patients with intracavernous aneurysms (Lapresle 1979, Picard 1983 personal communication, Yasargil 1984), many patients live for many years without treatment; the question arises as to whether a complete ophthalmoplegia should be treated since this symptom did not recover completely in any of our patients or those of Drake (Kupersmith 1984, Drake 1979, Jefferson 1938). Alternatively should treatment be performed prior to complete ophthalmoplegia, when the patient has a significantly higher chance of recovery (Kupersmith 1984).

Although the short course seems benign in most cases, cavernous aneurysms were responsible for five deaths among Jefferson's (1938) fourteen untreated cases, one of Morley's (1968) 11 patients, and 2 of 3 in Barr's (1971) reports.

Indications for treatment include intractable severe pain from pressure on the trigeminal nerve in the skull base, as it resolved in all of our cases (Kupersmith 1984) as well as partial ocular motor palsy which resolved or improved in 70% of ours and 44% of Drake's patients.

III. Aneurysms of the External Carotid Artery

Aneurysms of the external carotid artery are rare lesions. A review of all reported cases of cervical carotid aneurysms from 1687–1977 by Schechter (1979) revealed that only 2.2% affected the external carotid artery. The great majority were post-traumatic, usually secondary to penetrating injuries as reported by Hite (1966). Davies (1961) collected 115 patients with superficial temporal aneurysms from the world literature prior to 1935. 72% were post traumatic and secondary to fencing or therapeutic blood letting from the temporal region; both activities were in vogue at the time. Davies (1961) reported 2 traumatic pseudoaneurysms secondary to penetrating injuries and Wortzman (1963) reported the first angiographically documented pseudoaneurysm. In 1977, De Stephano reported a pseudoaneurysm of the lingual artery. In 1983, Gomori reported the angiographic and CT findings of a lingual pseudoaneurysm confirmed pathologically, although no history of trauma or infection could be obtained. We have seen pseudoaneurysms of the internal maxillary artery from a penetrating injury (gunshot wound) (Fig. 7.20) and of the facial artery after blunt trauma (fistulous pouch without bone fracture) (Fig. 7.21).

Nontraumatic aneurysms of the proximal middle meningeal artery were reported by Berk in 1961 and New in 1965 in association with Paget's disease. Mujica (1981) reported a 54 year old female presenting with subarachnoid hemorrhage in whom two aneurysms were found in the meningeal branch of the ascending pharyngeal artery. One sac was at the level of the foramen magnum immediately lateral to the medulla. The second one was found alone the side of the medulla. Although this is the only documented case of such an occurence. Lasjaunias's description

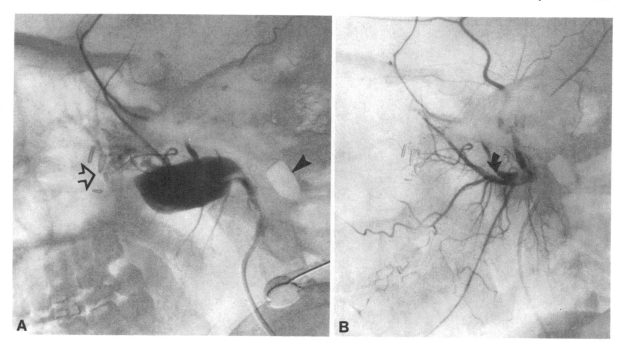

Fig. 7.20 A, B. Traumatic false aneurysm of the IMA following a gunshot wound. The patient presented with acute epistaxis which responded to surgical clipping of distal IMA branches. Delayed recurrence of epistaxis brought the patient to angiography. **A** Lateral subtraction angiogram of the proximal internal maxillary artery shows a large pseudoaneurysm of the IMA at the origin of the middle meningeal artery. Note the large caliber bullet *(arrowhead)* and the surgical clips *(open arrow)*. **B** Post embolization study. The aneurysm has been occluded *(curved arrow)* with a large piece of Gelfoam. In a previously healthy vascular system, the purpose of embolization is to produce hemostasis. Gelfoam accomplishes tempory mechanical occlusion that permits thrombosis

(1979) of the subarachnoid course of the ascending pharyngeal branches along the nerve roots supports this possibility.

We have personally observed pseudoaneurysms of the superficial temporal artery (Fig. 7.22) and middle meningeal artery after surgery, or in association with other vascular injuries (Fig. 6.9, and Chapter 6). Although the former may have little clinical significance if stable and expansile, the latter carries the potential of producing and extra-axial collection (Fig. 6.48). Extradural hematomas were seen in 70% of patients and subdural collections in 20% of patients reported by Treil (1977). In 80% of cases the lesion was secondary to skull trauma.

The position of the middle meningeal artery between the inner table of the skull and the dura mater makes it particularly liable to injury during head trauma. As in other areas, trauma may be followed by pseudoaneurysms or other vascular injuries, including damage of the pial vessels, or cerebral injury. Fractures at the site of the injury are seen in the great majority.

In Treil's (1977) series, the most frequent findings following trauma of the meningeal arteries were extravasation of contrast material followed by arteriovenous fistula formation and less commonly false aneurysms. It is interesting that pseudoaneurysms were associated with arteriovenous

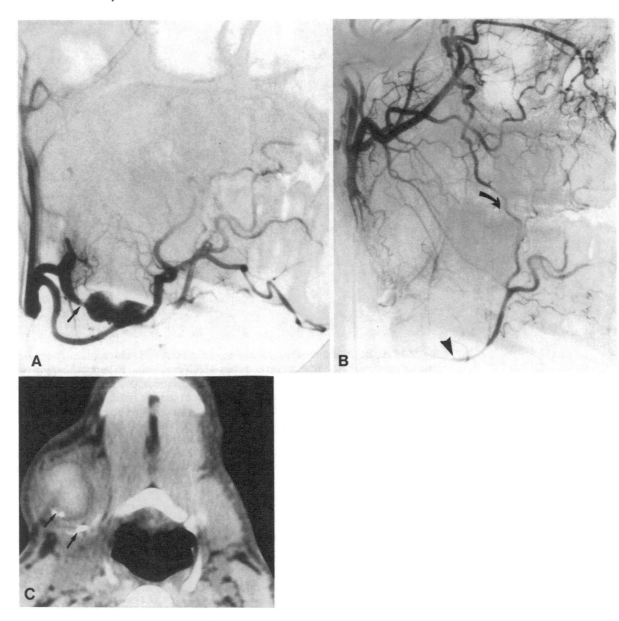

Fig. 7.21 A-C. False aneurysm of the facial artery following blunt trauma. **A** Lateral subtraction angiogram of the proximal external carotid artery. Note the bilobed aneurysm of the facial artery *(arrow)*. **B** Distal external carotid control after embolization with IBCA. Note the collateral circulation distal to the aneurysms *(arrowhead)* via the buccal artery *(curved arrow)*. **C** Axial CT image without contrast administration following embolization of the facial artery with IBCA. Clotted blood is seen within the false aneurysm. *Arrows* indicate the intra arterial IBCA

Fig. 7.22. 48 year old male with non surgical laryngeal malignancy s/p radiation therapy presented with significant oral bleeding from the larynx. Superselective catheterization of the superior thyroidal artery demonstrate a pseudoaneurysm. The pressure injection has produced a significant extravasation (*O* occiput; *M* mandible). It is important to remember when investigating hemorrhagic emergencies or looking for pseudoaneurysms, that superselective wedged injections carry the risk of rupturing a damaged blood vessel. Therefore superselective catheterization is done only after the diagnosis has been established and only if needeed for treatment

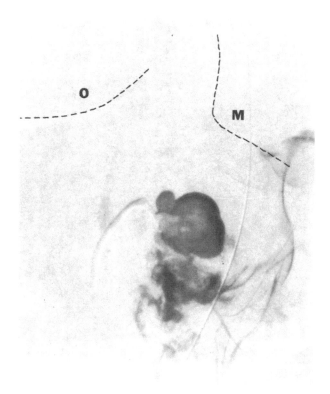

fistulas in more than half of the cases. In some, the fistula was at a different location from the fracture or pseudoaneurysm. These lesions were always associated with severe head trauma and the mortality rate was more than 50%. The clinical course of patients with pseudoaneurysms differs significantly compared to that of those with arteriovenous fistulas. False aneurysms frequently produce signs of delayed hemorrhage, and are one of the causes of coma following a typical lucid interval in patients with epidural hematomas and late intracranial hemorrhage (Roski 1981). Patients with traumatic AV fistulas, if untreated, often recover spontaneously.

Ericson (1981) described the frequent occurrence of extravasation from the middle meningeal artery and filling of diploic veins in patients with epidural hematomas during good quality external carotid angiography. The filling of diploic or dural veins following head trauma does not necessarily indicate a true arteriovenous fistula, but may be secondary to active extravasation into a closed compartment at high pressure. Traumatic middle meningeal aneurysms or dural AV fistulas may give acute Bell's palsy.

With the exception of the intracranial branches, traumatic lesions of the external carotid artery produces few symptoms, probably because of the rich local collateral circulation. In symptomatic patients the clinical diagnosis is usually based on a pulsatile mass in the distribution of one of the external carotid artery branches (Figs. 7.21, 7.23). Turbulent flow within an aneurysm may give the false impression of a "bruit" which suggests the presence of a fistula. Epistaxis may occur in sphenopalatine injuries, and may be intermittent (Figs. 10.33, 7.20). Late development of symptoms may occur as other false aneurysms may present with a pulsatile mass. Differentiation of true pulsations from transmitted pulsations through a

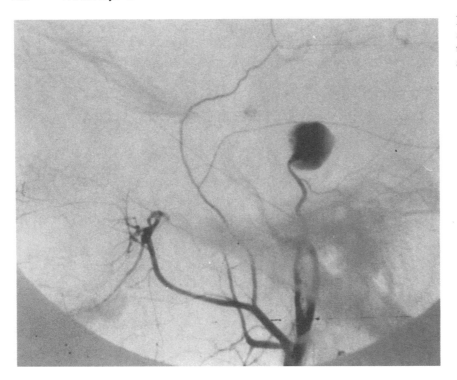

Fig. 7.23. Traumatic pseudo-aneurysm of the superficial temporal artery, presenting as a pulsatile mass

mass is important, but may sometimes be difficult. The diagnosis is made by CT followed by angiography. Extravasation of contrast material may be demonstrated during periods of active bleeding (Fig. 7.22). When performing angiography on an emergency basis after trauma, one should be prepared to embolize, as it may be lifesaving.

Other causes of pseudoaneurysms in the external carotid distribution include radiation therapy for malignant disease, vessel wall invasion by tumor (Fig. 7.22), and iatrogenic vessel injury during surgery or percutaneous biopsy. The evaluation of acute bleeding in a patient who may have a pseudoaneurysm is one of the few situations where superselective angiography is *not* indicated, as there is a real risk of rupture and hemorrhage if the catheter is wedged during injections (Fig. 7.22).

Mycotic aneurysms of the external carotid artery are extremely rare; we have had no personal experience with such.

Developmental or congenital aneurysms of the external carotid artery are seen in arteriovenous malformations (Fig. 10.15) and in some of the phakomatosis syndromes (Fig. 8.17).

Embolization of External Carotid Aneurysms

Aneurysms of the external carotid artery are usually easier to treat by endovascular occlusion, than those of the internal carotid artery, and the success rate is near 100%. Almost any technique that produces a mechanical obstruction is effective in traumatic lesions (Fig. 7.20).

IV. Extradural Vertebral Aneurysms

Extradural vertebral aneurysms are rare; in a review of 125 cases Killian (1950) reported that 17.5% involved the first or proximal segment, 70% the second portion, and 12.5% the third portion of the vertebral artery. Trauma is the most frequent cause. After its origin from the subclavian artery, the first segment of the vertebral artery is enclosed by fascia as it traverses the neck to enter the transverse foramen of the 6th cervical vertebral body. At this point it courses between tendons of the scalenus anterior, longus coli and scalenus media muscles. It then ascends through the transverse foramena of the upper cervical vertebra. It is accompanied by a plexus of veins, which communicate with the epidural lingitudinal vertebral sinus, the basisvertebral veins, and the prevertebral veins, which ultimately drain into the internal jugular vein. The third segment exists from the transverse foramena of the atlas and courses posteriorly and medially arround the lateral mass of the atlas to reach a groove on the upper surface of the posterior arch of the atlas. The fourth segment of the vertebral artery penetrates the oblique ligament of the atlas (inferior border of the atlanto-occipital membrane), pierces the dura of the spine and then courses upwards through the forament magnum to unite with the opposite side to form the basilar artery (Davis 1983).

Because the vertebral artery is significantly affected by neck motion, a description of head and neck kinetics is warranted (Davis 1983). Approximately 15° of the full 130° of cervical flexion and extension occurs at the atlanto-occipital joint. Motion at this joint is limited in part by the transverse ligament which attaches the odontoid process to the anterior arch of C1. The atlanto-occipital joint also allows approximately 12° of head and neck rotation from the midline with an additional 12° occurring at the lateral atlanto-axial joint. When the head starts to turn, the atlas pivots eccentrically on the ipsilateral atlanto-axial joint (Kapandji 1974). Because of this anatomical disposition turning the head may produce vertebrobasilar damage. Vertebral dissections and thrombosis have been reported following a variety of movements, especially chiropractic manipulations and sports.

Most traumatic pseudoaneurysms of the vertebral artery result from penetrating injuries, including osseous fracture fragments. Due to the close proximity between the vertebral artery and the paravertebral venous plexus, arteriovenous fistulas following trauma and direct puncture vertebral angiography are relatively more frequent than pseudoaneurysms (see Chapter 6, VAFs) (Davis 1983, Dutton 1970, Jamieson 1965, Lester 1966, McDowell 1971).

Nontraumatic aneurysms of the vertebral artery are more rare. Among 125 cases reported by Kilian (1951) 7 had mycotic aneurysms associated with osteomyelitis of the cervical vertebrae. A primary dissecting aneurysm of the vertebral artery resulting from degeneration of the media was described in a hypertensive 56 year old female by Bostrom in 1967. Newton (1968) reported an unusual case of bilateral saccular aneurysms of the vertebral arteries, internal carotid artery and brachial artery, probably the result of a congenital defect in the media. Enlargement of the adjacent neural foramena indicated that the lesions were longstanding. We have seen bilateral dysplastic aneurysms of the vertebral arteries in a young male who presented with supratentorial TIA's secondary to a third dysplastic aneurysm of the left internal carotid artery associated by a long proximal stenosis and/or dissection (Fig. 7.2).

The angiographic work up is the same as described for patients with cavernous aneurysms, and includes full angiographic work-up to rule out additional lesions, assessment of collateral circulation and tolerance testing. The treatment of choice for surgically inaccessible lesions is trapping of the aneurysm with preservation of supply to the ipsilateral posterior inferior cerebellar artery. The technique and principles are similar to those mentioned in the treatment of carotid artery aneurysms and vertebral artery fistulas (see Chapters 1 and 6).

V. Fibromuscular Dysplasia (FMD)

1. General

Fibromuscular dysplasia (FMD) is an increasing recognized angiodysplasia. Manelfe's (1974) review of 70 cases in France and more recently Mettinger's (1982) review of 37 patients demonstrated that FMD is often associated with high blood pressure and is more frequent in middle aged Caucasian females. The disease is characterized by multifocal dysplasia of vessel walls, involving branches of the aorta and is frequently associated with intracranial aneurysms. The lesions (Fig. 7.19) may be stable or progressive. Over 1/3 of patients have a family history of certain vascular disorders (stroke, high blood pressure, migraine, impaired hearing, cerebral hemorrhages etc.). It has been suggested that FMD is inherited as a dominant trait with reduced penetrance in males.

The morphological features in affected head and neck arteries are the same as those described in the renal artery, and include fibroblast like transformation of smooth muscle cells. Each of the three layers of the arterial wall may be dysplastic. The spectrum of lesions include the "beaded" type which is generally caused by medial fibroplasia (60–85%) with alternating ridges (fibroproliferative tissue or collagen disrupting the smooth muscle) and aneurysms (deficient smooth muscle or lamina elastica interna) in the media. Tubular stenosis (elongated narrowing of the lumen) and focal ring-shaped or eccentric stenoses may also occur. Macroscopic aneurysmal outpounchings and dissections present on angiographic and at gross pathological examination are thought to represent complications of FMD.

FMD of the brachiocephalic vessels characteristically occurs distal to the cervical bifurcations and is rarely found in the proximal portions of the carotid or vertebral arteries. The angiographic appearances were classified by Osborne in 1977 into 3 groups: ·

Type 1: present with the classical "string of beads" with multiple contrictions of the lumen in the affected segment; between the constrictions, the lumen appears normal or enlarged (Fig. 7.19B). A single constriction may exist.

Type 2A: tubular stenosis with or without further constrictions.

Type 2B: tubular stenosis with aneurysmal dilatations in the stenotic segment of the vessel (Fig. 7.20).

Type 3: Semicircumferential lesions concentrated on one side of the vessel wall, producing a diverticulum like smooth or corrugated outpouching, referred to as "atypical FMD".

The clinical presentation of FMD is includes frequent headaches in more than 90%, high blood pressure, high incidence of associated cerebral aneurysms with cerebral hemorrhages and frequent occurence of ischemic cerebral episodes. Associated Horner's syndrome and hearing impairment may occur. These symptoms, when present in a young patient (particularly a female) are highly suggestive of FMD.

2. Diagnosis and Treatment of FMD

When performing vascular studies for cerebral hemorrhage of ischemic episodes in young women with high blood pressure, we recommend a complete angiographic study, even if the characteristic angiographic pattern of FMD is not found in the symptomatic side. In patients with subarachnoid hemorrhage, it is often difficult to differentiate FMD from spam or flow artifacts which are frequently seen during angiography (especially after direct carotid puncture). Manelfe (1974) found involvement of the occipital artery to be a sensitive indicator of FMD.

Renal angiography should be done routinely in these patients to document stenosis. Stenotic lesions of the carotid arteries may be treated either by surgical resection of the involved segment or by progressive intraoperative dilatation (Ehrenfeld 1974). More recently, Hasso (unpublished data) has reported the use of angioplasty balloons to dilate single constrictions (Type 1) with apparently good results. The use of antiplatelet medications appears to be effective in preventing cerebral ischemic episodes.

When an extradural aneurysm associated with FMD is to be treated by embolization, the parent vessel probably should be sacrified, as in the treatment of aneurysms in other vascular dysplasias (Neurofibromatosis). If preserved the dysplastic wall may fail to support the hemodynamic changes, resulting in distal embolization. The issue is obviously controversial and therefore should be thoroughly assessed in each individual case.

CHAPTER 8

Dural Arteriovenous Malformations (DAVMs)

Dural arteriovenous malformations (DAVMs) represent abnormal shunts within the dura. Theoretically, they can occur at any site within the dura, but most frequently they develop near the venous sinuses. Venous drainage may occur via the venous sinuses or meningeal veins, via adjacent cortical cerebral or cerebellar veins, or a combination. Arterial supply is usually through adjacent branches of the neuromeningeal arteries although less frequently cutaneous or osseous (posterior auricular, deep temporal) branches may contribute.

The use of the term malformation is somewhat inappropriate, as it implies a developmental origin, while there is evidence that these lesions are at least partly acquired, probably secondary to venous obstruction (Figs. 8.1, 8.2). Although they frequently occur spontaneously, trauma, infection and hormonal changes have been implicated as etiologic factors.

I. Historical Review

Historically, these lesions have attracted considerable interest. DAVMs were first described by Sachs in 1931 and then by Tonnis in 1936 (Aminoff 1973).

Verbiest and Fincher (1951) first introduced the concept of the "spontaneous" dural fistulae. The early case reports described the slow flow lesions, and in 1964 van de Werf presented the first case of a spontaneous or congenital high flow dural arteriovenous malformation in a 3 year old child. The concept of the "spontaneous" DAVM has since stimulated much discussion and controversy.

The 1960's were marked by emphasis on the topography of individual cases (Hayes 1963, Laine 1963, Pecker 1965). Later reports demonstrated the role of angiographic analysis of these lesions using selective (Newton 1968, 1969, 1970) and supraselective (Djindjian 1968, 1973) techniques.

In the 1970's, major European and North American contributions further established the entity of spontaneous DAVMs (Houser 1972, Aminoff 1973, Obrador 1975).

Castaigne, in 1976, first emphasized the specific angiographic and clinical features of the DAVMs which drain into the cerebral veins.

The monograph of Djindjian (1978) illustrated most of the angiographic features of DAVM which can be demonstrated by supraselective techniques and presented the first large series of DAVMs treated by embolization; proposed a simplified classification based on the patterns of venous drainage (Table 8.1).

The late 1970's and early 1980's were marked by multiple individual case reports; more recently, the unusual potential for hemorrhagic complications with DAVMs of the anterior cranial fossa and tentorium (Ito 1983,

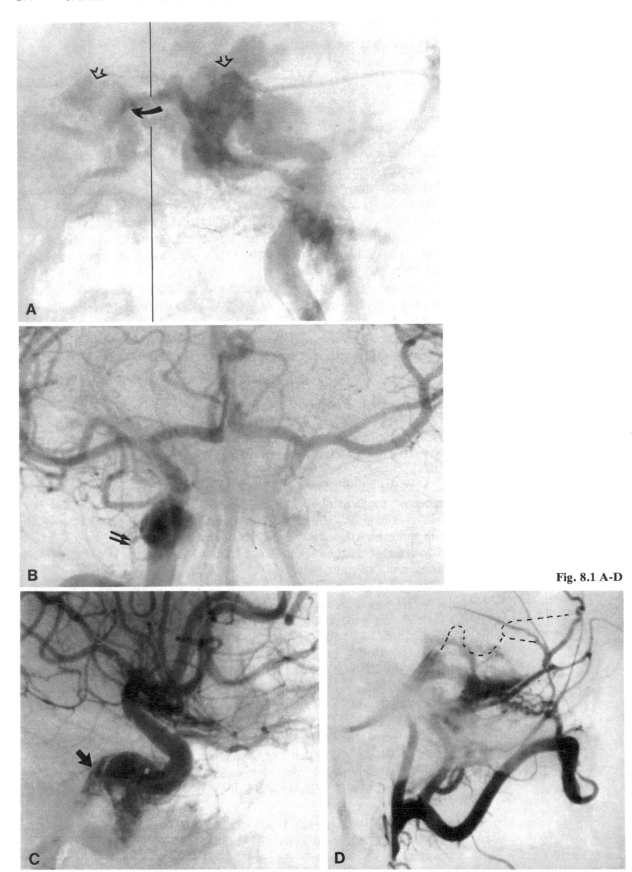

Fig. 8.1 A-D

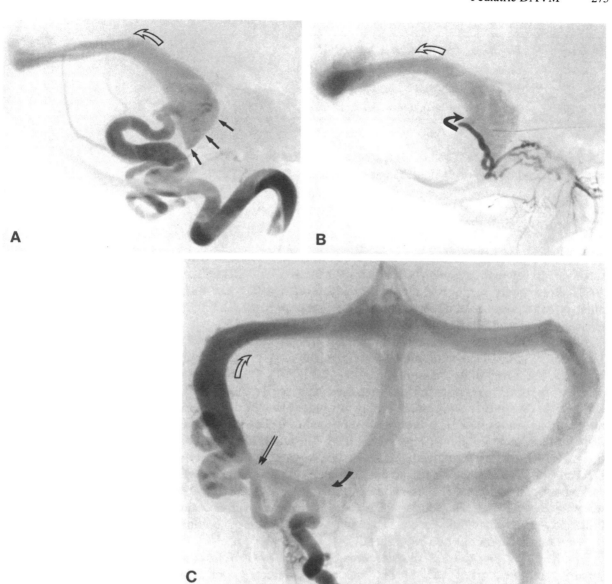

Fig. 8.2 A-C. 3 year old girl presenting with enlarged infraoccipital vascular channel, and an objective bruit in the right mastoid region with no history of previous trauma or other AVM. **A** Right selective occipital artery injection demonstrates a direct AVF between the mastoid branch and the sigmoid sinus. Note the distal sinus obstruction *(arrow)* and the retrograde drainage *(open curved arrow)* towards the opposite side. **B** Selective injection in the posterior branch of the ascending pharyngeal artery demonstrates the same AVF *(broken arrow)*. **C** The ipsilateral vertebral artery fills the fistula via the C_1 anastomosis with the occipital artery; note the drainage in the opposite jugular vein and the patency of the ipsilateral jugular foramen distal to the sigmoid sinus obstruction *(double arrow)*, filled via a medial occipital venous sinus *(curved arrow)*

◄ **Fig. 8.1. A** Left internal carotid angiogram in a patient with a traumatic CCF. Note the bilateral venous outflow *(curved arrow)* and opacification of both superior ophthalmic veins *(open arrows)*. **B** Opposite internal carotid angiogram. Note the visualization of ILT *(double arrow)* without evidence of shunt. **C** Right internal carotid angiogram. 3 months after successful embolization of the left CCF. The patient had complained of right-sided pulsatile tinnitus. A dural AVM is seen at the level of the cavernous sinus *(arrow)*. **D** Internal maxillary artery branches also supply the lesion. Note the unique drainage posteriorly

Table 8.1. Classification of DAVMs by venous drainage (Djindjian 1978)

Type I	Drainage into a sinus (or a meningeal vein)
Type II	Sinus drainage with reflux into cerebral veins
Type III	Drainage solely into cortical veins
Type IV	With supra or infra tentorial venous lake

Terada 1984, Grisoli 1984) and the characteristic features of DAVMs in the pediatric population (Albright 1983) were established (Table 8.7).

II. Pathophysiology

DAVMs are generally considered to be acquired lesions which develop secondary to venous obstruction (Djindjian 1978, Houser 1981, Chaudhary 1982). Presumably micro AV shunts normaly present within the dura enlarge in the presence of increased arterial or venous pressure leading to clinically significant arteriovenous shunting (Table 8.4).

A variety of causes of venous obstruction may be associated with DAVMs, including congenital anomalies (hypoplasia, aplasia), trauma, infection, and cerebral or craniofacial AVMs (Table 8.2). DAVMs have also been reported to occur following intracranial surgery (Watanabe 1984, Bitoh 1982, Aminoff 1973) presumably due to venous thrombosis or other alteration in venous flow. It is possible that the induced changes in dural flow (ie the dural AV shunt) may persist after the provocative process (venous obstruction) has resolved, this accounting for cases of spontaneous DAVMs, or DAVM which appear to present remote in time from possible causative events. However, if one considers that DAVMs are relatively uncommon, and that the factors which are felt to be causative occur frequently in the population (Table 8.2) it appears that factors in addition to venous obstruction must be implicated.

Djindjian (1978) reported the development of DAVMs following surgery in remote parts of the body (ie hysterectomy, varices) as well as in the post partum period. In 9 of 23 patients reported by Lasjaunias et al. (1984), DAVMs were associated with unusual circumstances, early childhood, pregnancy, premenstrual augmentation of symptoms, coincidental brain and palpebral AVM (Fig. 8.3) and developmental aneurysms (Fig. 8.4). Among the 23 patients, 9 had a history of trauma, but the trauma involved the head in only four. Fifteen patients were found to have some form of vascular disease, including hypertension and congenital anomalies of arteries and/or veins. Only one patient had a history of previous infection (brain abscess). More recently we have observed a DAVM in a patient with Rendu Osler Weber disease. Other authors have also reported an association between DAVMs and vascular abnormalities such as aneurysms and vascular malformations involving brain, skin and bone (Debrun 1972, Heishima 1977, Djindjian 1978, Robinson 1970) (Table 8.3). These observations suggest that DAVMs develop in the presence of a structural "weakness" in the dura which is activated by a trigger factor. It seems reasonable to postulate even in the pediatric population that DAVMs represent not the primary anomaly, but an

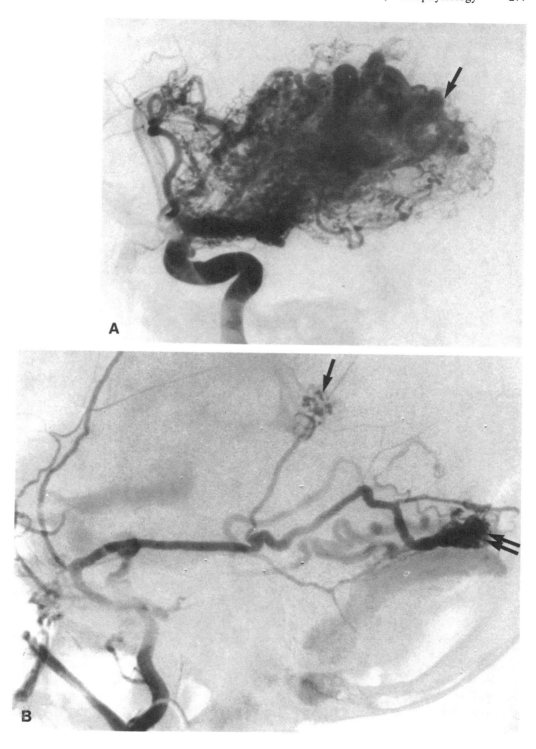

Fig. 8.3 A, B. Cerebral AVM in a 54 year old female which bled twice prior to this angiogram. **A** Left internal carotid angiogram. The posterior portion of the lesion *(arrow)* is supplied by dural vessels as seen during the ipsilateral internal maxillary artery injection **(B)**. In addition a DAVM of the transverse sinus *(double arrow)* is demonstrated; it lies separate from the brain AVM and drains both into the transverse sinus and temporal veins. Although no thrombosis could be demonstrated, the venous drainage of the high flow brain AVM showed indirect evidence of venous obstruction (venous ectasias)

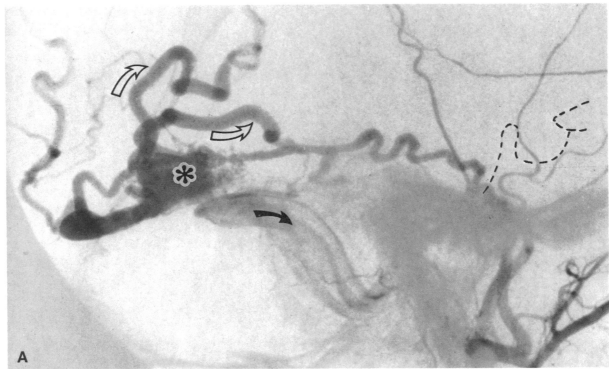

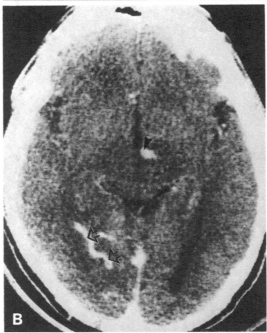

Fig. 8.4 A-D. 65 year old patient presenting with visual seizures. **A** Right distal external carotid angiogram demonstrates a DAVM of the lateral sinus *(asterisk)* draining both into the sigmoid sinus *(curved arrow)* and occipito-temporal *(open curved arrows)* venous systems. **B** CT examination demonstrates both the venous drainage of the lesion deep in the calcarine fissure *(open arrows)* and a premesen- cephalic enhancing mass *(arrowhead)*, which was shown to be a basilar tip aneurysm on the right vertebral angiogram *(arrow)*. **C** The DAVM was embolized with radiopaque IBCA before treatment of the basilar tip aneurysm to control one of the two possible causes of intradural bleeding **(D)**

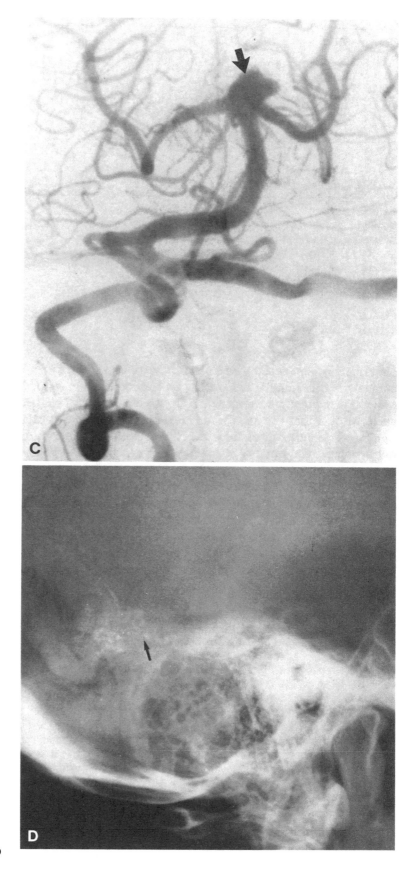

Fig. 8.4 C, D

Table 8.2. Venous abnormalities associated with DAVMs

Developmental anomalies:	– aplasia – hypoplasia
Venous thrombosis due to:	– trauma – infection – intracranial or cervical surgery – meningiomas – cerebral arteriovenous malformation

Table 8.3. Associated vascular diseases in DAVMs

Cerebral AVM
Maxillo-facial AVM
Intra- or extradural arterial aneurysms
Multiple DAVMs
Rendu Osler Weber disease
Bone AVM (local invasion or metameric expression?)

abnormal communication which has developed secondary to a venous anomaly or other similar defect. The secondary communication may have even occurred in utero, producing a "congenital lesion". From our experience, we feel that the most frequent triggering factor is a transient but significant venous obstruction, which transforms a clinically quiescient dural vascular abnormality into a clinically significant DAVM. However, obstruction or thrombosis alone cannot explain the infrequent presence of DAVMs in association with tumor invasion of major sinuses (see meningiomas and paragangliomas). We do not fully understand the nature of the underlying dural vascular "weakness" but it appears that increased pressure on the arterial or venous side can significantly alter local dural hemodynamics. The alteration can regress with the disappearance of the local hypertension, or can persist as a latent or as a clinically apparent DAVM (Table 8.4).

The clinical behavior of cavernous sinus DAVMs illustrates some of these proposed hypotheses. These lesions are supplied by the internal carotid artery and by branches of the internal maxillary artery (IMA) and are usually drained by the superior division of the ophthalmic vein which also drains the nasal mucosa. They can be associated with Rendu Osler Weber disease, pregnancy and hormonal changes, all of which involve nasal congestion. Some cavernous sinus DAVMs regress following bilateral particle embolization of IMA (Lasjaunias 1975). Aside from the occlusion of IMA branches to the cavernous sinus, the major effect of IMA embolization is a significant decrease in the arterial flow to the nasal mucosa and therefore in the superior orbital vein flow (Moret, personal communication). It is felt that the decrease in the nasal venous congestion is effective in decreasing the secondary hypertension in the cavernous sinus. Similarly, cavernous sinus DAVMs may respond to estrogen therapy, possibly also on the basis of a decrease in nasal venous hypertension; this mechanism remains so far speculative.

Table 8.4. Pathophysiological hypothesis for the development of "spontaneous" DAVMs

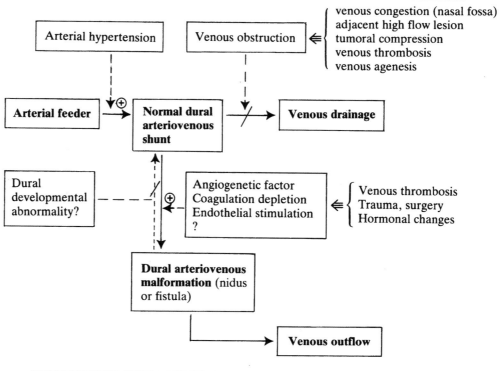

III. Classification

Although the topographical classification of DAVMs is useful in the planning of the endovascular therapeutic approach, we feel that it is more practical to classify these lesions according to their venous drainage (Table 8.1). DAVMs may drain solely into meningeal veins (in locations without dural sinuses such as the anterior cranial fossa or free margin of the tentorium) or into dural sinuses (Djindjian Type I); or into adjacent cortical veins (Djindjian Types II and III). As will be discussed later, it is of paramount importance to distinguish between those lesions without and those with cortical venous drainage. The symptomatology of these two groups of lesions differs and those with cortical venous drainage may be associated with life threatening complications, requiring a more agressive therapeutic approach (Lasjaunias 1984, 1986) (Fig. 8.5).

IV. Clinical Behavior of DAVMs

The symptomatology of DAVMs is variable, depending upon the location of the defect, the type of venous drainage, and the flow characteristics (Lasjaunias 1986). The possible effects are summarized in Tables 8.5–8.7, 8.9, 8.10, and include bruits, cranial nerve deficits, ophthalmologic complications, focal cerebral deficits, intracranial hypertension, hemorrhage, hydrocephalus and congestive heart failure.

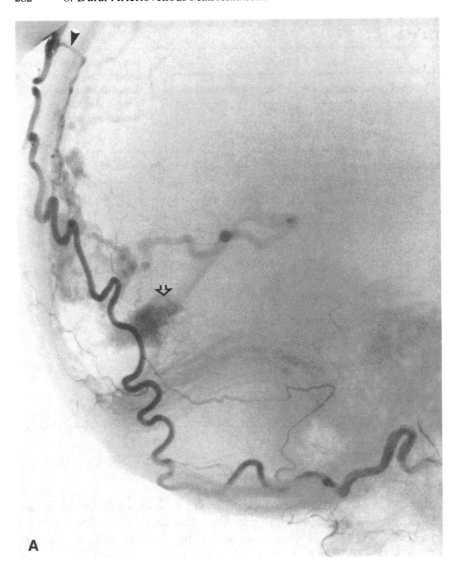

Fig. 8.5 A

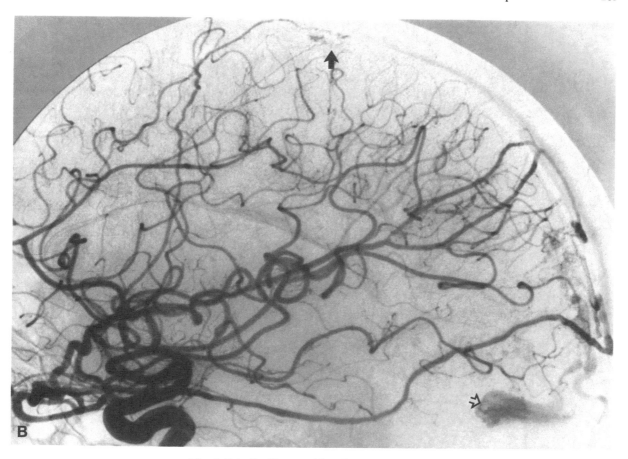

Fig. 8.5 A-C. 45 year old male presenting with visual seizures and headaches. **A** Right occipital angiogram demonstrates a dural AVM of the superior sagittal sinus fed by a transosseous artery *(arrowhead)*. Note the ectasia of the draining cortical veins *(open arrow)*. **B** Left internal carotid artery angiogram demonstrates the same DAVM and pouch *(open arrow)* fed by the middle meningeal artery which arises from the ophthalmic artery. In addition note the other DAVM involving the superior sagittal sinus *(arrow)*

Table 8.5. DAVMs of the cavernous sinus: neuro-ophthalmological symptoms

Cranial nerves palsies; III, IV, VI, V (partial or complete)
Proptosis
Conjunctival hyperemia
Hypertensive glaucoma
Decreased visual acuity

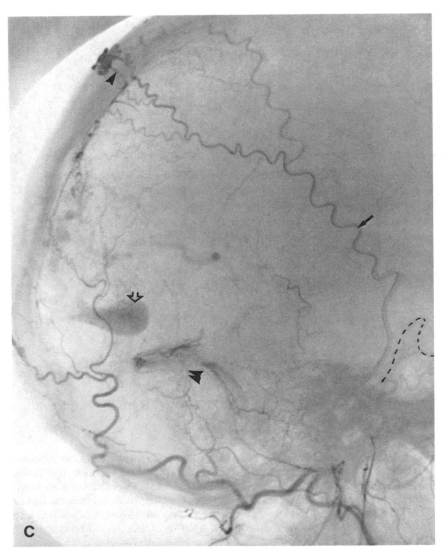

Fig. 8.5. C Right occipital artery angiogram 2 years after incomplete embolization with PVA particles and IBCA. Although the previous branches have been partially controlled, collateral circulation via the superficial temporal artery *(arrow)* via the transosseous branch *(arrowhead)*, still opacify the DAVM and its venous pouch *(open arrow)*. In addition a new DAVM at the sigmoid sinus is demonstrated *(double arrowhead)*

Table 8.6. General symptoms related to the DAVMs

Pulsatile tinnitus	Papilledema
Objective bruit	Craniomegaly
Mass effect (venous lake)	Optic atrophy
Hydrocephalus (communicating)	Heart failure

Table 8.7. Characteristics of pediatric DAVMs

High flow (communicating hydrocephalus)
Venous lakes (non communicating hydrocephalus Djindjian type IV)
Cardiac decompensation
Cortical atrophy
Involvement of the posterior circulation (venous)
Sinusal drainage
Poor prognosis
CSF reabsorption impairment (communicating hydrocephalus)

Fig. 8.6. 35 year old woman who presented during the last trimester of her first pregnancy with a spontaneously regressive left facial nerve palsy. 3 months post partum she developed a pulsatile bruit on the left side. She was blind in the right eye due to a congenital cataract. The middle meningeal angiogram demonstrates a DAVM at the level of the foramen spinosum fed by the petrous artery. Note the arterial ectasia *(double arrow)* and the posterior venous drainage

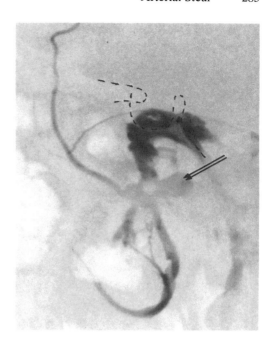

1. Symptoms Related to Arterial "Steal" Phenomena

Most DAVMs are relatively slow flow lesions with little or no significant supply from the internal carotid artery or vertebral artery. Therefore arterial "steal" is probably not responsible for cerebral symptoms. On the other hand the cranial nerves are perfused by the meningeal arteries and ischemia due to an arterial "steal" phenomenon may well contribute to the cranial nerve palsies sometimes encountered in these lesions (Lasjaunias 1984, 1986). The fact that cranial nerve symptoms may be relieved following selective arterial embolization supports the concept of an arterial steal phenomenon. Figure 8.6 illustrates a cavernous sinus DAVM with meningeal arterial supply, which was associated with facial nerve palsy. Other authors have suggested that venous occlusive or mechanical factors are responsible for the cranial nerve symptoms produced by DAVMs (Brismar 1976, Vinuela 1984). Possibly either or both mechanisms play a role, depending upon the location.

Table 8.8. Causes of the venous dilatation

Venous ectasias	– vascular mural dysplasia – arterial compression (post stenotic ectasia) – subdural-dural venous junction stenosis
Venous lakes	– intra sinusal dilatation – extra dural (diploic) dilatation

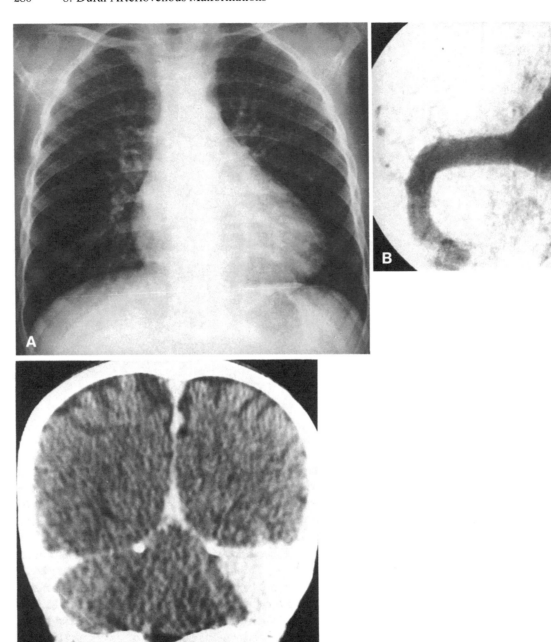

Fig. 8.7 A-G. 5 year old boy who presented with a failure to thrive, an objective intense bruit of which he did not complain, moderate macrocephaly, dyspnea with effort, and poor school performance. **A** Chest X-ray shows moderate enlargement of the cardiac silhouette (cardiac output measurement was 9 L/mn). **B** Intravenous digital angiography demonstrates a large supratentorial venous lake derived from the left lateral sinus. **C** Frontal enhanced CT

Fig. 8.7 (continued). Selective injections in the left internal carotid **(D)** occipital **(E)** and ascending pharyngeal **(F)** arteries demonstrate the multiple feeders to the pouch (supratentorial) *(arrow and double arrow)*, infratentorial *(arrowhead)*, and transosseous *(double arrowhead)*. The same vessels on the right side supplied the lesion (not shown). The shunt was well controlled by incomplete embolization and the systemic effects of the shunt on growth and school performance abated within one year. **G** Follow up showed a moderate decrease in the size of the venous mass

Fig. 8.7 D-G

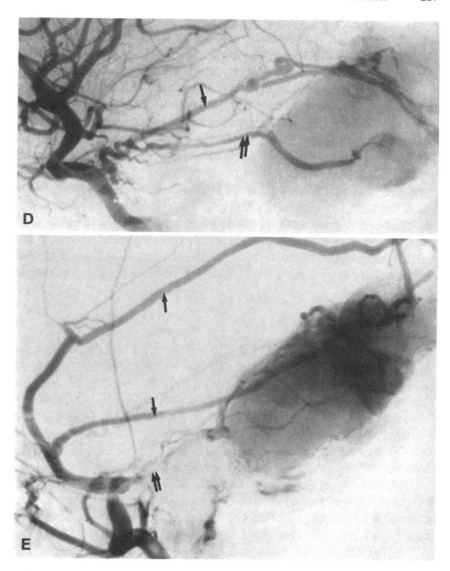

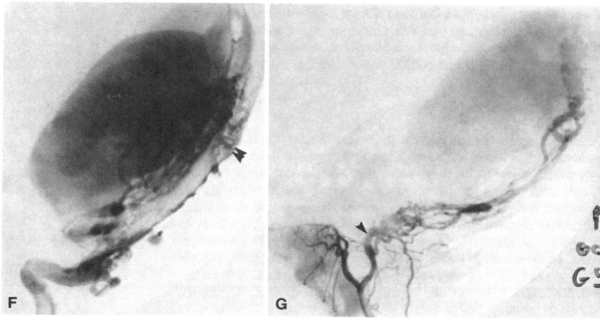

2. Factors Involved in the Production of Tinnitus and Objective Bruits

At angiography two distinct types of nidus morphology can be recognized: those with a single arterial feeder and an AV fistula and those with a complex arterial network and multiple AV shunts. Pulsatile tinnitus occurs in both types and is produced by turbulent flow in the nidus and adjacent draining vein. However, DAVMs in some locations are more commonly associated with this symptom than others (Table 8.6) and it appears that tinnitus is most frequently perceived when the drainage involves a venous sinus which is in direct contact with the petrous pyramid. The higher the flow in the nidus, the more intense is the tinnitus. 40% of patients with pulsatile tinnitus have objective bruits (Lasjaunias 1986). They are constant in the pediatric population, presumably because DAVMs in children are usually high flow lesions (Albright 1983). It is important to realize that children with DAVMs and objective bruits may not complain of tinnitus if the lesion has been present since birth as they perceive the sound as normal.

3. High Flow Lesions

As described above, high flow DAVMs are usually associated with intense tinnitus and objective bruits and are characteristic of the pediatric population. Especially in infants, these lesions may lead to cardiac decompensation and death (Table 8.7). In addition, the large draining dural venous lakes may have significant mass effect (Fig. 8.7, Table 8.8) (Albright 1983, Gursoy 1979, Van de Werf 1964). Torcular ectasia secondary to adjacent DAVM may occur to the same degree as is seen with the vein of Galen "aneurysms" secondary to brain AVMs, with the same local effects.

Other effects of high flow DAVMs in children include increased intracranial pressure and communicating hydrocephalus with secondary macrocephaly. Analogous effects occur in the adult population, manifest as papilledema and optic atrophy (Kuhner 1976, Sundt 1983).

These effects are felt to be secondary to chronic impairment of CSF absorption (Sundt 1983) which may be produced by two mechanisms: venous sinus hypertension (Lamas 1977) or repeated episode of minor subarachnoid hemorrhage with subsequent meningeal reaction (Kosnick 1974). The former mechanism is more frequent, as hemorrhage in general occurs only with lesions with cortical venous drainage.

4. Venous Thrombosis (Fig. 8.8)

Although increased flow in the venous sinuses secondary to the AV shunt is sufficient to produce increased intracranial pressure, the problem is aggravated by obstruction to venous outflow, and sigmoid sinus thrombosis (Sundt 1983). Focal thrombosis of dural venous sinuses which are less important for craniofugal drainage generally does not produce raised intracranial pressure but, because it modifies the direction of flow from the AV shunt, may affect the clinical manifestations of the lesions; for example partial cavernous sinus thrombosis is frequently (Brismar 1976, Viñuela 1984) present with cavernous sinus DAVMs, but raised intracranial pressure has not been reported in patients with these lesions. A thorough

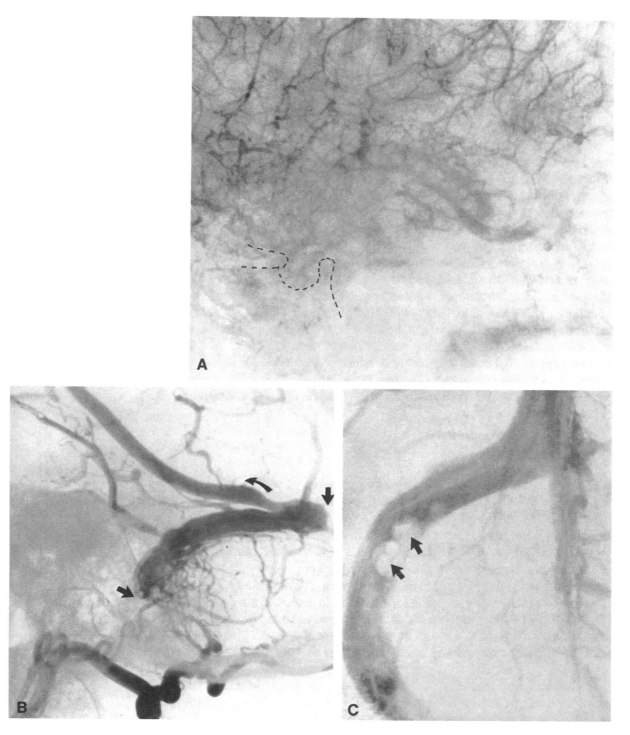

Fig. 8.8 A-C. 60 year old male presenting with intermittent temporal aphasia. **A** Note on the venous phase of the internal carotid arterial injection the venous hypertension of the left hemisphere. Most of the venous drainage is via the superior sagittal sinus. **B** The injection in the occipital artery demonstrates a DAVM of the transverse sinus, draining into the vein of Labbé *(curved arrow)*. Note the proximal and distal thrombosis of the sinus *(solid arrows)*. **C** Venous phase of the opposite internal carotid artery injection confirms the patency of the contralateral sigmoid sinus and demonstrates two defects *(arrows)* inside the lateral sinus, interpreted as thrombi or cavernous nodules

knowledge of the anatomic variations of venous drainage of the head is necessary to fully appreciate all the changes associated with DAVMs (Dora 1980). In our experience, DAVMs of the posterior fossa (sigmoid or transverse sinus), presenting with papilledema often developed on a dominant or single draining sinus.

5. Venous Ischemia

In addition to this generalized effects of increased venous pressure described above, patient with drainage of DAVMs into cortical veins may manifest focal CNS symptoms (Castaigne 1976, Lasjaunias 1986). The symptomatology depends upon the topography of the lesion and especially the draining veins and may include aphasia, motor weakness, transient deficit and seizures (Miyasaka 1970). These symptoms are ischemic in nature and are related to chronic increased pressure in the veins which drain both the DAVM and underlying normal brain (Kosnick 1974) (Fig. 8.8). This phenomenon is well demonstrated by angiography. Prior to embolization, the venous phase of cerebral angiography shows absence of opacification of the cortical veins which drain the DAVM, and rerouting of drainage to adjacent territories. Following successful embolization of the dural arterial supply of the lesions, cerebral arteriography typically shows a return of the drainage of the involved brain into the veins previously opacified by the DAVM. At the same time the focal cerebral symptomatology may be reversed.

6. Venous Mass Effect

Mechanical compression of CNS structures by enlarged venous channels draining the DAVMs has been suggested as a cause of some symptoms (Kosnick 1974). Although it is conceivable that a large venous lake may exert a significant mass effect (Table 8.8) (Castaigne 1976, Lepoire 1963, Van de Werf 1964) we feel that in general the mechanical effect is less important than the secondary raised venous pressure. Figure 8.13 illustrates a patient in whom the mechanical compression of the visual pathway appeared to be the best explanation for a visual field defect. In this example of a DAVM of the floor of the anterior cranial fossa, the olfactory vein and basal vein of Rosenthal were dilated, but there was no angiographic evidence of a hemodynamically significant venous obstruction.

Mechanical phenomena may also be responsible for the pseudoextraocular motor nerve palsies in patients with cavernous sinus DAVMs draining into the orbital venous system; diplopia and restricted ocular motor function may be secondary to the proptosis and altered muscle tension rather than nerve dysfunction. An interesting feature of cavernous sinus DAVMs is the occurrence of "paradoxical" symptoms, when ipsilateral cavernous sinus thrombosis causes rerouting of venous drainage to the contralateral orbital veins (Fig. 8.9).

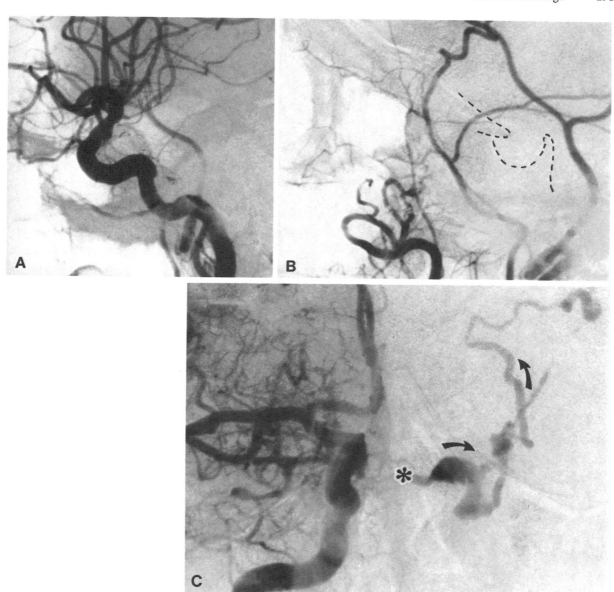

Fig. 8.9 A-C. 68 year old female presenting with progressive left exophthalmus associated with conjunctival hyperemia. Contrast injections in the ipsilateral internal carotid **(A)** and in the internal maxillary **(B)** arteries failed to demonstrate an abnormality. **C** The contralateral internal carotid angiogram injection demonstrates a DAVM *(asterisk)* draining into the left cavernous sinus and ophthalmic vein *(curved arrows)*

7. Venous Rupture

Intradural hemorrhage is a specific complication of DAVMs with cortical venous drainage (Castaigne 1976, Lasjaunias 1986) and is one cause of focal CNS manifestations. In a review of patients with all forms of venous drainage, Obrador (1975) reported an incidence of hemorrhage of 20%. Castaigne (1976) reported that 42% of DAVMs with cortical venous drainage were complicated by intradural homorrhage. These figures may underestimate the true incidence of bleeding, as episodes of headache,

Fig. 8.10 A-F

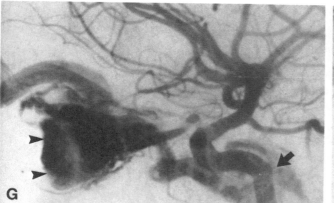
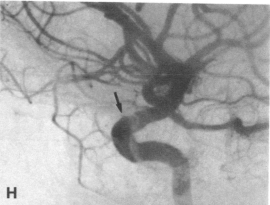

Fig. 8.10 A-H. 30 year old male with progressive left exophthalmus conjunctival hyperemia and occular pain following hypertensive glaucoma, without a history of previous trauma. At the time of the initial study he had been blind for 4 months. **A** Internal carotid angiogram demonstrates a DAVM of the optic nerve *(solid arrow)* with an intraconal venous pouch draining into the ophthalmic vein anteriorly and also into the cavernous sinus posteriorly. Note the enlarged C_5 collateral of the carotid siphon *(broken arrow)* which appeared to contribute to the intracavernous shunt in the early phases (not shown). Injections in the middle meningeal artery in lateral **(B)** and frontal **(C)** projections demonstrate shunts both in the orbit *(arrow)* and in the cavernous region *(double arrow)*. **D** Distal internal maxillary artery injection demonstrates two additional feeders to the DAVM from the infraorbital *(arrow)* and anterior deep temporal *(double arrow)* arteries. Plain skull films **(E)** and **(F)** postembolization show the radiopaque IBCA in both the orbital nidus *(arrow)* and the cavernous sinus nidus *(double arrow)*. **G** The immediate postembolization control angiogram in the left internal carotid artery shows a decrease in flow in the orbital lesion with a fluid level into the pouch *(arrowhead)*. The C_5 internal carotid branch is no longer visible. The patient was asked to perform manual compression of his left carotid artery with the right hand for 1 minute each hour. **H** Five days later a control angiogram shows complete disappearance of the lesion. The ophthalmic artery is not seen *(arrow)*

which may be due to minor hemorrhage are common (Sundt 1983). Cortical venous drainage occurs with a high frequency in DAVMs in several locations; those in the anterior cranial fossa (Ito 1983, Terada 1984) and in the tentorium (Grisoli 1984), accounting for the higher incidence of hemorrhagic complications in these locations. Bleeding may occur in the subarachnoid and subdural spaces and intracerebral structures but does not occur in the epidural space. The incidence of repeated hemorrhages is not known; one patient reported by Grisoli (1984) experienced two episodes of hemorrhage within a twelve day period.

V. Evolution of Symptoms

Secondary thrombosis of the venous outlet of a DAVM which initially drained only into sinus may lead to rerouting of the venous drainage into cortical veins, leading to potential focal CNS symptoms and/or hemorrhagic complications. The disappearance of pulsatile tinnitus preceding

Table 8.9. Major symptoms related to the anatomic type of venous drainage (DAVMs in adults) (Lasjaunias 1986)

Sinusal venous drainage	Cortical venous drainage
Proptosis	Intradural bleeding
Cranial nerve palsy	Focal CNS deficits
Visual symptoms	Seizures
ICP changes	Transient CNS symptoms
Bruits	

ICP, intracranial pressure

the development of ICH or focal CNS manifestations, implies a change in the venous drainage (Castaigne 1976). Thrombosis may also lead to the so-called spontaneous cure of a DAVM, but probably only if the thrombosis extends into the nidus. Spontaneous regression has been reported following hemorrhage (Katoaka 1984, Olutola 1983), and is more frequent in slow flow lesions. It has not been reported to occur in children (Albright 1983) and also appears to be infrequent in lesions with cortical venous drainage. Hypertensive glaucoma and retinal detachment may be observed in the evolution of some cavernous sinus DAVMs, but the mechanisms which produce these complications are not well understood. Both occur in the presence of slow flow lesions which drain into the ophthalmic venous system. Probably, glaucoma is the result of a disorder of vitreous reabsorption and retinal detachment is secondary to venous rupture. Visual impairment is related primarily to congestive venous ischemia of the optic nerve and may progress acutely following venous thrombosis, since collateral venous drainage of the orbit is poor (Fig. 8.10).

In summary, with exception of cranial nerve involvement, the symptomatology of DAVMs can all be related to the nature of, and temporal changes in, their venous drainage (Fig. 8.11).

Table 8.9 summarizes the relationships between the clinical symptoms and the type of venous drainage seen at angiography (Gaston 1984).

Table 8.10 lists the symptomatology related to the location of the nidus, as determined from a series of 192 patients (Lasjaunias 1986). DAVMs in two locations have the highest incidence of hemorrhage: the floor of the anterior cranial fossa (84%) and the tentorial area (70%). The same locations having the highest incidence of cortical venous drainage (compare with the lower incidence of hemorrhage in other areas: cavernous sinus 0–1%, posterior circulation 15%), reflect the fact that the draining veins in these locations cannot enlarge significantly in response to changes in AV shunting.

The greater potential for venous dilatation on the surface of the spinal cord is remarkable since spinal DAVMs have not been reported to bleed, while intracranial DAVMs do (see Vol. 4).

In comparing the two groups of DAVMs with sinus or cortical venous drainage it is interesting to note the difference in the distribution between the genders; in general DAVMs occur more frequently in males (with a male to female ratio of 1.5 : 1) but in the group with cortical venous drainage females predominate (female to male ratio 3:1 reported by Gaston 1984).

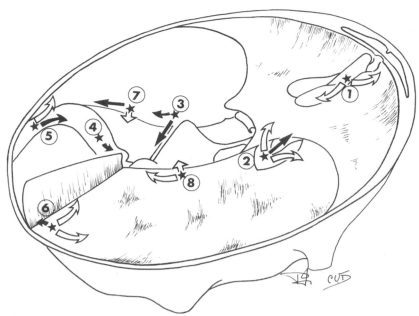

Fig. 8.11. Schematic representation of the most common DAVM locations *(asterisk)* with their possible venous drainage; the *plain arrows* correspond to sinus drainage, and *open arrows* to cortical (or intradural) venous drainage. *1* Anterior cranial fossa: frontal vein and olfactory vein. *2* Anterior cavernous sinus: ophthalmic vein, Breschet's sinus and deep sylvian vein. *3* Posterior cavernous sinus: superior and inferior petrosal sinuses. *4* Sigmoid sinus: sigmoid sinus and internal jugular vein. *5* Transverse sinus: sigmoid sinus and temporal veins (vein of Labbé). *6* Torcular: medial occipital and infratemporal veins. *7* Basal tentorial: superior petrosal sinus and petrous vein. *8* Marginal tentorial: tentorial veins, vein of Rosenthal, lateral mesencephalic veins

VI. Natural History

The natural history of DAVMs is unknown as insufficient numbers of well documented cases have been followed without treatment.

However DAVMs are not static lesions: they may *regress*, either spontaneously or following hemorrhage or angiography; manual compression of the cervical vessels by the *opposite* hand may be useful in stimulating thrombosis of slow flow DAVMs. Regression following direct puncture angiography may involve the same mechanism. Spontaneous regression should not be expected in patients with high flow lesions, cortical venous drainage, or in children.

Spontaneous *progression* may also occur; the severity of symptoms depends upon the topography and the type of initial venous drainage (Fig. 8.11, Tables 8.10, 8.11): cavernous sinus, blindness; sigmoid sinus, CSF malabsorption; torcular, tentorial and anterior cranial fossa: focal CNS symptoms.

The changes which produce progression in lesions with initial cortical venous drainage are venous rupture with hemorrhage and venous thrombosis. The factors which induce progression of lesions which initially drain into dural sinuses or meningeal veins include thrombosis, with rerouting of venous drainage or increased ICP. Increase in the AV shunt may affect both types of lesions.

Table 8.10. Major manifestations of pure spontaneous DAVMs

Anterior fossa		Cavernous sinus		Tentorial		Lateral sinus, sigmoid sinus and torcular	
Intradural bleeding:	84%	Intradural bleeding:	0%[a]	Intradural bleeding:	70%	Intradural bleeding:	15%
SAH	63%	Bruit	42%	SAH	80%	Bruit	70%
ICH	50%	Visual symptoms	28%	ICH	60%	Visual symptoms	12%
SDH	25%	Proptosis	83%	SDH	10%	Papilledema	22%
		CNS	3%	CNS	42%	Headache	46%
		PNS	44%	PNS	14%	CNS	13%
						PNS	7%

PNS, Peripheral nervous system deficits; CNS, Focal central nervous symptoms; SAH, Subarachnoid hemorrhage; ICH, Intracerebral hematoma; SDH, Subdural hematoma

[a] In the large series selected no bleeding was found; however intra cerebral hematomas have been observed as a rare presentation in a DAVM of the cavernous sinus.

Table 8.11. Most common type of drainage of intracranial DAVMs in adults

Location	Sinusal venous drainage	Cortical venous drainage
– Cavernous sinus	Almost constant	Rare
– Sigmoid sinus	Almost constant	Rare
– Superior sagittal	Depending on type	Depending on type
– Transverse sinus	Depending on type	Depending on type
– Torcular	Depending on type	Depending on type
– Anterior cranial fossa	Not described	(Almost?) constant
– Tentorium	Rare	Almost constant

VII. Hormonal Influences

The onset of symptoms during pregnancy due to DAVMs has been reported several times (Doyon 1973, Toya 1981, Lasjaunias 1984). We have also noted premenstrual augmentation of symptoms in females.

One such patient, a 48 year old woman, had acute visual symptoms each month before the onset of her menses. Embolization of the cavernous sinus DAVM (ipsilateral ECA and ICA) was incomplete, leaving a small amount of flow from the opposite ICA system. She initially showed a marked clinical improvement but symptoms recurred in the premenstrual period one month later. After one 8 week course of oral dihydrostilbestrol her lesion regressed completely and has not recurred.

The exact target of action of hormones in patients with DAVMs is unknown. We have not observed distinguishing angiographic features of the vascular architecture. However, these cases do illustrate a definitive relationship between hormonal changes and clinical symptoms in some patients, and of this group some may benefit from a trial of estrogen therapy prior to more aggressive treatment.

Table 8.12. DAVM-Angiographic protocols

Region to explore: ipsilateral pedicles	Internal carotid artery (ICA)	Internal maxillary artery (IM)	Middle meningeal artery (MM)	Ascending pharyngeal artery (AsP)	occipital artery (OA)	Vertebral artery (VA)	Other arterial pedicles
Anterior cerebral fossa	A/P and L (+)	A/P (+) L (+)	L (+)	–	–	–	– Contralateral ICA: A/P (+), Distal IM:A/P (+) and MM:A/P (+)
Anterior part of cavernous sinus	L (+)	L (+)	L (+)	L (+) cavernous ramus	–	–	– Contralateral ICA: A/P (+)
Posterior part of cavernous sinus	L (+)	L (+)	L (+)	L (+)	L (±)	L (+)	– Contralateral ICA: A/P (+), As.P. (clival anastomoses): A/P (+) and IMA: A/P (±)
Insicura tentorii	L (+)	L (+)	L (+)	L (+)	L (+)	L (+)	– Contralateral ICA: A/P (+), As.P. (clival anastomoses): A/P (+)
Transverse and sigmoid sinuses	L (+)	–	L (+)	L (+)	L (+)	A/P + L (+)	– Posterior auricular (±) (see confluens sinuum)
Confluens sinuum	A/P (+) contro-lateral compression	–	L (+)	L (+)	L (+)	A/P + L (+)	– MM and contralateral OA: A/P (+) – Contralateral AsP: L (+) and dominant VA A/P (+)
Superior sagittal sinus	L (+)	–	L(+)	–	L (+)	A/P (+)	– Contralateral ICA: A/P (+) – MM: A/P (+) – Occipital: A/P (+) – Superfic. temporal artery bilaterally
Foramen magnum	A/P (±)	–	L (±)	L (+)	L (+)	A/P + L (+)	– Contralateral As.P.: A/P (+) – Contralateral occipital: L (+)

(+) artery should be injected in all cases; (±) should be injected according to anatomical variation; (−), injection unnecessary; A/P, anteroposterior films; L, lateral films

VIII. Pretherapeutic Evaluation

Although routine skull radiographs may demonstrate prominent vascular markings and enlarged foramen at the base (foramen spinosum) due to increased flow in the meningeal vessels, as well as signs of increased intracranial pressure (Brismar 1976, Newton 1968) CT or MRI examinations are necessary in the early evaluation of the patient (Chiras 1982, Myasaka 1980, Solis 1977, Waga 1977). In patients with pure peripheral dural sinus or meningeal venous drainage, these examinations may be

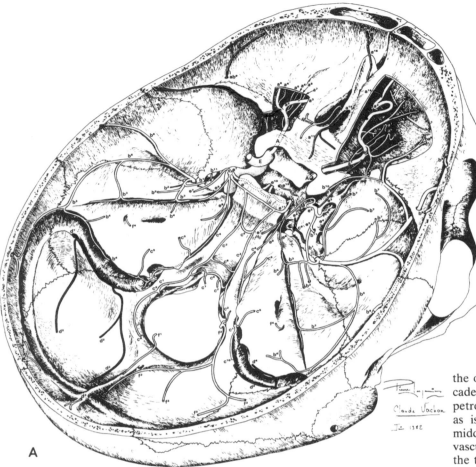

A

Fig. 8.12 A-C. Illustrations showing the meningeal arteries at the base of the skull (right posterolateral view). All of the dural meningeal envelopes and the right carotid siphon have been removed. The roof of the right orbit and optic canal, and posterior part of the left orbital roof have been opened to show the branches of the ophthalmic artery

A Localization on the right of the meningeal branches of the anterior and posterior ethmoidal arteries and the anastomotic branch between the ophthalmic artery and the infero lateral trunk of the carotid siphon (passing through the superior orbital sissure). The carotid branch of the ascending pharyngeal artery passes trough the foramen lacerum while a collateral of the occipital artery can be seen to run to the sigmoid sinus. The left half of the base of the skull shows the ophthalmic origin of the frontal and parietal branches of the middle meningeal artery, as well as a mastoid branch of the occipital artery supplying all of the posterior fossa on the left side. Note also the transosseous artery at the level of the confluens sinuum

B The branches of the carotid siphon. On the left, these branches arise from a common trunk originating from the posterior vertical portion of the carotid siphon while on the right, the branches to the petrosal apex and dorsum sellae arise separately. Note also on the right the lateral clival arteries which (when present) originates from the horizontal part of the carotid siphon. The following branches of the vertebral artery are also shown: a meningeal artery supplying the right posterior cerebellar fossa; an artery supplying the falx cerebelli arising from the posteroinferior cerebellar artery (not shown); the subarcuate arteries, both of which lie behind the internal auditory canal

C The branches of the internal maxillary and ascending pharyngeal arteries. On the left, only the occipital and squamous divisions of the middle meningeal artery are shown, since on this side the frontal and parietal branches can be seen to arise from

the ophthalmic artery. The arcade lying along the superior petrosal sinus is clearly visible, as is the contribution of the middle meningeal artery to the vascularization of the walls of the transverse sinus. Also visible on the left is the meningeal territory of the hypoglossal branch of the neuromeningeal division of the ascending pharyngeal artery. Note in particular the contribution of the hypoglossal branch to the dural vascularization of the foramen magnum and its anastomoses with the ipsilateral medial clival artery. On the right are shown the branches of the accessory meningeal artery passing through Vesale foramen medial and slightly anterior to the foramen ovale. The artery of the foramen rotondum and the branches running along the sphenoid ridge on the right side are also clearly shown. The territories of the jugular branch of the neuromeningeal division of the ascending pharyngeal artery are also illustrated, i.e. the inferior petrosal sinus, sigmoid sinus and lower part of the cerebello pontine angle

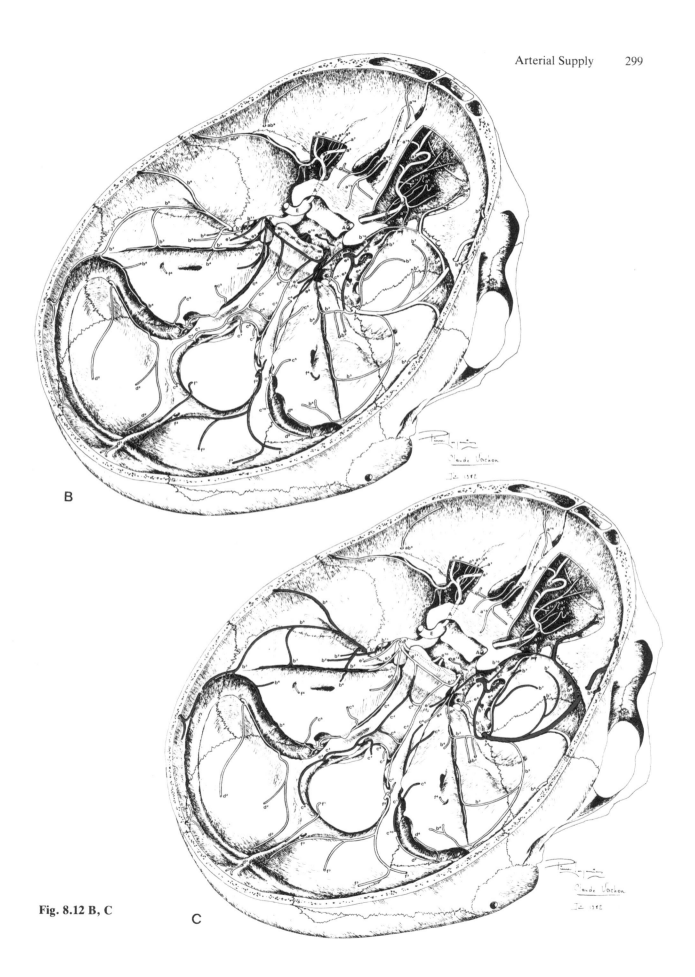

Fig. 8.12 B, C

B

C

within normal limits or may show only nonspecific secondary changes, such as focal or generalized atrophy or dilatation of the CSF spaces (hydrocephalus) (Chiras 1982). In patients with cortical venous or central dural sinus drainage, the enhanced CT or MRI scans frequently demonstrate dilated vessels, similar to the findings in brain AVMs (Fig. 8.4). If a DAVM is suspected clinically, selective angiography should be performed, even in the presence of a normal CT examination: to confirm the diagnosis of a vascular malformation, the dural origin of the nidus, and to outline its arterial supply and venous drainage. Global arteriographic or intravenous studies should be avoided, as they do not provide sufficient information for the basis of therapeutic decision.

Angiographic evaluation should be superselective (Djindjian 1973, Newton 1970) and should follow a precise topographical protocol (see Table 8.12, Fig. 8.18; see also Vol. 1, Chapters 15, 16).

The presence of patent dangerous anastomoses, the nature of the venous drainage of the DAVMs, and the arterial supply and venous drainage of the adjacent healthy territories must all be demonstrated before the therapeutic approach can be planned. The need to identify associated venous or dural sinus thrombosis or anomalies and other associated vascular malformations necessitates a complete study of the head, neck and brain vasculature. Finally, one must remember that neither the falx nor the tentorium cerebelli constitute a barrier to dural arterial supply, so that all possible infra and supratentorial arterial feeders must be evaluated.

IX. Therapeutic Aspects

1. Objectives and Strategy

The use of IBCA in DAVMs has dramatically improved the quality and stability of the result of embolization. Liquid agents however are more difficult to use than particules (PVA). To be effective and complication free, both techniques require training, skill and a thorough understanding of the local anatomy and nature of DAVMs.

Although Djindjian' series in 1973 was very illustrative, it can hardly be compared with the results of embolization after 1980, because of recent improvements in both embolization and microsurgical techniques. In a personal, small series of patients (23 cases between 1980 and 1983), the complication rate was low, with no permanent complications directly related to embolization. However, we did observe transient problems, some of which required specific management which will be discussed later.

The combination of embolization and surgery was used in three patients; once to develop a collateral circulation (IMA) to make the lesion accessible to transvascular techniques (ethmoidal artery clipping) (Fig. 8.13), once to resect the mastoid artery to compensate for proximal embolization, and once to treat an insufficiently embolized DAVM draining into the cortical venous system (Fig. 8.5).

Several other therapeutic approaches have been proposed: Irradiation (Bitoh 1981), electrothrombosis (Ishikawa 1982, Nishijima 1984), oestrogens (Suzuki 1981), and surgery (Sundt 1983, Malik 1984, Grisoli 1984) (see below).

However, DAVMs in most instances constitute a benign disease. Spontaneous regression can be expected in many cases of cavernous sinus DAVMs. Active treatment should only be considered when the clinical

Table 8.13. DAVM therapeutic approach

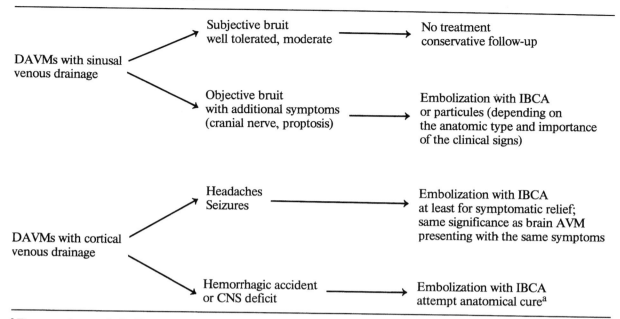

DAVMs with sinusal venous drainage

→ Subjective bruit well tolerated, moderate ⟶ No treatment conservative follow-up

→ Objective bruit with additional symptoms (cranial nerve, proptosis) ⟶ Embolization with IBCA or particules (depending on the anatomic type and importance of the clinical signs)

DAVMs with cortical venous drainage

→ Headaches Seizures ⟶ Embolization with IBCA at least for symptomatic relief; same significance as brain AVM presenting with the same symptoms

→ Hemorrhagic accident or CNS deficit ⟶ Embolization with IBCA attempt anatomical cure[a]

[a] The anatomic cure of a DAVM corresponds to a stable disappearance of an arteriovenous shunt within the dura and to the sequentially and morphologically normal filling on cerebral angiography of what use to be its venous outlet (sinus or cortical vein)

symptoms and the potential risks of the lesion affect (or may affect) the patient's life. As a general principle, the therapeutic strategy and degree of aggressiveness will be based on the pattern of venous drainage of the lesion (Table 8.13). The morphological goal, whenever treatment is indicated, is the permanent occlusion of the shunt at the site of the abnormal AV communication (Fig. 8.14), with preservation of the venous outlet. Depending on the angioarchitecture of the lesion (network or direct single hole fistula), particles or liquid agents will be used. However, in most instances when particles are used stable complete occlusion is not obtained (Lasjaunias 1984). In general, if a well trained surgical neuroangiographic team is available, DAVMs that have an arterial supply reachable by an endovascular approach should first be managed by embolization.

2. Topographic Considerations

The topography of an individual DAVM has little influence in the decision for or against intervention. However, specific anatomic features make some locations more challenging than orthers. For example, DAVMs in the anterior cranial fossa must be treated quickly and effectively because of their potential hemorrhagic complications; however, they are usually readily accessible following ethmoidal artery clipping. DAVMs of the superior sagittal sinus are technically challenging because of the distal location of the nidus in relation to the embolic delivery device. Those in the tentorium require perfect embolization of the nidus to avoid collateral circulation from the internal carotid artery branches.

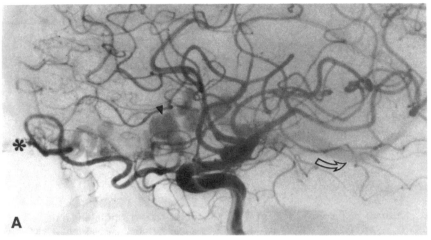

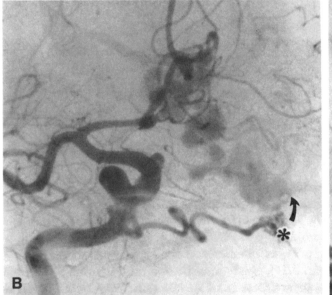

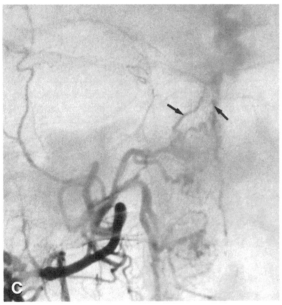

Fig. 8.13 A-H. 50 year old male presenting with moderate spontaneous epistaxis and right inferior quadrantanopsia. **A** Right and **B** left internal carotid angiograms demonstrate DAVM of the anterior cranial fossa *(asterisk)* draining into the left olfactory vein *(curved arrow)*, the deep sylvian vein *(arrowhead)* and posteriorly into an ectatic basal vein of Rosenthal *(open curved arrow)*. Both left anterior ethmoidal arteries supply the DAVM. **C** Internal maxillary artery injection frontal projection shows poor filling of the DAVM although direct feeders are visualized *(arrows)*. One month following intraorbital anterior ethmoidal artery clipping the DAVM is no longer seen on internal carotid angiograms **(D)** and **(E)** and internal maxillary artery branches *(open arrows)* seen in the early phase **(F)** and late phase **(G)** of the angiograms constitute the only supply to the nidus *(arrowheads)*. The lesion was then embolized with PVA particles (160 μm) and has been stable for 3 years; the lesion could not be demonstrated during the last follow-up angiography **(H)**

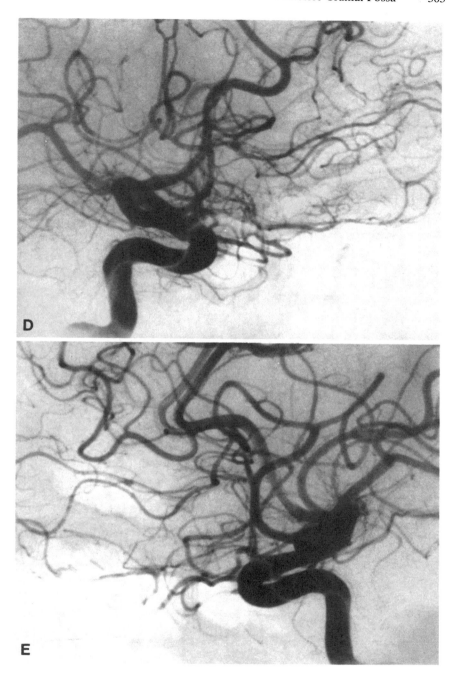

Fig. 8.13 D, E

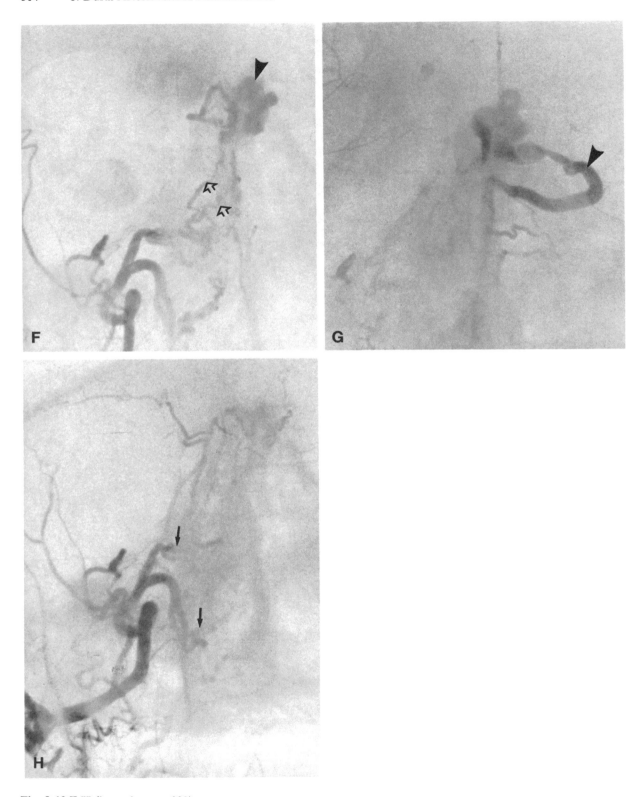

Fig. 8.13 F-H (legend see p. 302)

Lesions of the foramen magnum are fed by arteries which are hazardous to embolize because of patent anastomoses with the posterior fossa and spinal cord arteries (i.e. occipito or pharyngo-vertebral anastomoses; lateral spinal artery). Preservation of vision may be difficult or impossible when treating large orbital lesions (Fig. 8.10). In these situations, the goal should be to prevent the systemic effects of the hypertensive glaucoma and to preserve the globe (even if sightless) for cosmetic purposes.

3. Technical Aspects

The most appropriate delivery system is a coaxial one which preserves the flow since the site of embolization is almost always far from the nidus (see also Chapter 1).

Vinuela (1983) proposed to use a calibrated leak balloon, however in our experience only one high flow DAVM in a child required flow control for safe delivery of the IBCA. We do not recommend the use of large embolic devices such as detachable balloons, coils or large particules as these do not have a lasting effect on the flow; they serve only to induce collateral circulation to the nidus. They may, in selected circumstances, be used to redirect flow into a feeding vessel which more safety allows the delivery of an embolic agent to the nidus. Resorbable agents are also not appropriate (Ahn 1983) especially in the pediatric age group, except for the transient protection of a normal vessel (Chapter 1, XII).

4. Embolization Timing

In many patients, the embolization of a DAVM can be performed at a single session. *Staged procedures* may be necessary in the face of technical problems during the initial approach, such as arterial spasm or patency of dangerous anastomoses which add to the risk of the procedure. Situations in which one should anticipate multiple sessions include: DAVMs in children, where the severe systemic effects of the disease (i.e., cardiac failure) as well as the technical challenges (contrast and fluid limitation, hypothermia in small infants, the small size of the vessels to be embolized) may limit the possible length of the procedure to preserve femoral artery patency.

In the case of severe congestive heart failure, the goal of the initial procedure is to decrease the shunt sufficiently to palliate the cardiac symptoms, with the intention of completing the embolization when the patient is more stable.

Emergency or *urgent treatment* is most often required following hemorrhagic complications of lesions with cortical venous drainage. Lesions with multiple thrombosis or venous ectasia are more likely to bleed acutely. DAVMs of the cavernous sinus, middle cranial fossa and orbit with rapid visual deterioration should also be treated urgently; they require agressive therapy to preserve vision.

The management of incompletely *embolized DAVMs* must be discussed after weighing the risks of further intervention against the risk of leaving a potentially progressive lesion. DAVM presenting with pulsatile tinnitus in eldery patients can probably be treated conservatively if following an initial incomplete embolization symptoms have improved. Absence of cortical venous drainage and/or venous thrombosis will further support the conservative approach.

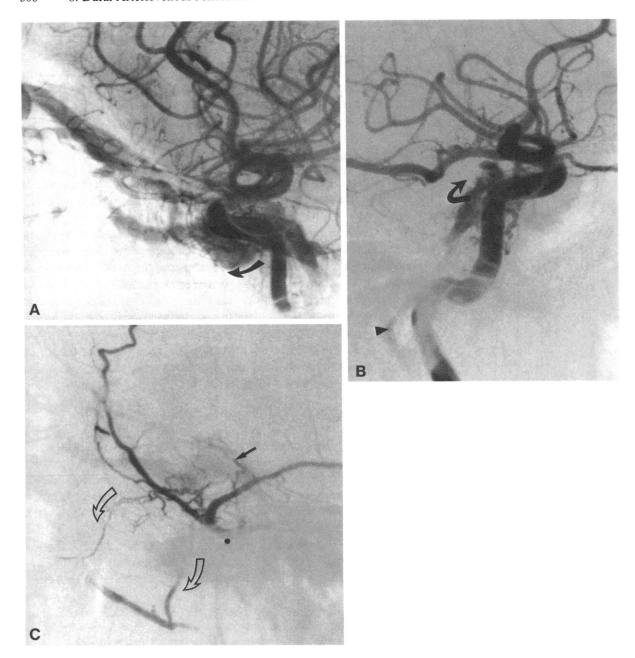

Fig. 8.14 A-K. 50 year old male presenting with progressive left exophthalmus, conjunctival hyperemia, diplopia and retro occular pain

A left cavernous sinus DAVM is demonstrated on the left **(A)** and right **(B)** internal carotid angiograms. The drainage is anterior into the left cavernous sinus *(curved arrow)* and ipsilateral ophthalmic vein, and posterior *(broken arrow)* into the left jugular vein *(arrowhead)*. **C** The middle meningeal artery injection at the foramen spinosum *(asterisk)* demonstrates the DAVM *(arrow)* and reflux into the accessory meningeal and foramen rotondum arteries *(open curved arrow)*

D, E Contrast injections in the posterior branches *(asterisk)* of the ascending pharyngeal bilaterally demonstrate the posterior component of the DAVM *(arrows)*. Note the odontoid process arterial arch *(curved arrow)*. Following PVA particle embolization of the left middle meningeal and ascending pharyngeal arteries the angiographic control **(F)** into the internal carotid artery the immediate

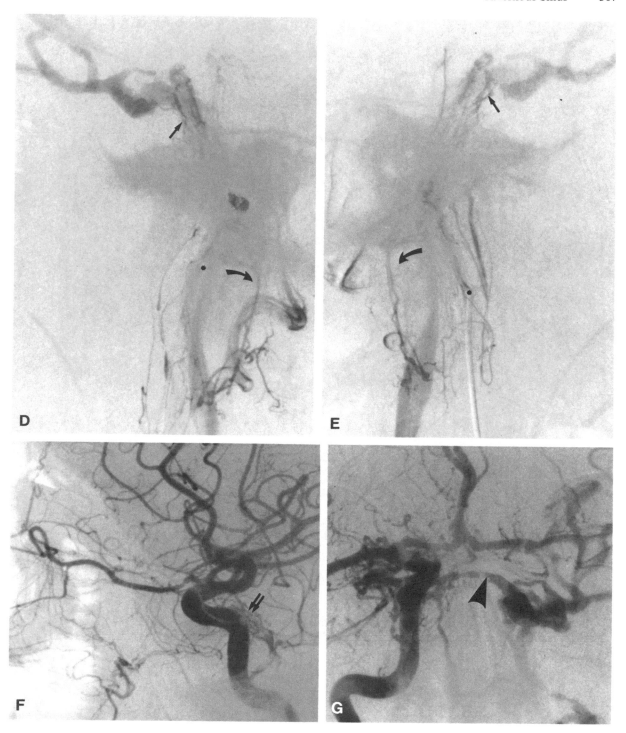

Fig. 8.14 (continued)
clinical changes were satisfactory (double arrow indicates almost no residual shunt
into the DAVM). The patient's symptoms improved dramatically but recurred one
month later. Repeat right internal carotid **(G)** and ascending pharyngeal **(H)**
angiograms demonstrated a prominent posterior component of the DAVM *(arrowhead)*. Ipsilateral ascending pharyngeal and middle meningeal arteries were still
occluded (not shown). IBCA embolization via the opposite *(right)* ascending
pharyngeal artery was achieved following a negative provocative test (Chapter 1,
XIII)

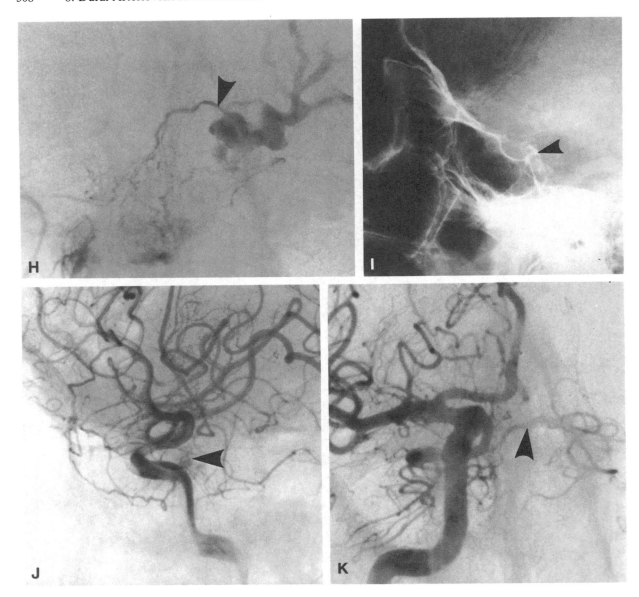

Fig. 8.14. (continued)
I Note the radiopaque glue in the posterior cavernous sinus *(arrowhead)*. **J, K** Final control angiogram shows no supply *(arrowhead)* from either internal carotid siphon

A short period of observation may be useful, in some patients with slow flow lesions where IBCA has been used, as the shunt may thrombose secondarily. Thrombosis is likely to occur if the embolic agent has reached the nidus (Fig. 8.15). DAVMs with cortical venous drainage presenting with neurological symptoms require further treatment following incomplete embolization. If embolization is not feasible an alternative mode of treatment such as surgical resection or estrogen therapy must be considered, as in this group of patients the therapeutic goal is an anatomic cure (see below).

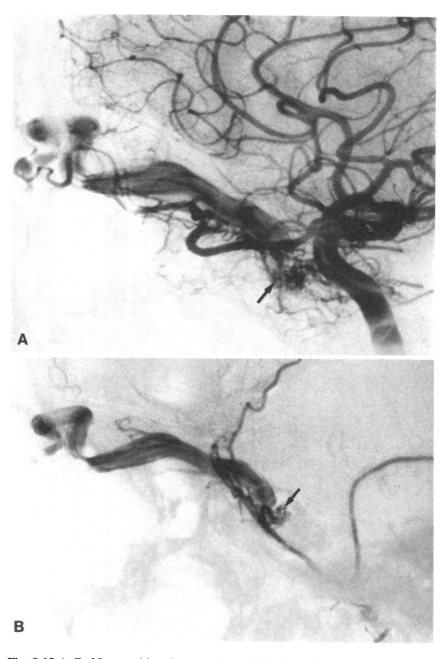

Fig. 8.15 A-G. 35 year old male presenting with left exophthalmus, conjunctival hyperemia and diplopia. Internal carotid **(A)** and middle meningeal **(B)** arterial injections demonstrate a DAVM *(arrow)* of the inferior lip of the superior orbital fissure draining into the superior ophthalmic vein

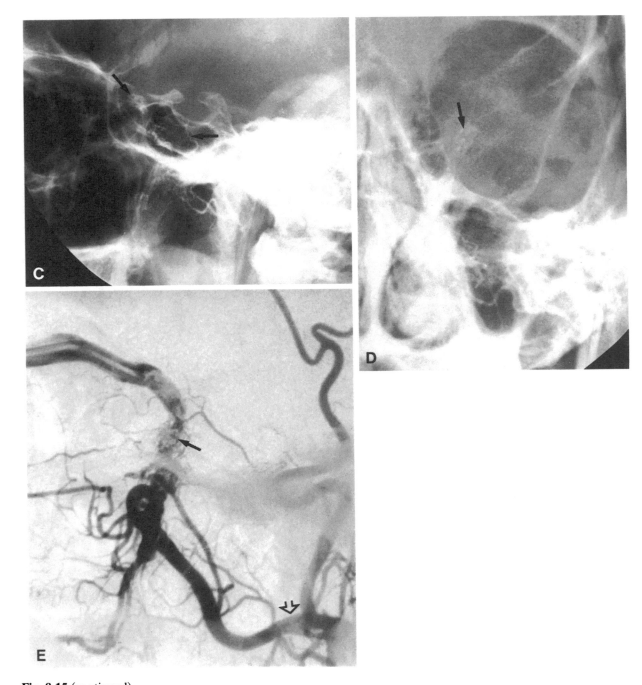

Fig. 8.15 (continued)
Following middle meningeal (and accessory meningeal) embolization with radio-paque IBCA *(arrows)* **(C)** and **(D)**. A control angiogram in the left distal external carotid artery shows a persistant nidus *(arrow)* fed directly by branches of the distal internal maxillary artery. Satisfactory embolization of these branches was impossible because of arterial spasm. 3 days later the distal internal maxillary **(F)** and the internal carotid **(G)** artery angiograms demonstrated secondary thrombosis of the nidus *(arrows)* and the draining vein *(open arrow)*. Symptoms cleared in a week; the result has been stable for 2 years

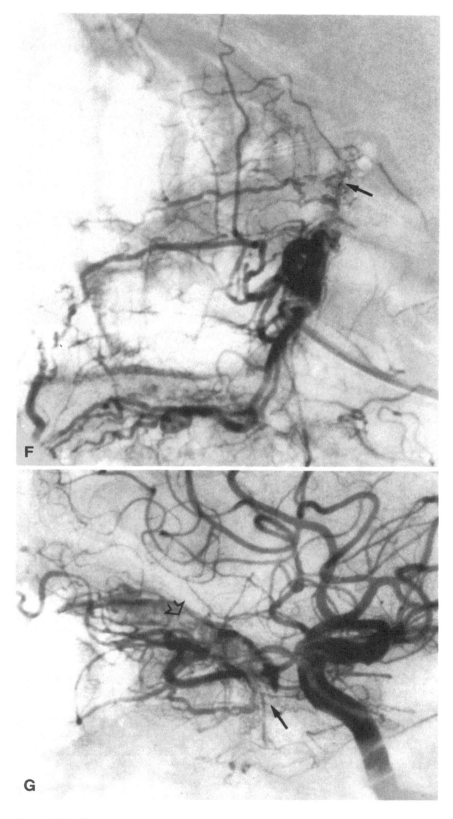

Fig. 8.15 F, G

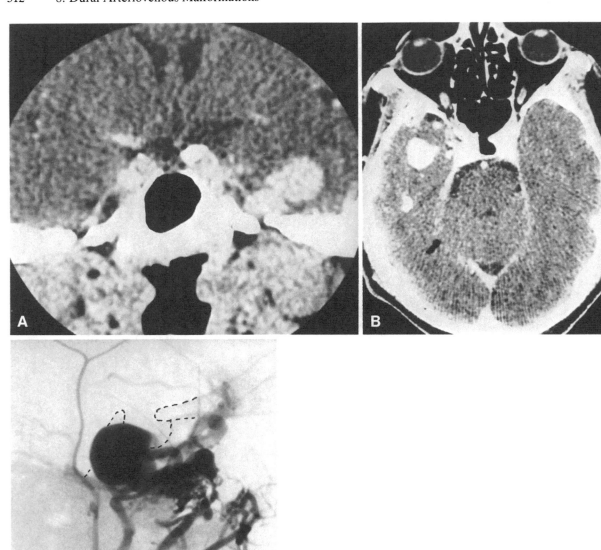

Fig. 8.16 A-E. Osteodural AVM of the middle cranial fossa in a 57 year old male presenting with temporal seizures. Note the venous ectasia *(arrow)* on the CT section in axial **(A)** and coronal **(B)** views. The supply to the nidus is seen on distal external carotid injection **(C)**, however selective catheterization of the middle deep temporal artery **(D)** and middle meningeal system **(E)** allowed even better visualization, and safer embolization. *Arrowhead* distal temporal branches, *open arrow* accessory meningeal artery

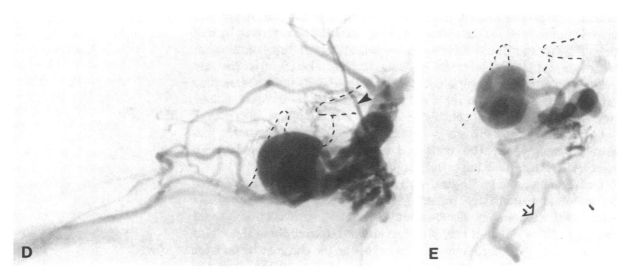

Fig. 8.16 D, E

5. Complications of Embolization

The potential hazards of embolization of DAVMs are related to the neurological territories or anastomoses of their feeders (see Chapter 1, and Vol. 1). We have noted three types of complication (Lasjaunias 1984).

α) Orbital. Transient non pulsatile proptosis developed in two patients, following secondary thrombosis of the superior ophthalmic vein. This problem has also been noted by others (Edwars 1977, Keplach 1978, Merlis 1982, Sugar 1979). The symptoms disappeared after a few days of steroid and heparin therapy, and no visual impairment occurred. Thus aggravation of symptoms following embolization of cavernous sinus DAVMs does not necessarily indicate recurrence, and can be managed medically.

β) Intracerebral. Spontaneous intracerebral hematoma occurred in a patient who was treated with systemic heparinization for 8 days in an attempt to prevent further thrombosis after inadvertent IBCA embolization of the superficial sylvian vein. Hemiplegia produced by the hematoma resolved slowly following evacuation of the clot. Active heparin therapy, a controversial issue, should not be used after the endovascular treatment of DAVMs, drainage into the cortical venous system.

γ) Cranial Nerve Palsy. This occurred in one patient following PVA embolization of the middle meningeal artery. The palsy regressed spontaneously in few hours. The procedure resulted in complete cure of the cavernous sinus DAVM. A provocative test should be performed in awake patients prior to embolization (see Chapter 1).

6. Surgery

Surgery should be considered whenever a complete cure is felt to be indicated and endovascular techniques are not feasible. Possible surgical approaches include direct intraoperative meningeal arterial embolization, resection of the abnormal dura, sinus endoluminal packing and clipping of the vein immediately at the nidus. When embolization is performed by well trained operators, it carries a lower complication rate than the surgical management of DAVMs (Malik 1984, Sundt 1983). Therefore, we feel that even in cases with difficult anatomy, embolization should be attempted first; even if complete control of the lesion cannot be achieved, embolization does not impair, but actually facilitates a future surgical procedure.

Other modalities, such as radiation therapy, electrothrombosis, and estrogen therapy should be considered only after embolization and surgery have been shown to be impossible or inadequate.

Occasionally, one has to deal with a patient with an acute subdural or intracerebral hemorrhage requiring surgical decompression, in whom emergency angiography demonstrates a DAVM with cortical venous drainage. Some surgeons may prefer to attempt to control the DAVM at the time of surgical decompression, even though the clot may be far from the dural lesion. We suggest embolization at the time of the diagnostic arteriography. The route taken for the individual patient however, will depend upon the availability of the technical expertise at the time.

A similar problem is produced by the simultaneous occurence of a DAVM and a second lesion such as a tumor or aneurysm which requires surgical managment. If both lesions are treated surgically during the same procedures, the surgeon must take care to completely remove the DAVM, as partial removal may transform a lesion with sinusal drainage into one with cortical venous drainage.

In general, simple ligation of feeding arteries should be avoided, as it will induce collateral circulation and make the lesions less accessible to future embolization. In children, ligation does not significantly change the flow in the lesion or the outcome; in Albright's series four of nine children treated this way died. For this reason we do not recommend the use of detachable balloons, coils or large particules; these agents occlude only the proximal vessels and have no effect on the lesion (nidus) itself.

Venous ectasias on the cortical venous drainage of a DAVM also represents a potential danger of secondary rupture since it reflects a downstream obstacle (Figs. 8.16, 8.17). Their presence indicate an active treatment, aiming for their disappearance with anatomic care of the DAVM.

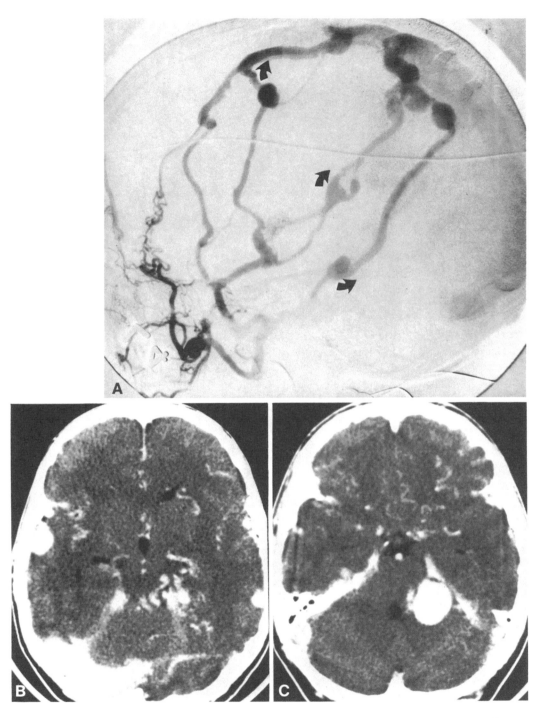

Fig. 8.17 A-C. 28 year old patient with a family history of Ehlers-Danlos disease, which presented with multiple SAH. Angiography **(A)** demonstrates DAVM with cortical venous drainage. **B** Enhanced CT. Study shows the venous ectasias both supra- and infratentorial

CHAPTER 9

Craniofacial Vascular Lesions: General

I. Introduction

A diversity of complex and often confusing classifications of head and neck vascular lesions may be found in the literature. The majority of these are descriptive, based on clinical appearances and pathological (histologic) features, and are not useful in modern clinical practice. Pretherapeutic pathologic examination is difficult or even hazardous to obtain; significant hemorrhagic complications have been known to occur following biopsies of these lesions. The specimen obtained may not reflect the various components of the lesion, and does not take into consideration the type of flow present.

The most useful classification would be one that could predict the clinical behavior of individual lesions, and lead to the selection of the most appropriate, currently available mode of therapy. At present the best available clinicopathologic classification is that of Mulliken and Glowacki, which includes tissue culture, histochemical and electron microscopic studies (Table 9.1). It enlightens some of the most difficult aspects of these lesions and is based on the separation of vascular lesions into two groups: those with a proliferative and sometimes potentially involutive behavior (hemangiomas); and those without (vascular malformations) which can be further classified according to the morphology of the abnormal channels present. From our clinical and angiographic experience we have reached a similar type of classification.

II. Postulated Embryogenesis

The mechanism of formation of vascular lesions has been deduced from the work of Woolard in 1922 on the maturation process of the capillary network of the limb bud of the pig. However, the analogy between the development of the limb and that of the head and neck must be reconsidered as several important differences in the embryogenesis of these two regions exist.

The progressive centrafugal development of the limb around a fixed arterial source, requires a constantly growing vascular bed similar to a growing tree. The various forms of vascular lesions have been considered by some authors to be caused by the arrests occuring at different stages of vascular development. For example, Kaplan, who based his conclusions on the vascular development of the extremities, related the capillary hemangiomas to an early stage 1 (undifferentiated capillary network) abnormality; later in the same stage, the lesion would be a cavernous type hemangioma. An arrest in the second stage (retiform stage) will produce a form of arterio-venous fistula (single hole or true AVM with a nidus).

Table 9.1. Modified from Mulliken et al. (1982)

	Hemangiomas	Vascular malformations
Mast cells per high power field (microscope)	25	0,8
Factor VIII antigen	+	+
Tissue culture	easy	almost impossible
In vitro angiogenesis	yes	no
Capillary formation		
– cell culture	1–2 months	no
– clot culture	5 days	no
Present at birth	30%	90%
Female/male ratio	5/1	1/1
Vascular walls	Thick basement membranes	Thin basement membranes
Cellular stroma	+	–

Finally, at stage 3 (maturation stage) arrest would lead to venous or lymphatic malformations.

The development of the head and neck area involves different and more complex changes (rotations, invaginations, migrations) of the tissues which locally crumple or blossom during the first weeks in utero.

We know from Paget's work (1948) that during normal development of the head and neck, the vasculature undergoes a series of changes in its branching patterns. Regressions and annexations of some arterial sources or territories account for the unique bidirectional flow in every branch of the head and neck area and for the variability in the territories supplied by a given artery. The relationships between the development of the facial buds and the changes in the arterial tree are difficults to establish. Both the ICA and the VA result from the persistance of several consecutively independent segments during the final maturation of the main head and neck vessels (see Vol. 1, Chapter 1).

Woolard's work (1922) has shown that in the limb bud of the pig, the veins are located in the periphery of the bud, whereas the arterial system is in the central portion. If one considers the traditional mechanisms evoked to explain the various types of vascular lesions, one can predict that malformations with a predominant arterial component should be located deep within the extremity while venous malformations should be more peripheral. Although this generalization is frequently true it is not constant: patients with Klippel-Trenaunay syndrom often have deep venous malformations of the lower extremities. In the maxillofacial area, each facial bud can be related to an embryonic vessel. However, during secondary development, bridges that modify the hemodynamic characteristic of their boundaries are established. Due to the nature of the specific modelling of the maxillofacial buds, it may be predicted that the vascular system of adjacent buds will overlap and eventually compete, leading to the annexations and regressions mentioned above. It becomes then almost impossible to find what could correspond to the initial central or peripheral portion of the maxillofacial buds.

The folds between adjacent buds represent critical areas for capillary maturation, primarily on the venous side. After this has occured, the arterial system can establish the necessary hemodynamic balance providing the nutritional equilibrium of the final dispositions. Delay in bud fusion produces specific arterial anatomical variation because the usual bridging tissue has been omitted. If the maturation of the capillary network is simultaneously delayed, vascular lesion may be seen in association with the arterial variations without clefts (see Vol. 1).

On a practical basis, the classical embryonic folds are not helpful in predicting the morphology or channel predominance of maxillofacial vascular lesions. Facial clefts and their various locations may be more helpful since it is possible to relate one artery to every single meridian described by Tessier (1976). This will be specifically discussed with the Sturge Weber syndrom (see Chapter 10. II. 3).

The study of the arterial vaculature of the palatine clefts (Fredericks 1973) shows that the clefts behave like anatomic barriers to vascular development and that their margins are highly vascularized (Ricbourg 1981 unpublished data). If this embryonic abnormality (the cleft) is associated with persistance of the embryonic state of the capillary network, vascular malformations should be found on the margin of the clefts or on the upper and lower corresponding meridian of Tessier (1976).

In the conclusion of her analysis of the palate cleft arterial supply, Fredericks rejected an ischemic phenomena by lack of vessel as a cause of the morphological gap. The author strongly suggested that due to the specific pattern of their blood supply, the existence of the clefts may be due to a "hematogeneous factor". The capillary arrangement of the cleft margins, which can be regarded as a pre-angiomatous state, may illustrate another aspect of the same factor. This "hematogeneous factor" could be responsible for the development of the vascular lesions with or without clefting or its equivalent.

Depending upon its nature, this developmental vascular disorder may manifest as a lesion which is:
– quiescent
– clinically expressed but reversible
– expressed but stable
– progressive.

The evolution or enlargement of the abnormal nidus will be due to proliferative cellular activity with tumor-like growth (Hemangiomas), or to a hemodynamic process, which increases the flow into the nidus (vascular malformations) (Table 9.1). Both mechanisms are believed to exist and they lead to the development of lesions with entirely different clinical behavior.

In summary:

1. Maxillofacial vascular lesions may be related to abnormal capillary maturation.
2. Their topography can in part be correlated with the facial buds.
3. Facial clefts constitute important landmarks of the critical areas of the developing maxillo facial area.
4. Vascular lesions with arterial predominance should theoretically occur on the margin of a meridian with no necessary cleft.
5. Venous malformations in the area should bridge two adjacent buds over the meridian.
6. Compartments within vascular lesion may account for the absence of apparent folds or clefts.
7. Neither sites of the disorder which gives rise to a vascular lesion nor the mechanisms reponsible for its development are known.

III. General Classification
Clinical Behavior and Treatment Strategy

The classification that we use is similar to that of Mulliken and Glowacki (1982). Under a generic name of vascular anomalies, two types of lesions will be differentiated: vascular malformations and vascular tumors (Table 9.2). Complex vascular anomalies (Table 9.3) will be presented as a separate group, but belong to the vascular malformations.

Table 9.2. Craniofacial vascular lesions (primary lesion)

1. Vascular malformations	*2. Vascular tumors*
a) Arterial with or without fistula	a) Hemangiomas
b) Capillary	• capillary in children (potentially involutive)
c) Capillaro-venous	• cavernous in adults (non involutive)
d) Venous	b) Hemangiopericytoma
e) Lymphangiomas	c) Hemangioendothelioma
f) Hemolymphangiomas	d) Kaposi
	e) Angiosarcoma

Table 9.3. Complex head and neck vascular anomalies

Multifocal AVM
Multifocal ectasias
Associated AVM and ectasias
Angiodysplastic syndromas
    • Sturge Weber
    • Rendu Osler Weber (systemic)
    • Wiburn Mason (functional)
    • von Recklinghausen
    • Ehlers Danlos
    • Fibro muscular dysplasia
    • Blue Rubber bled naevus

The predictable difference in clinical behavior in the two major categories of vascular lesions, hemangiomas and vascular malformations, dictate entirely different therapeutic approaches.

The treatment strategy that we propose is based on a ten year experience with vascular malformations and hemangiomas in different parts of the body. Each territory carries specific therapeutic risks which will affect the choice between conservative management and the search for a complete cure. The understanding of vascular lesions and progress in their treatment is one of the most rapidly changing areas in medecine. Therefore, the possibility that therapeutic techniques may be improved in the future dictates against the use of unnecessary potentially mutilative procedures now.

1. Hemangiomas (See Fig. 9.1)

Hemangiomas are tumors that enlarge by proliferation of endothelial cells and some (infantile hemangiomas) may involute by progressive cellular death and dropout. At histologic examination, potentially involutive hemangiomas of childhood consist of masses of endothelial cells with or without vascular lumens. The stimulus for involution is unknown. Possible mechanisms include occlusion of the vascular bed by endothelial cellular proliferation or by humoral factors. What we see histologically as the lesion involutes is a lack of thrombosis or infarction. However, there is nothing in the vessels or stroma that would predict involution. We feel that the non involuted cavernous hemangiomas of adults are also tumors which evolved by cellular proliferation. However, their clinical behavior and histologic appearance are quite different from that of infantile hemangiomas. They often contain evidence of thrombosis in the vascular lumen.

Potentially involutive hemangiomas of childhood have characteristic angiographic features which are similar to other benign tumors. They include mass effect, an organized pattern of arterial supply from adjacent arteries, drainage into dilated superficial veins which empty into normal veins, and parenchymal stains which are often lobulated (Fig. 9.2). Arteriovenous shunting may be present. Non-involutive cavernous hemangioma of adults typically appears as avascular masses on angiography, although, some parenchymal blush and filling of vascular spaces may occur in the late venous phase, if sufficient contrast material is injected. They grow like tumors and should not be considered as vascular malformations.

Conservative treatment is the rule for most patients with involutive *hemangiomas*. These lesions, which have a strong female predominance (5:1) are present at birth in only approximatively 30% of patients. The majority appear in the first three months of life. They typically demonstrate a period of rapid growth (proliferation phase), usually in the first 6 months of life followed by a period of gradual involution which generally begins at about 12 months of age and is complete by 7 years (Pitangy 1984). Involution can be expected to occur in over 95% of patients (Bowers 1960, Bingham 1979, Blackfield 1957) (Fig. 9.1). Unfortunately, it is not possible to predict the 5% of patients in whom involution will not occur. Active therapy to increase the rate of involution is indicated in selected patients including those with functional impairment (orbital, oral, subglottic), complications (hemorrhage, congestive heart failure, hypoprothromi-

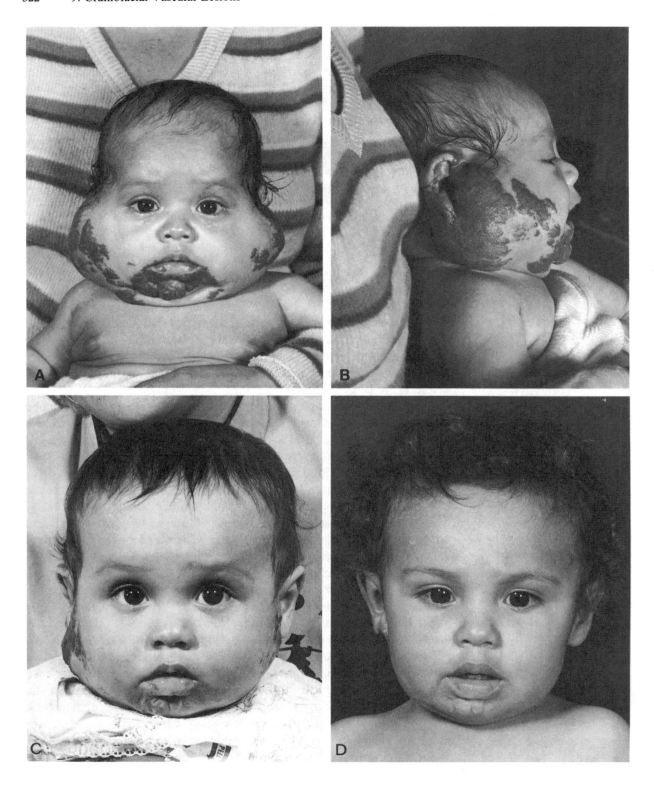

Fig. 9.1 A-H. Sequential pictures of a spontaneous evolution of a capillary hemangioma, the pictures cover a period of 5 years

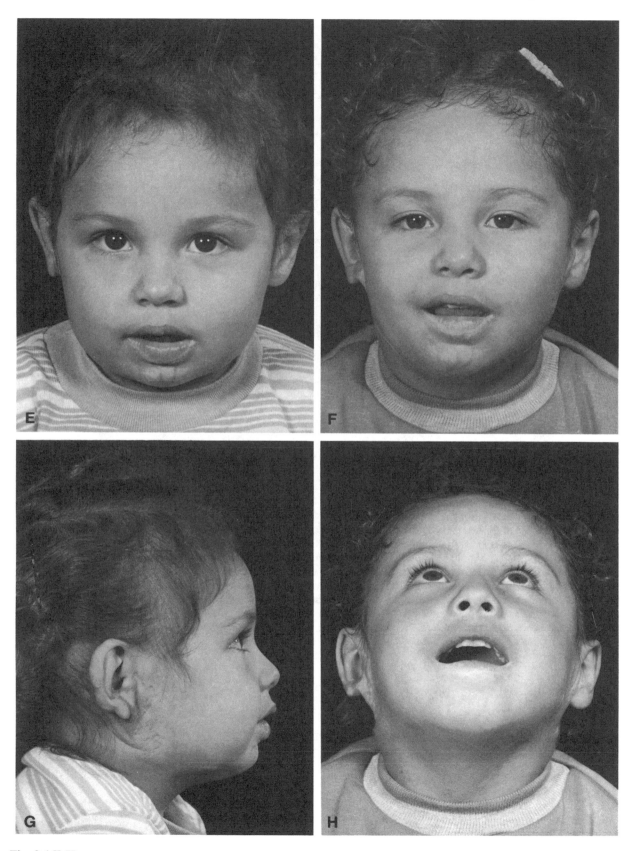

Fig. 9.1 E-H

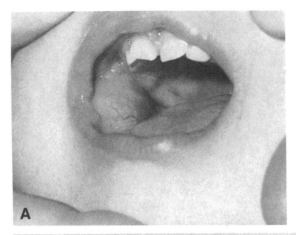

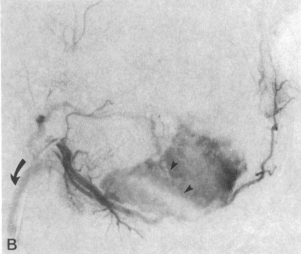

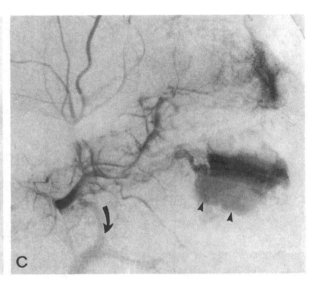

Fig. 9.2. Capillary hemangioma of the cheek in a 6 month old child **(A, B** and **C)**; angiographic aspect of the facial **(B)** and the internal maxillary **(C)** arteries, note the sharp margin between the two compartments of the lesion *(arrowhead)* and the rapid venous shunting *(curved arrow)*. **D, E** Follow up angiogram one year later when the mass was compromizing the teeth eruption, note the intralesional changes associated with the disappearance of the arteriovenous shunts within the tumor; at this point periodic swelling led us to embolize with particles. **F** Control angiogram one year later shows disappearance of the capillary blush. This angiographic improvement correlates with the clinical decrease of the mass; this result is still stable with 5 years follow up **(G)** and there are no teeth eruption problems

nemia; see Kasabach Merritt syndrome) and extremely large lesions. The most effective nonsurgical treatments are:

– systemic corticosteroid therapy and/or
– embolization.

Corticosteroids should be tried first, but unfortunately are not always effective and may not be well tolerated, especially where long term treatment is required with steroid dependent lesions. Hemangiomas are at

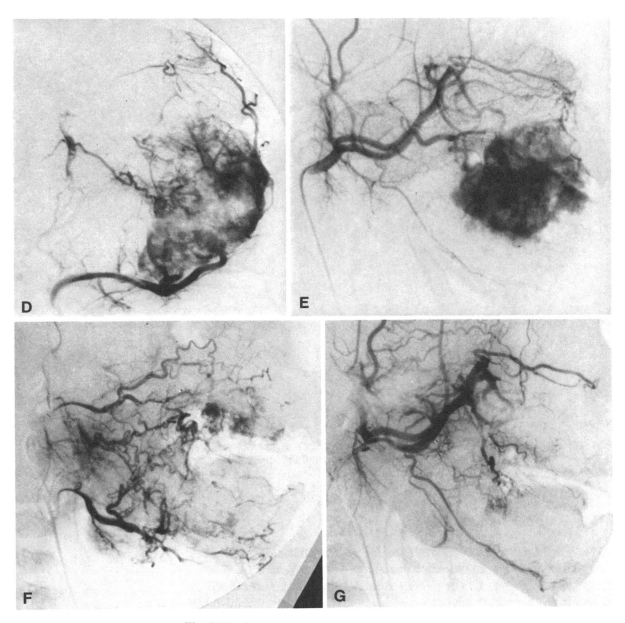

Fig. 9.2 D-G

least theoretically responsive to radiation therapy, but this modality is not currently considered acceptable due to its long-term side effects (malignancy, regional growth impairment, and scarring). Streptokinase, heparin and aspirin have been used with mixed results. Aminocaproic acid has been used in some patients, but is also not an innocuous drug (Neidhart 1982). In selected patients, embolization using small particles can be expected to be effective in arresting the proliferation phase and speeding the onset of involution (Fig. 9.2).

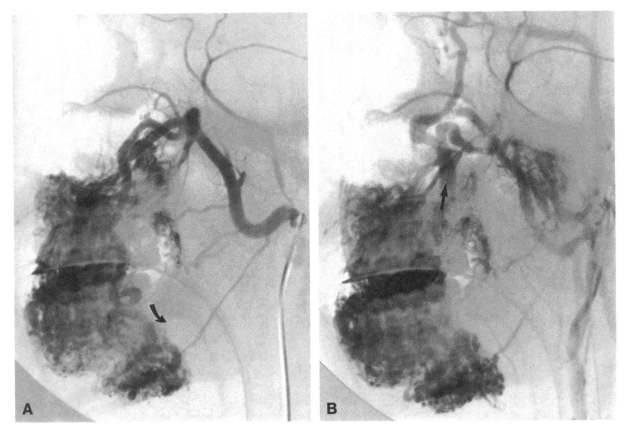

Fig. 9.3 A, B. High flow arteriovenous malformation of the cheek. Note the rapid filling of the buccal artery territory *(curved arrow)* **(A),** and the important venous drainage through the same system *(solid arrow)* **(B)**

2. Vascular Malformations

Vascular malformations are inborn errors of vascular morphogenesis. They may be formed by any combination of abnormal capillary, arterial, venous, or lymphatic channels with or without shunt. Changes in size are secondary to rheologic (hemodynamic) changes. They are neither proliferative nor potentially involutive. They are almost always present at birth, they may expand but they do not have cellular proliferation. At histologic examination, they consist of channel of varying morphology without an endothelial cellular stroma (Table 9.1).

A wide spectrum of angiographic appearances exists for the vascular malformations and correlates with the underlying channel abnormalities. The positive angiographic differences include the opacification of channels which do not normally exist whereas the relevant negative angiographic differences, include the absence of a well defined parenchymatous "tumoral blush" (although some small vessel malformation may show a blush) (Figs. 9.3, 9.4).

Lymphangiomas and hemolymphangiomas of the oral regions are considered to be malformations rather than true neoplasms (Batsakis 1979). Pure lymphatic malformations do not regress spontaneously. They often communicate with adjacent systemic veins and may be combined with

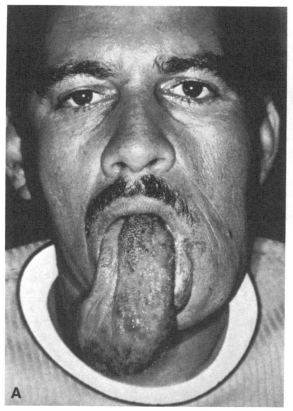

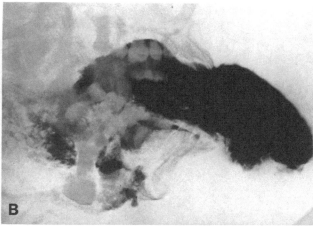

Fig. 9.4. A Venous malformation of the tongue with extension to the lower lip and the upper neck. **B** In situ injection of 30 cc of contrast demonstrates the deep and floor of the mouth extension of the malformation. Note the stagnant flow (see Fig. 1.24)

venous or arteriovenous malformations (hemolymphangiomas). Hemolymphangiomas may expend acutely, secondarily to infection, hemorrhage or venous thrombosis, and may then uncompletely regress (spontaneously or after embolization), leaving behind some hypertrophic area involved (tongue, floor of the mouth, cheek, lips) (Fig. 9.5).

Port wine stain is a vascular malformation and consists of small capillaries, venous or venular channels located within the dermis. Port wine stains are frequently present in the mesodermal dysplastic syndromes and when isolated in the face, may represent a minor expression of Sturge Weber syndrome (Fig. 9.6).

The clinical behavior of *vascular malformations* varies according to the morphology of the channel abnormalities, their secondary hemodynamic effects and locations. They differ significantly from hemangiomas because of the absence of proliferative and involutive potential. Certain lesions may exist in a dormant state (Table 9.4), until stimulated to expand by a trigger factor (Figs. 9.7–9.9, Table 9.5). The majority enlarge gradually in proportion to the growth of the patient. Their effects vary from minor cosmetic blemishes to major deformity or functional impairments (Table 9.6). The treatment of these complex lesions requires careful planning by a multidisciplinary team. In general, treatment of vascular malformations in children, should be conservative in the absence of significant functions or life

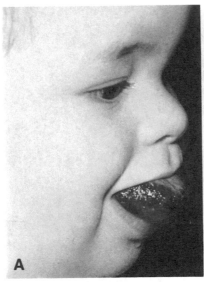
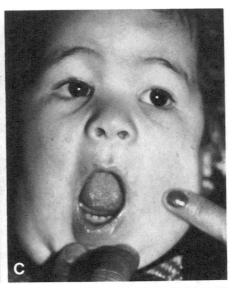
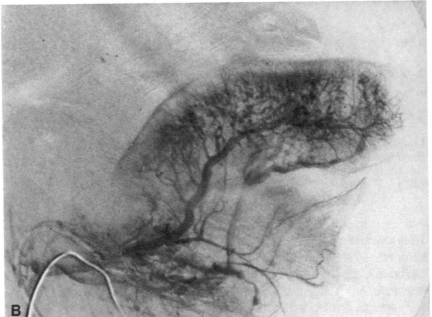

Fig. 9.5 A-C. Hemolymph-angioma of the tongue in a four and half month old child. **A** Spontaneous protraction of the tongue. **B** Selective injection of the lingual artery before embolization with microparticles (PVA 140 microns) (bilateral). **C** Clinical result obtained after two sessions of embolization four months after **A**; the patient remained stable (4 years follow-up)

Table 9.4. Dormant AVM clinical manifestations

Mass effect
- facial difformity (cosmetic)
- functional disturbance (swallowing, breathing, vision, mastication)
- maxillofacial growth disturbance
- teeth eruption disturbance

Skin discoloration

Fig. 9.6. Port wine stain in the territory of the V$_2$ and V$_3$ nerves, no venous abnormality could be found on the intracranial study

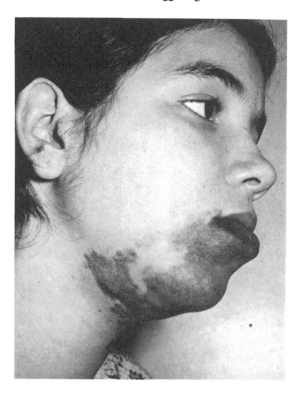

threatening complications. Radiation therapy has no therapeutic role at present, unless all other modalities endovascular, surgical or a combination of these fails. Incomplete surgical resection should be avoided as it is frequently ineffective, may aggravate the problem, and makes future endovascular therapy difficult or impossible. Mulliken (1982) proposed a rheologic basis for the therapy of vascular malformations which is in accordance with our current philosophy and embolization techniques. In adults, the aggressiveness of the therapeutic approach may depend more on the team skills, cultural environment (as it relates to the goal of treatment and possible complications) rather than to the characteristics of the vascular malformations.

Table 9.5. Triggering or aggravation factors of maxillofacial AVM

Direct trauma: • Mouth hygien
• Feeding
• Blunt
• Iatrogenic (biopsy, surgery, teeth extraction, oral prosthesis proximal ligations, or embolizations)
Regional infection
Teeth eruption
Hormons and contraceptives
Psychological stress
Venous and arterial hyperpressure
Excessive sun exposure

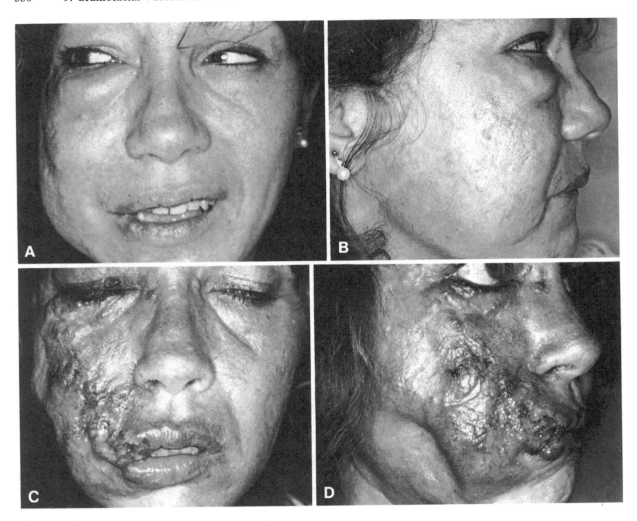

Fig. 9.7. High flow arterio-venous vascular malformation of the right cheek; the lesion became apparent after the third pregnancy **(A, B)**. Note the clinical evolution with ulceration of the lip, cheek and palate areas **(C, D)**

Table 9.6. Evolutive AVM, additional clinical manifestations

Bleeding	Bruit
Swelling	Glaucoma
Growth (nidus)	Heart failure
Pain	Thrombophlebitis
Ischemic ulceration	

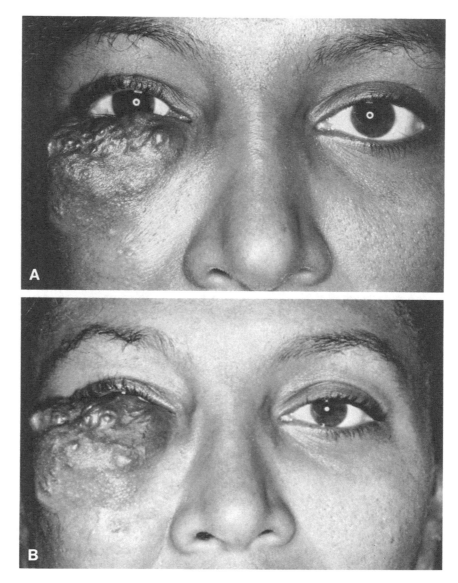

Fig. 9.8 A, B. 32 year old female with a high flow vascular malformation of the lower eyelid. **A** Presenting appearance. **B** Clinical aspect during menstruations. Same patient as Fig. 1.21

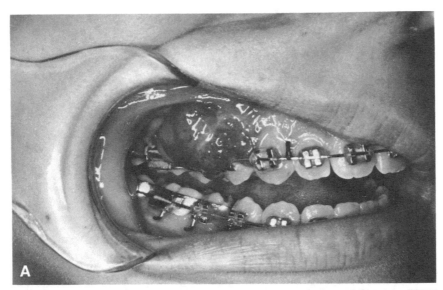

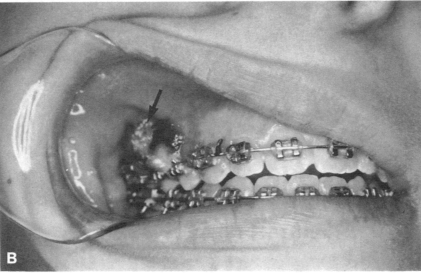

Fig. 9.9 A, B. 17 year old female. Capillary vascular malformation of the maxilla and gum, the malformation became active following braces placement **(A)**. The lesion was embolized for recurrent severe bleed (IBCA). Note the significant shrinkage of the lesion and the white discoloration in relation to the use of white tantalum powder. She had surgical resection of the AVM following the embolization, with no recurrence 3 years later

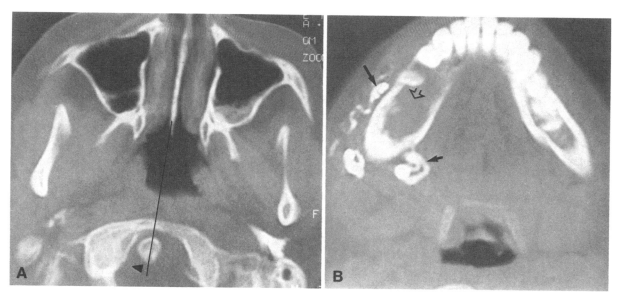

Fig. 9.10 A, B. 11 year old young male presenting a high flow malformation of the horizontal portion of the mandible. Note the *(left)* displacement of the ondontoid process to compensate the mandible translation **(A)**. The lesion has been embolized with IBCA *(arrows)* **(B)** for recurrent hemorrhagic complications. Note the bone enlargement at the level of the draining vein into the inferior dental canal *(open arrow)*

IV. Pretherapeutic Evaluation of the Vascular Lesions of the Head and Neck Area

Due to the complexity of these lesions a multidisciplinary approach is necessary to optimize the analysis and treatment strategy by a given team in a specific case. Therefore, the expertise of the various physicians (otolaryngologists, head and neck surgeons, oral surgeons, pediatricians, plastic surgeons, neurosurgeons, ophthalmologists, orthodontists) will help us in determinating the clinical, psychological and technical problems or challenges related to the managment in a specific instance.

The pretherapeutic evaluation of a vascular lesion of the head and neck must start with a thorough clinical examination of the lesion, the surrounding areas and the rest of the body. The past medical history of the patient and of his family must be noted as well as any triggering factor in the evolution of the lesion. Once this has been established, the differentiation between a hemangioma and a vascular malformation can be made. If it is decided that no treatment should be given, further studies are not usually needed, and a conservative follow-up can be done. Good photographs of the head and neck areas and body should be taken at the initial examination and at subsequent consultations. If treatment is indicated additional evaluations may be made.

Pretherapeutic evaluation will include some noninvasive radiological studies: Chest X-ray, panoramic view of the maxillomandibular area, axial and coronal CT without or with enhancement. Neither plain skull films nor complex motion tomography have proven in our experience to be of any significant value in most solitary vascular lesions of the head and neck. They

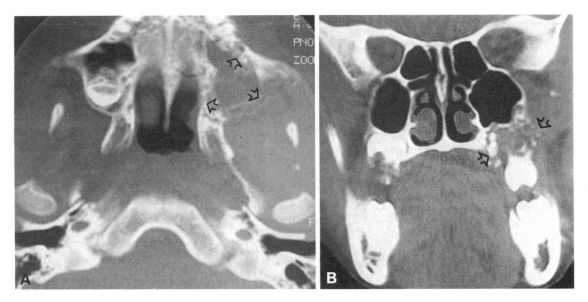

Fig. 9.11 A, B. 11 year old female presenting with a high flow vascular malformation of the maxillar gum. Note the bone destruction of the maxillar *(open arrows)*, studied with axial **(A)** and coronal **(B)** CT sections

may be useful to the plastic surgeon for specific needs in presurgical evaluation. MRI has not yet shown any major advantages in the appreciation of bony or soft tissue extension. Intravenous digital angiography, as in other lesions of the head and neck area, does not provide enough information to contribute to the decision making process. It reproduces in best of cases informations given by a good quality enhanced CT study. Ultrasound is reserved for cervical and parotid masses, to differenciate the vascular nature of the lesion from other masses (hygroma, branchial cyst or adenopathies). Doppler has not proven to be useful in our experience, although it might demonstrate nonperceptive bruits which would further contraindicate any attempt to biopsy.

With the above information, bony and soft tissue extension, and extension to the orbit or cavernous sinus can be assessed; they represent the key necessary to appreciate the future evolution and technical difficulties in dealing with a deep seated malformation or hemangioma (Figs. 9.10, 9.11).

Clinical suspicion of angiomatosis from the family history, the examination of the skin or complaints in another territory (digestive system, respiratory system etc...) should probably lead to additional tests. Family examination will be mandatory in some cases (Rendu-Osler-Weber, von Recklinghausen, von Hippel Lindau, Blue Rubber naevi) to appreciate the penetrance of a hereditary angiomatosis.

Finally, specific laboratory tests will be requested with specific attention to coagulation tests (Kasabach Merritt syndrome).

Fig. 9.12 A-C. 3 month old female presenting with a capillary hemangioma of the eyelid and parotid region **(A)**. Due to the eye occlusion, and to prevent amblyopia, angiography and embolization with PVA particles were carried out. **B** Early and **C** late phase of the distal external carotid artery angiogram. Note the multilobulated capillary blush and the venous shunt draining into the ophthalmic vein

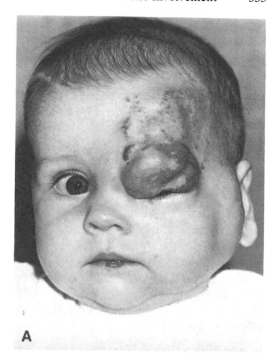

A

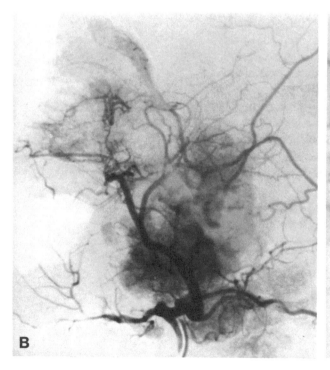

B

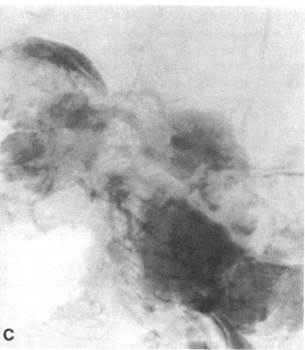

C

V. Urgent or Emergent Pretherapeutic Evaluations

The pretherapeutic evaluation of vascular lesions is usually not urgent except for subglottic or eyelid hemangiomas (Fig. 9.12), hemorrhagic episodes usually associated to ischemic ulcerations, and dental arcade AVM (Fig. 9.13) with bleeding complications. Severe consumption coagulopathies (see Kasabach and Merritt 1940) or heart failure caused by large lesions in neonates or infants will constitute emergency situations. The great majority of vascular lesions of children will be treated conservatively, waiting until complete regression or maxillofacial maturity. However, appreciation of the secondary consequences of a deeply located dormant lesion and its potential complications (vision, cranial nerves, hemorrhages) following triggering factors, may require complete pretherapeutic evaluation to further establish prognosis and eventually consider prophylactic treatment.

Oral cavity lesions with their consequences on the maxillofacial growth represent the best indication of prophylactic treatment; even in the absence of airway or digestive disfunction, bleeding or cosmetic problems (Figs. 9.14, 9.15).

More difficult are the lesions in the orbital wall (maxilla, malar, ethmoid, sphenoid region) without visual symptoms which will require pretherapeutic studies probably including selective angiography. Careful attention has to be paid to the school performance of affected children, as it may detoriate with impairment of the vision, compromises of hearing, or attention, with the onset of a bruit. Children usually do not complain about these changes, therefore proper and direct questioning may be relevant. In this population in particular, but in the adult one as well, appreciation of the psychological consequences of the lesion is sometimes difficult to acess. Pure cosmetic problems represent a difficult therapeutic challenge and whenever possible attempt at complete resolution or cure should be made by combined treatment (Fig. 9.16). As already mentioned, partial surgery should be avoided.

Asymptomatic pulsatile bruit discovered during clinical examination will invariably lead to pretherapeutic evaluation, to precisely demonstrate the venous channels involved in the drainage of the lesion, and the retrograde congestive consequences that it may induce.

Finally, true port wine stains in the trigeminal territory should only be investigated with CT for diagnostic and prognostic purposes (see below).

VI. Angioarchitecture

Our description of angioarchitecture of vascular lesions of the head and neck is based on our experience collected by superselective studies of more than 600 patients over the past 10 years. The precise angiographic protocol is based on the topography of the lesions. It is necessary to accurately demonstrate the angioarchitecture of the nidus, the feeding arteries and draining veins, the flow characteristics of the lesion and the collateral circulation through the nidus and surrounding healthy tissue; the angiographic features which must be analyzed in every case include:

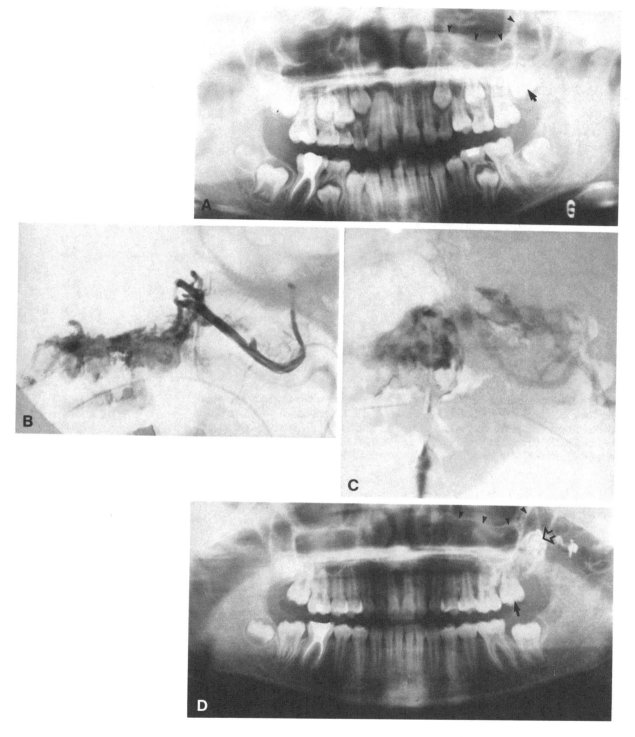

Fig. 9.13 A-D. Same patient as Fig. 9.11. **A** Panoramic radiogram performed at the time of hemorrhagic complication related to molar eruption *(arrow)*. Note the density of the lower portion of the adjacent maxillary sinus *(arrowheads)*. **B** Selective injection of the internal maxillary artery before embolization. **C** Direct injection into the maxillary extension of the lesion for in situ IBCA deposition. **D** Panoramic radiogram one year later. Note the satisfactory eruption of the teeth, disappearance of the maxillary sinus extension and the radiopaque IBCA *(open arrow)*

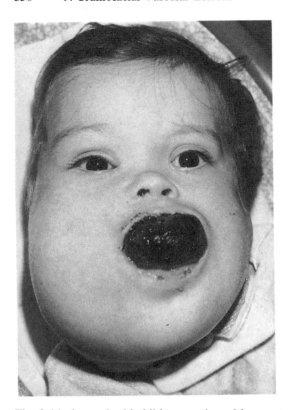

Fig. 9.14. 6 month old child presenting with an extensive hemolymphangioma of the tongue, cheek, upper neck extensing to the mediastinum which required tracheostomy. He presented with repeated hemorrhages. PVA embolization with particles in the tongue failed to produce significant changes on the volumen of the tongue. However, spontaneous bleeding decreased dramatically

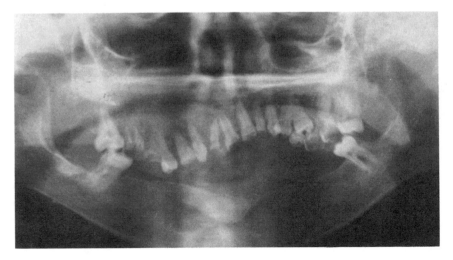

Fig. 9.15. Panoramic radiogram demonstrates secondary changes in the teeth and mandibular growth due to hemolymphangiomatous macroglossia, in a 13 year old male

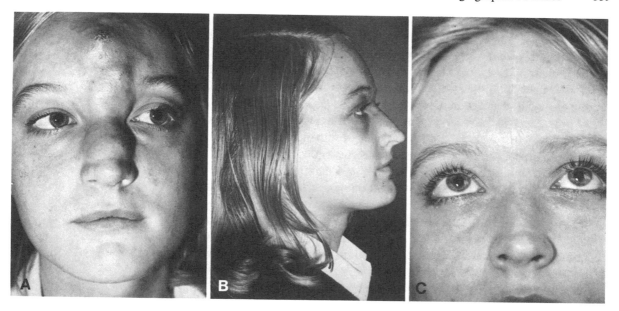

Fig. 9.16. High flow arteriovenous malformation of the forehead and nose before (**A**) and after (**B** and **C**) combined endovascular and operative surgery. No recurrence with 6 years follow up

- topography
- nidus angioarchitecture
- secondarily induced high flow
- collateral circulation (arterial and venous)
- iatrogenic changes (surgery, radiation therapy, previous embolizations)
- angiographic changes (evolutive factors)
- arterial ectasias
- mass effect and parenchymal component (hemangiomas, and other vascular tumors)

In practice all of these features may not be defined in each patient but the information obtained represents irreplaceable in vivo information that neither direct vision (surgery) nor pathology can give. The capability to identify in specific cases what may correspond to the active portion of the lesion, as opposed to what represents the reversible induced phenomena of surrounding tissues may lead to a limited treatment. The data gathered from the vast quantity of angiographic work has contributed greatly to the understanding and treatment of vascular lesions in the head and neck areas.

Feeding arteries are usually enlarged in the presence of arteriovenous shunting but may be normal in size in the presence of highly vascularized lesions without an arterio venous shunt (as seen in most hemangiomas) (Figs. 9.2, 9.3). Rarely increased size with slow flow circulation will correspond to a normal flow pattern. The classical concept of arterial "steal" and its related symptoms may be difficult to demonstrate; typically the selective angiogram shows preferential flow to the lesion while the feeding arteries to the surrounding tissues are poorly or not visualized. However, the complete examination of the area and the surrounding healthy territories, shows that no vessels are absent. One can demonstrate that the ischemic phenomena noted clinically are not at the level of the arterial "steal" seen at angiography; the venous drainage affects the normal territories by retrograde venous congestion, leading to decreased tissue perfusion and ischemia. By analogy, venous hypertension can explain: the ischemic ulcer of the Klippel Trenaunay disease, the ischemic deficits of the dural AVM draining into the central nervous system venous channels or leptomeningeal vascular malformation in Sturge Weber syndrome, the visual symptoms of "slow flow" dural AVM draining into the ophthalmic vein, and the usual asymptomatic character of the angiographic "steal" of the entire hemisphere seen in some carotid cavernous fistulas. These lead us to believe that ischemic ulcers in head and neck AVMs represent an excellent indication for arterial embolization to decrease the strain on the venous system.

Acute (post traumatic) arteriovenous fistulas may create an arterial "steal", however, it has not been our experience that clinically ischemic phenomena were related to arterial deprivation. A different situation exists in the postembolization trismus which always relates to arterial ischemia induced by embolization of the normal muscular vascular territory. The same arterial mechanism is involved when ectopic emboli reach the capillary level of a cutaneous territory (distal to the last possible collateral channel) and produce cutaneous necrosis.

Traumatic transformations (iatrogenic or not) typically manifest as evolution in vascular malformations and regression in hemangiomas. The triggering factor behaves differently in these two major categories. But in some other instances endothelial trauma of an arterial feeder to an AVM may stimulate an angiogenetic activity, which will become secondarily active by an angioectatic effect dependent on the type of AVM (see Vol. 1).

As previously discussed, the precise mechanism involved in the evolution of vascular lesions and their reaction to trauma and hormones are not known. Although definitive changes in the architecture of normal nasal mucosa are known to occur with hormonal changes, we have observed no specific angiographic features in the vascular malformation of patients who presented clinically with increased bleeding during their menstrual period. Humoral angiogenetic factors probably play a role in the evolution of certain neoplasm (Folkman 1981) but their role in the evolution of vascular malformations is not at all clear. At this time, we feel that the trigger effect of the hormonal changes on the vascular malformation is a rheologic (angioectatic) one. Trauma clearly plays an important role in the evolution of vascular malformations probably related to non proliferative changes in the endothelium in addition to the development of new shunts, or thrombosis with some impairment in drainage.

CHAPTER 10

Craniofacial Hemangiomas, Vascular Malformations and Angiomatosis: Specific Aspects

Following the general comments on the vascular lesions and our classification, some specific features should be studied either for their clinical, topographical or technical specificities. We shall first analyze specific problems within the hemangiomas and then the various types of of vascular malformations.

I. Hemangiomas

1. Subglottic Hemangiomas

The subglottic hemangioma represents the pediatric pedunculated equivalent of the flat supraglottic vascular lesion of the adult (Ohi, 1979). Bommel reviewing 26 cases found 20 females for 6 males. Dyspnea developed before the age of 6 month, usually with a normal interval following birth, but occuring after nose or throat infection. Associated hemangiomas were noted in 60%; one patient had a Sturge Weber syndrome. Ohi in 1979, presented the clinical profile of these lesions (Tables 10.1, 10.2). Dyspnea is a frequent symptom, but biphasic or inspiratory stridor was noted in 84.7% of cases, and cyanosis in 16.5%. These subglottic hemangiomas are capillary lesions composed of the proliferation of endothelial cells with no definitive capsule but separated from the epithelial layer. In 2/3 of patients they are posterior or lateral on the left side. In this subglottic localization they are constantly or exclusively fed by the inferior thyroidal artery. Inspite of their small size, these lesions can cause asphyxia and require emergency therapy to prevent airway obstruction (endotracheal intubation or tracheostomy). Even when these lesions begin to spontaneously involute they may demonstrate the rebound growth following infection or discontinuation of therapy. Subglottic hemangiomas usually involute by the age of 2 years.

Corticosteroid therapy is usually the first treatment used (prednisone 2 mg/kg per 24 hours). Among 17 patients (Bommel) 35% did not respond

Table 10.1. Subglottic hemangiomas period from birth to onset of symptoms (Ohi 1979)

	No. of cases	%
At Birth	21	26,3
Within 1 month	25	31,2
Within 3 month	33	41,2
Within 6 month	1	1,3
After 6 month	0	
Not stated	24	

Table 10.2. Symptoms of subglottic hemangiomas (Ohi 1979)

	No. of cases	%
Cases with symptoms	85	
Stridor	72	84,7
Dyspnea	37	43,5
Retractions	29	34,1
Wheezing	16	18,8
Cyanosis	14	16,5
Feeding problems and weight-loss	10	11,8
Hoarseness	8	9,4
Tachypnea	2	2,3
Cardiac arryhthmia	1	1,2
Not stated	19	

to corticosteroids. Among 9 patients who had to be intubated for immediate respiratory distress, and 8 additional patients for steroid resistance or dependence, after 10 days of tracheal intubation 30% of the patients did well and were stable (1 stabilized after 20 days and 2 after 30 days). 60% of the patients required intubation and radioactive phosphorus (450 rads). One child required 2 month of intubation and only 10 cures were observed after one application of phosphorus. As mentioned by Bommel, the therapeutic goal is to gain time since the hemangiomas always regress. Therefore, there is no indication for mutilating treatment unless every conservative one has proven ineffective.

Embolization in our experience, has proven to be immediately effective on the obstructive symptomatology of the hemangioma. In two cases (6 and 7 kg infants) immediate discontinuation of the corticosteroid therapy could be achieved and extubation was possible immediately after embolization. One patient required corticosteroid therapy and antibiotics for a few days after a throat infection 4 month after the embolization. In each case, the procedure was easy and expeditious, one single artery had to be embolized (the inferior thyroidal) with PVA particles (140 microns in size) (see Vol. 1, p. 402).

As a strategy we think that each time an infant has to be intubated or corticosteroid therapy needs to be increased or repeated (corticosteroid resistance, corticosteroid dependence), embolization should be tried. Although no complications were reported in Bommel's series, we feel that a properly performed embolization and 3 days hospitalization has to be balanced against the 10 days or more of hospitalization in an intensive care unit required for intubation and corticosteroid therapy considering that the clinical results are similar.

2. Eyelid Hemangiomas

Children presenting with complete occlusion of the eye due to a potentially involutive hemangioma require rapid treatment to preserve future vision. Thompson (1979) considers that blindness will follow one week occlusion of the palpebrae in infants. Pasyk (1984) could not preserve the vision in one of her 9 patients with two sessions of steroid treatments, although the hemangioma seemed to respond to treatment (Fig. 9.12). In fact, visual acuity is extremely difficult to assess in infants, therefore, the decision has to be made on the clinical picture. Some favorable situations, particularly in the upper lateral eyelid locations, permit complete embolization of the nidus.

Pasyk (1984) reviewed all the therapeutic modalities used in capillary hemangiomas since the eyelid localization is one of the few which may force early treatment. Cryotherapy with carbon dioxide or liquid nitrogen can be useful for superficial lesions, however it does not penetrate deep enough in eyelid lesions to produce rapid resolution. Injection of sclerosing agents, radiation therapy, and surgical ligation are either noneffective or dangerous for the future growth of the maxillofacial skeleton and may produce secondary carcinogenesis. Systemic or local steroid treatment with the exception of Kasabach Merritt syndrome (Brown 1972) is not always effective in capillary hemangiomas (Haik 1979) and some rebound growth may be observed after discontinuation (Lasser 1973). However, it may take 1 or 2 weeks to observe a response with a too rapid involution with necrosis and ulceration leading to considerable problems of reconstruction (Pasyk 1984). Argon laser has been used with some sucess by Apfelberg (1981). However, its indication remains more for the port wine lesions and cutaneous portions of other (vascular malformations), than for capillary hemangiomas. In cases where we used particle embolization shrinkage was obtained in 2–4 days, if at least 70% of the lesion was reached by the particles.

3. Oral Hemangiomas

These rarely involve the bone, but may present with rapid osseous deformity and spontaneous bleed. Surgical treatment may be needed in combination with embolization (Fig. 10.1). Soft tissue hemangiomas of the cheek are usually well tolerated; when necessary embolization can fasten the involution to avoid any consequence on the teeth eruption (Fig. 9.2) or psychological development (Fig. 10.2).

In adults, tongue hemangiomas are usually of a cavernous type and may present with pain or mass syndromes; they are poorly vascularized at angiography, however, particle embolization produces a stable relief of the pain syndromes and may decrease their size (see Vol. 1).

4. Salivary Gland Hemangiomas

Parotid gland hemangiomas are the most common type of tumor of the parotid gland in children (Wisniski, 1984). The facial nerve is usually not involved, facial asymmetry may be noticed following rapid growth of the lesion. These hemangiomas seem to present the same potential for involution as other proliferative lesion of the same kind, however, vascular masses in the same location, which present later in young adults (capillary vascular malformations) do not regress and may require invasive treatment (Hidano 1972, 1977).

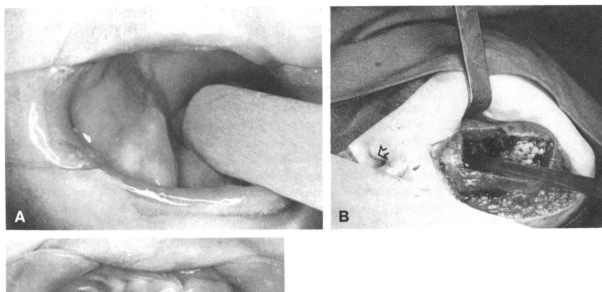

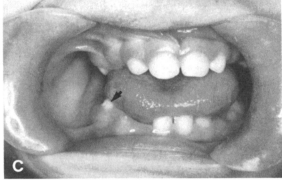

Fig. 10.1. 6 month old female presenting with a (potentially involutive) hemangioma of the mandible **(A)**. Following embolization intraosseous curetage could be achieved **(B)** with preservation of the mandibular cortex. Pinna indicated for orientation *(open arrow)*. **C** Follow up examination 8 month later shows normalization of mandibular size and normal tooth eruption from the segment of the mandible previously involved with the hemangioma

5. Bone Hemangiomas

Vascular tumors of the maxillofacial bones in adults represent less than 1% of all osseous neoplasms (Dorfman 1971). As Batsakis stated, these figures may be even smaller if we exclude the bony changes associated with adjacent vascular malformations. Osseous hemangiomas are rare, and are more frequent in the calvarium (Wike 1949) where they represent 10% of benign neoplasms of the skull (Bridger 1976). Recently Glassock (1984) reported three cases of temporal hemangiomas and reviewed the literature. Forty-two cases of skull base hemangiomas have been reported and most of them arose from the temporal bone. Neither the symptoms nor the radiological investigation are specific for this slow benign entity. The diagnosis is therefore usually made at surgery. No specific angiographic patterns has been reported. In the jaw, they behave like slowly growing benign tumors; they usually occur in females (2:1) in the second decade (2/3 of cases reported by Batsakis 1979). Spontaneous hemorrhage is rare, however, tooth extraction may provoke a profuse bleeding as with mandibular vascular malformations. Bony hemangiomas are usually of the

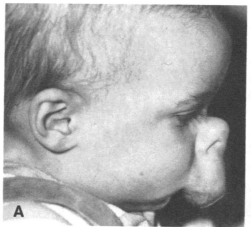
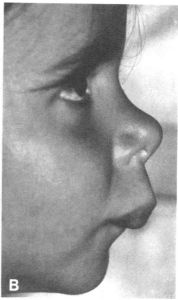

Fig. 10.2. A (Potentially involutive) hemangioma in a 6 month old girl. Due to cosmetic problems and parental pressure, embolization was undertaken. **B** One year later the result is satisfactory although the rate of regression had stabilized, note the normal nasal development

capillary type and are highly vascularized; however, some may not be visualized during angiographic studies (cavernous or fibrous type).

Mandibular or aneurysmal bone cyts are very rare and make up only 2% of lesions occuring in all bones.

Hemangiopericytomas and malignant vascular tumors are also extremely rare in the facial skeleton and usually result from the bony invasion of adjacent soft tissue lesions. In each case, there are few specific clinical or radiological findings (which will confirm the nature of these rare lesions). Any slow growing bleeding mass which changes with hormonal events or which is associated with a cutaneous telangiectasia should be explored angiographically.

6. The Kasabach and Merritt Syndrome

This is a rare condition in which hemangiomas are associated with a consumption coagulopathy characterized by thrombocytopenia (Kasabach 1940), fibrinogenopenia and accelerated fibrinolytic activity (Blix 1961). Coagulation studies in patients with this disease frequently reveal a profile similar to that of disseminated intravascular coagulation (DIC) (Inceman 1969). ^{131}I fibrinogen or ^{51}Cr-labelled platelets injected in some of these patients (Straub 1972, Brizel 1965, Warrel 1985) has been reported to accumulate within the tumor, pointing to localized clotting and fibrinolysis within the hemangioma rather than "disseminated" intravascular coagulation, secondary to a localized consumption of platelets and clotting factors within the tumor. The process that is responsible for the coagulopathy is still not clear; various theories have been suggested, including a deficiency

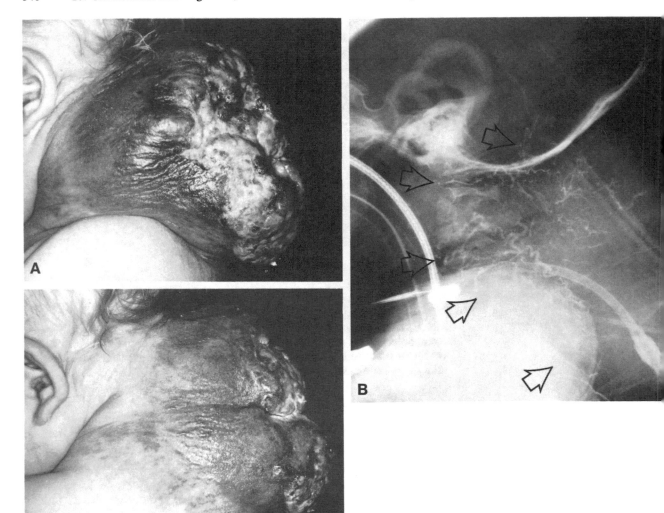

Fig. 10.3 A-C. Kasabach and Merritt syndrome (KMS)

A 45° view of a midline capillary hemangioma in an 8 month old girl with KMS after failure of radiotherapy (3000R) which resulted in necrosis and infection but no improvement in the coagulopathy. High IV doses of steroids and antibiotics, produced no regression or increase in platelet count nor improvement in D.I.C. During embolization in 5 stages, each procedure was followed by a temporary aggravation of the D.I.C. which responded to cryoprecipitate. Platelet consumption responded only temporarily but became more stable with each procedure, although platelet transfusions were still necessary to keep levels in the 20,000 to 30,000 range. 3 weeks after the last embolization the platelets increased to over 50,000 and the D.I.C. resolved, permitting easy removal and reconstruction. Selective angiography (not shown) demonstrated in mid arterial phase a capillary type (potentially involutive) hemangioma with a dense blush without AV shunting

B Lateral plain film showing the IBCA cast after 5 different procedures in which multiple branches of both sides were superselectively catheterized and embolized with IBCA, using an 0.038 open end guidewire

C Clinical picture during the staged embolization. Note the reduction in size primarily in the anterior, superior and inferior aspects, which correlates with the cast shown on *B*. The skin discoloration was markedly improved. At this point, the child could lift her head, and lie on her back and an anterior margin of the mass could be felt on physical examination, thus permitting easy surgical excision of the hemangioma and resolution of the coagulopathy

of the production of prostacyclin by the endothelial cells, and adhesion of thrombin to these cells. Alternatively, neoplastic endothelium within the hemangioma may initiate contact activation of the intrinsic coagulation pathway (Awbrey 1979). Interaction between thrombo-modulin and protein C (Owen 1981) or secretion of plasminogen activator could allow the formation of platelet fibrin thrombi (Luskutoff 1977). Stasis of blood in the hemangioma may lead to an accumulation of activated coagulation factors and increased local fibrinolysis. Coagulation in the hemangioma could then become autocatalytic resulting in thrombocytopenia and depletion of coagulation factors.

The syndrome usually occurs in children. In some patients the coagulopathy is mild and does not affect survival, but in others it is more severe and in the absence of treatment can result in fatal hemorrhage. Complete erradication of the hemangioma by surgery or radiation has been reported to eliminate the coagulopathy (Shim 1969, Hill 1962). More recently, Neidhart in 1982 and Warrell in 1985 have reported the control of this coagulopathy with aminocaproic acid alone or in conjunction with cryoprecipitate in extensive nonsurgical lesions. Although successful in controlling the consumption coagulopathy, the treatment required very high doses over a long period of time and has been associated with episodes of acute thrombosis at sites distant from the tumor which required temporary suspension of treatment. In addition, minor paraesthesias of the lower extremities were noted in Warrell's (1985) patients.

Corticosteroids (usually in high doses) may be effective in the control of the platelet consumption (Brown 1972) and heparin therapy has also been suggested (Rodriguez 1971). However, in our personal experience, the platelet count often rises at the onset of steroid therapy but falls again when the medication is tapered or stopped, suggesting some dependence; or they are not effective, and unless the first problem (the hemangioma) is corrected, the consumption persists.

The syndrome is uncommon and there is no large experience with the disease. Patients with multiple or very large non surgical lesions and those with sufficiently severe coagulopathy to prevent surgery represent a difficult therapeutic challenge. In this instance, an intervention which produces local thrombosis should decrease flow within the tumor resulting in involution. Such intervention include fibrinolytic inhibitors such as aminocaproic acid as described above and radiation (Shim 1969; Hill 1962).

We have had experience with 2 children with this syndrome who responded to embolization. One was steroid dependent and responded readily to extensive microembolization with IBCA. A second child (Fig. 10.1) had failed therapy with corticosteroids, heparin and radiation (which was followed by significant necrosis) and was finally embolized in 5 stages with IBCA. Each embolization session was followed by temporary aggravation of the D.I.C. requiring cryoprecipitate transfusions, but also by incremental shrinkage and devascularization and after 2 weeks the platelet count rose and the D.I.C. resolved, permitting surgical removal of the lesions with complete resolution of the coagulopathy (Fig. 10.3).

Due to our limited but positive experience with aggressive embolization to reduce the size of the lesions or to convert them to surgically accessible ones, we believe that endovascular embolization may be an effective adjunct in such difficult situations.

The principles of pretherapeutic strategy and techniques of embolization are similar to those described for other lesions with the additional technical problems of catheterization of pediatric patients (small vessels, contrast limitation). It may be necessary to perform the embolization in multiple stages, with careful monitoring of the coagulopathy until stabilization has occured.

Special precautions include the use of intraoperative and immediate postoperative transfusions of platelets and cryoprecipitate to obtain proper hemostasis at the arteriotomy site. In the postoperative period as the lesion is thrombosing and/or involuting, careful monitoring and treatment of the coagulopathy is needed.

II. Vascular Malformations

In the head and neck region, the oral cavity represents the pivotal area in the maxillofacial growth. At birth the viscerocranium has given rise to the upper maxillofacial (facial buds) and the mandibular (first branchial arch) skeleton. Muscular derivatives are linked to specific bones or a specific portion of the bone (see Vol. 1, Table 6.1). Therefore, it is possible to establish multiple functional (static and dynamic) musculoosseous relationships.

The role of these muscles will be to permanently adjust the position of the mandible in relation to the maxilla. Since the latter is fixed to the base of the skull, adjustments can only be achieved by the muscles acting on the position of the mandible.

Maxillofacial growth is peculiar in that it occurs relatively late, compared with that of the base of the skull and calvarium. Breathing, sucking and swallowing are important activities which affect the development of the maxilla and mandible during infancy and childhood. Muscle action on the mandibular subunits generates osseous growth (calcium deposition or reabsorption). The facial motor and sensory activities are established early in life, and normally from the corporeal scheme (unconscious maxillofacial praxis) which is maintained. The sensory motor system which adjust the maxillomandibular contact and stimulates growth includes:
1. the bilabial contact
2. the tongue to palate contact
3. the alveolar contact (with or without teeth)

Any alteration in these activities produces a non harmonious growth of the mandible and will result in additional deformity which may later require treatment (malocclusions including micrognathia, prognatism, open bite syndromes etc.) furthermore the "normal state" imprinted by the corporeal scheme will be in fact pathological (Table 10.3).

If a spontaneous or therapeutic regression restores normal morphology of the oral cavity, the corporeal scheme may identify it as an "abnormal state" and its motor orders and motor coordination will effect certain movement to return oral structures to the previous state thought to be "normal" and therefore opposed to the morphological correction achieved.

This is to emphasize that lesions which involve the growing face pose multiple functional problems in addition to morphological ones. The anatomical reconstruction of the oral cavity must be followed by the proper

Table 10.3. Sensory motor relationships

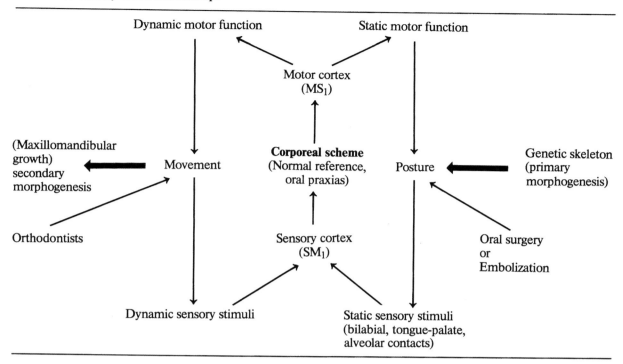

re-education of the corporeal scheme. For this purpose, the analytical and therapeutic contributions of the orthodental member of the team is essential (Lasjaunias 1984).

1. Oral Vascular Lesions

a) Dental Arcade AVMs

Vascular malformations involving the dental arcade represent the most challenging of the maxillofacial AVMs. Anderson in 1981 reviewed 60 cases of mandibular AVM published in the american literature since 1859. He found that:

A. They often manifest or worsen secondary to hormonal changes (puberty, pregnancy, menses) (Figs. 10.4–10.6).
B. They are usually of an arterial type with high flow (Fig. 10.6).
C. They are exposed to frequent trauma specific for the area (tooth eruption, eating, hygiene or dental treatments which frequently reveals the AVM) (Figs. 10.6, 10.10).
D. They bleed frequently and often require emergency treatment for hemostasis (Fig. 10.6).
E. Radical surgery is often cosmetically mutilating.
F. Secondary functional disturbances are very disabling (trismus, speech problems, swallowing, facial deformity, etc.)
G. Pain, bruit, subcutaneous invasion and ischemic ulceration are related to local evolution of the lesions sometimes accelerated by local infection (i. e. the so called "pyogenic granuloma") or surgical intervention.

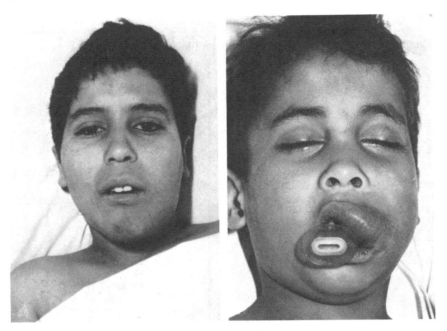

Fig. 10.4   **Fig. 10.5**

Fig. 10.4. High flow vascular malformation of the left hemimandible in a 14 year old boy (same patient as Fig. 9.10). Note the hemifacial hypertrophy

Fig. 10.5. High flow vascular lesion of the maxillar bone extending across the midline in a 9 year old male. Note the cutaneous telangiectasias and the soft tissue difformity

Fig. 10.6 A-O. 13 year old female **A** seen as an emergency for acute spontaneous ▶ bleeding from the right hemimandible. **B** Panoramic radiograph taken at the time of bleeding. Note the enlarged inferior dental canal *(arrowheads)*, and the wisdom tooth (No. 48) *(arrow)*. **C** Ipsilateral internal maxillary artery injection. The arteriovenous shunt arises near the wisdom tooth and drains into the inferior dental vein *(broken arrow)*. Note the decreasing size of the inferior dental artery *(arrowhead)*. **D** Opposite internal maxillary artery injection. Branches crossed the midline *(curved arrow)* to join the nidus of the malformation and drain into the enlarged inferior dental vein *(arrowhead)*.
E (see p. 352) Ipsilateral facial artery. **F** Opposite side facial artery. **G** Ipsilateral lingual artery. **H** Contralateral lingual artery. To obtain hemostasis each feeder illustrated above had to be embolized with PVA particles. The bleeding stopped only after the last embolization. 3 months later the panoramic radiogram **(I)** shows the radiopaque PVA *(open arrow)* and a slightly larger wisdom tooth *(arrow)*. At that point the patient was noted to have a necrosis of the anterior third of the tongue which required antibiotics to avoid infection. **J** Panoramic radiograms 6 month after the embolization show a decrease in size of the inferior dental canal *(arrowheads)*. However, there is destruction of the roots of tooth 45 *(arrowhead)* which was very mobile at the clinical examination. 9 month after embolization the patient complained of moderate bleeding. The panoramic study **(K)** demonstrates a slightly enlarged space with bone destruction between the teeth 47 and 48 *(open arrowhead)*. Selective injection of the ascending pharyngeal artery **(L)** shows the arteriovenous shunt around tooth 48, its venous drainage *(arrowheads)* and the venous outlet into the inferior dental vein *(curved arrow)*. At this point the artery could not be embolized with particles and fluid material was not desirable due to the

Fig. 10.6 A-D

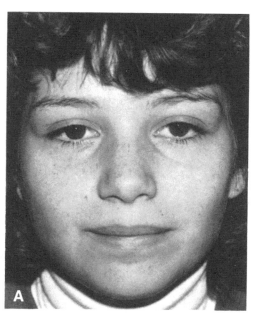

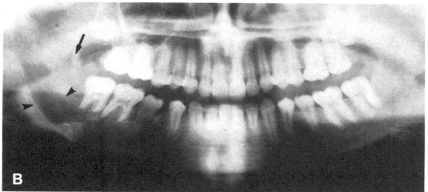

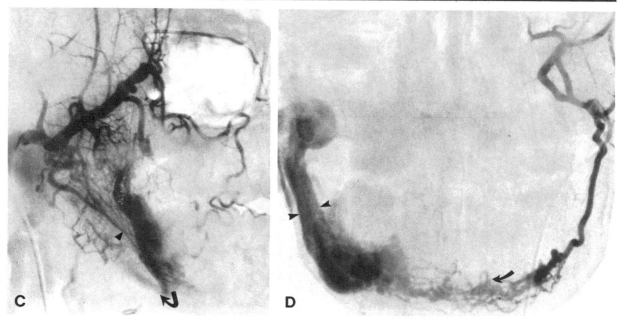

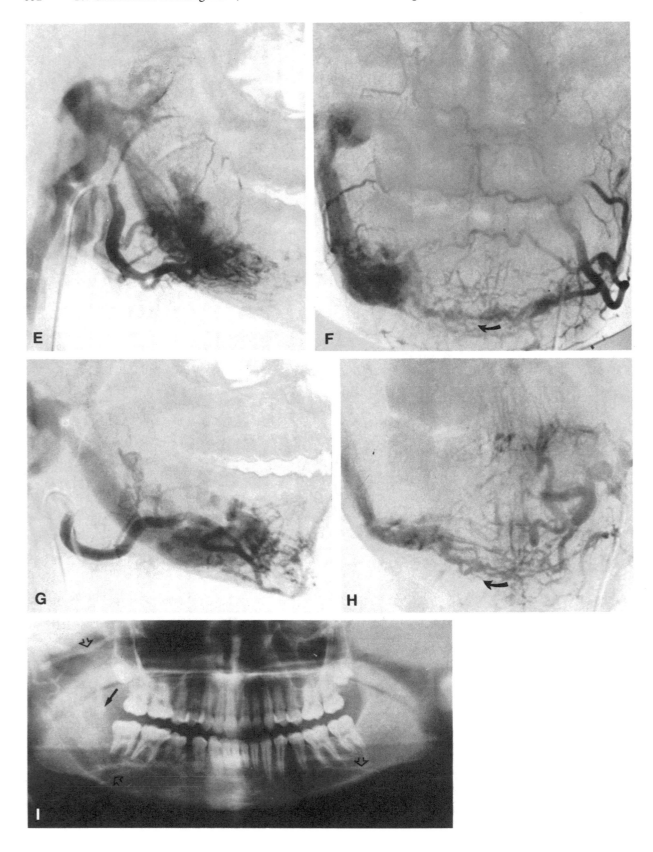

Fig. 10.6 E-I (legend see p. 350)

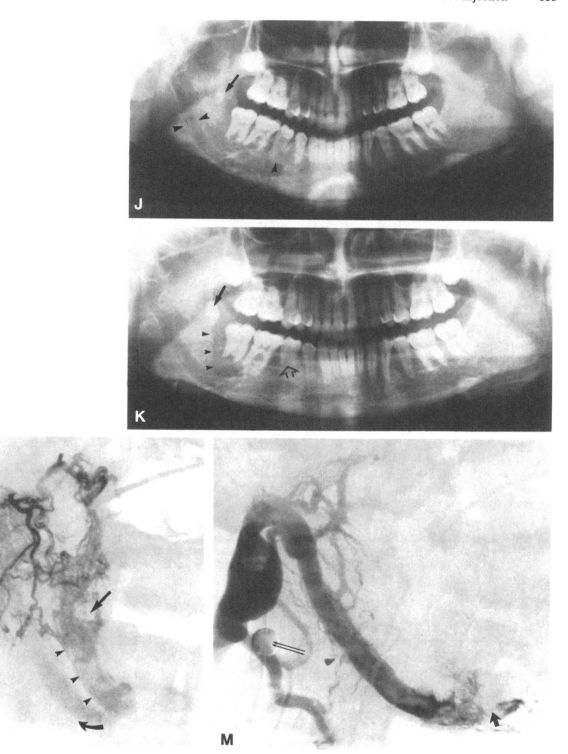

Fig. 10.6 (continued)
previous therapeutic complication. A direct approach was chosen to allow removal of the tooth 45. **M** Selective injection of contrast material into the nidus by transcutaneous direct puncture. The needle has been inserted into the nidus *(solid arrow)* and a double lumen balloon catheter is placed into the venous system of the neck in an attempt to diminish the venous outflow. Radiopaque IBCA was injected in this position

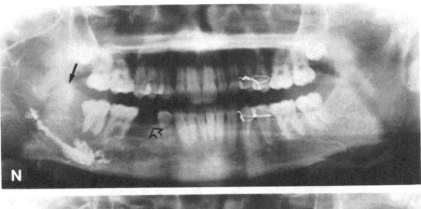

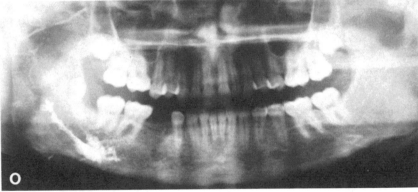

Fig. 10.6 (continued). **N** On the panoramic control 2 days after the IBCA injection and tooth extraction, the glue is seen to be properly located. Note the braces which were placed for 36 hours, after the tooth extraction to guarantee mechanical hemostasis. **O** Final control after 6 months after the extraction. Note the recalcification of the bone between the teeth 47 and 48 and in the 45th position. Spontaneous healing of the necrotic tongue occurred rapidly; there is no speech disturbance 3 years following this complication

Patients who are afraid of bleeding may try to avoid the primary source of trauma by decreasing oral hygiene. The resulting local infection produces in fact the same trauma and secondarily generates an ischemic and infected ulceration leading to further complications.

b) Treatment Strategy of Oral Vascular Lesions

The facial skeleton should be maintained whenever possible. If complete intraosseous curretage preserving the bony cortex can be achieved, radical surgery following embolization can be performed (Fig. 10.1). Otherwise, the radical surgery should be reserved for after the maxillofacial growth is complete, at least a few years after puberty. Embolization alone represents the best non mutilating method to obtain immediate hemostasis. Embolization should be planned before every tooth extraction on the side of the AVM or on the site of its venous drainage. During tooth eruptions, antibiotics and anti-inflammatory treatment is indicated each time mouth infections do not respond to local antiseptic gargles. In general, radiographic evaluation with a panorex study once per year in children and every 18 month in adults (Fig. 10.6) is sufficient, if no urgent treatment is needed.

Technically, embolization of lesions of the oral cavity must be carried out bilaterally in most cases. The tongue represents a difficult territory because

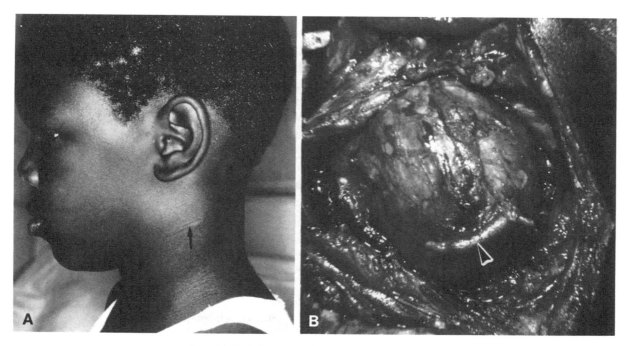

Fig. 10.7. A 9 year old black boy presenting with a subcutaneous infraauricular capillary hemangioma. Embolization of the ipsilateral occipital artery was performed before surgery. **B** A well encapsulated and circumscribed lesion was found at operation and removed

of its muscular nature and particularly sensitive response to ischemia; therefore, we prefer the use of particles rather than IBCA, whereas in floor of the mouth AVM, IBCA may be better.

Results of embolization in the oral cavity can be extremely rewarding, particularly in children with vascular malformations of the tongue which respond in a spectacular fashion to bilateral particle embolization (Figs. 10.2, 10.10).

c) Salivary Gland AVMs

Salivary gland AVMS seem rare; in our experience, we have encountered only two parotid gland vascular lesions whose character seem to correspond to an arterial type of malformation. Both were embolized only and decreased in size by about 50% with PVA particles. They are stable with 5 and 2 years follow up. Some lesions seem to present the same clinical characters (rapid growth, young adults, high flow) with no obvious link with the glands themselves (Fig. 10.7) but have a tumoral appearance at surgery.

d) Lymphatic Malformations

Wisniski in 1984, in his review discussed several embryological hypothesis to explain or understand the lymphangiomatous vascular malformations. Huntington in 1907 proposed an absence of anastomosis between the lymph sacs and the venous system (cavernous and cystic hygromas). Other hypotheses are lymphatic blockage with upstream dilatation (Bill 1965). In fact the lymphatic system is linked to the venous circulation and for that reason, purely lymphatic lesions or cystic lymphangiomas are not anatomically reachable by transarterial embolization.

However, mixed lesions like hemolymphangiomas of the face and of the tongue are different lesions that usually present immediately after birth and evolve by acute swelling; they may be partially regressive. In the tongue area, the mucosa becomes dark, the mouth is permanently opened, bleeding may occur following desquamation of the constantly protruding dry tongue (Fig. 10.8). Some extensive lesions compromise the airway or alimentary tract and require intubation or tracheostomy; swelling is usually induced by local infections (Fig. 10.15).

Although potentially regressive these acute changes of hemolymphangiomas always leave a mass effect even after maximal regression of the symptoms. These lesions are frequently corticosteroid resistant, and in the acute phase, embolization can be useful. In our experience, complete resolution or swelling and stabilization can be obtained after embolization. Moderate shrinkage of the lesion can usually be followed by conservative treatment with orthodontic assistance.

It seems to us that particularly in the tongue situation; bilateral embolization with particles must be considered when glossectomy, even cuneiform, appears to be the only alternative. Hemolymphangiomas behave as a mixed lesion: capillary that can be reached and the lymphatic malformation that is unreachable. Pure lymphangiomas of the tongue are clinically different as they present with swelling but with normal pinkish or pale appearance to the mucosae. Embolization is not effective in this lesion. They are noninvolutive (Fig. 10.9).

Some lymphangiomas of the cheek can be associated with other vascular malformations of the head and neck, particularly port wine stains in Sturge-Weber syndrome. Traumatic transformation of the hemolymphangiomas in this territory may sometimes require endovascular control of an acquired arteriovenous fistula.

2. Cutaneomuscular Vascular Lesions

a) Face and Scalp AVMs

α) **Introduction.** Since the first report by Dandy in 1946 in which he proposed the use of pieces of muscle to treat a post-traumatic AVM of the face, confusion in congenital versus traumatic AVM has remained. The confusion also extends to the distinction between superficial AVM of the scalp fed by the middle meningeal artery and the dural AVM fed by the occipital or superficial temporal arteries. In his discussion, Dandy individualized the type I scalp vascular lesion fed by the middle meningeal artery (which is common in our experience) and a type II lesion in which he shows a dural AVM draining into the cortical venous system as well as the suboccipital region via the mastoid emissary vein. This differentiation emphasizes the contribution of superselective angiography (Djindjian, 1978) to understanding the vascular architecture and the hazards related to the treatment of AVMs of the scalp.

One of the important diagnostic questions is the significance of the transosseous supply to a scalp AVM: does it correspond to a bony and dural invasion or to a purely cutaneous AVM fed by an emissary artery? In

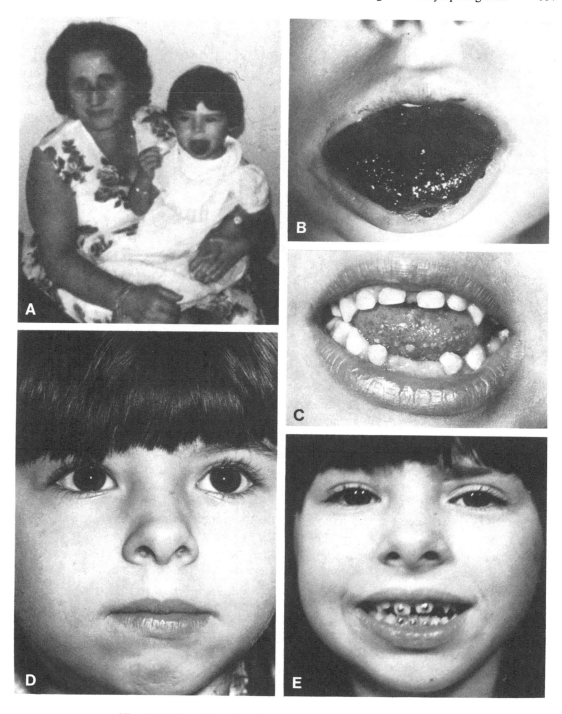

Fig. 10.8. Hemolymphangioma of the tongue in a 3 year old female (**A** and **B**). **C, D** One year after embolization of both lingual arteries with PVA, she could close her mouth but still had an open bite syndrome. **D** This was corrected later by a course of orthodontic therapy. Using this combined approach, the tongue and dental function were preserved and mutilating surgery was avoided. **E** Follow-up 5 years after the initial embolization

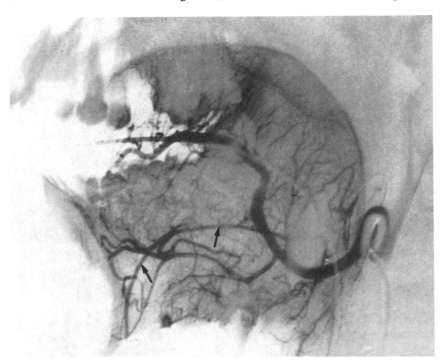

Fig. 10.9. Pure lymphangioma of the tongue and the floor of the mouth. Note the mass effect produced by the extension into the floor of the mouth *(arrows)* shown on the lingual artery injection

general, the venous drainage of the nidus will give its topography, especially if a compartmental analysis is made. The calvarial lesions draining into a sinus is a dural lesion whereas a lesion draining into a subcutaneous vein of the scalp arises in the scalp. Both lesions can receive their arterial supply from either dural or cutaneous sources (but bony foramen can usually be seen, and partial reconstruction after careful superselective analysis gives the best analysis). The mastoid area is the most difficult to evaluate since a strong muscle insertion (sternocleido-mastoid muscle, nuccal muscle) brings superficial arteries deep into the bone. Therefore, some dural lesions involving the inner table, may recruit a shower of small scalp arteries without any cutaneous involvement (see Vol. 1, Chapter 20).

The presence of an emissary vein with suboccipital pulsatile venous ectasia may also complicate the analysis. However, if the lesion is dural, the ascending pharyngeal or the vertebral artery will participate in its supply. If the lesion is superficial, the superficial temporal or cutaneous branches of the occipital arteries will contribute to its supply.

Surgical and pathological confusion between intrinsically normal, but transformed veins draining an arteriovenous shunt, and the truly abnormal vessels within the nidus of an AVM, has led to incorrect description of the extent of lesions; the normal draining veins, although enlarged, were considered to be part of the primary abnormality, and were sometimes described as a cavernous component. The removal of these enlarged normal veins was even recommended and it took a long time before the normal hemodynamic transformation of these draining veins and the reversibility of their status was appreciated. Many recurrences occured because of the partial removal of the enlarged but normal venous drainage, leaving behind part of the nidus.

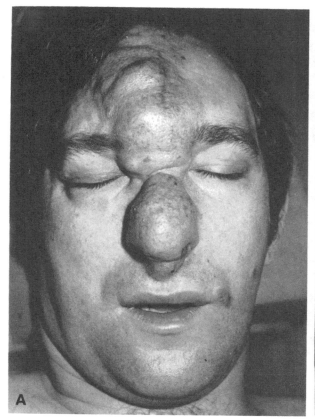
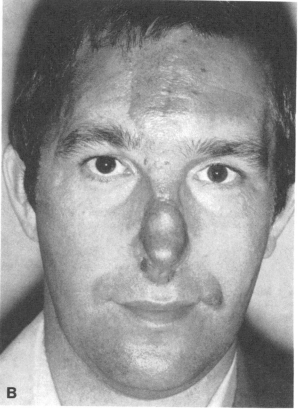

Fig. 10.10. A High flow malformation of the forehead and nose which had recurred after previous surgery. Embolization and reoperation accomplished complete removal of the lesion **(B)**. A skin graft was needed for the crest of the nose

One must be aware of the facial vascular deformities which are associated with intracranial or intraorbital AVM draining into maxillofacial veins (like in Bonnet Dechaume and Blanc syndromes). In these instances, the visible dilated vessels and palpable thrill do not represent the malformation itself but the venous drainage of the deeper shunt.

Many types of vascular lesions are encountered in the face and scalp:

– the port wine stain related to Sturge-Weber syndrome
– the telangiectasias of Rendu Osler Weber disease
– the isolated AVM which can be of any type: capillary, arterial, venous, lymphatic or a combination of different channels (hemolymphangiomas, capillary venous, arteriocapillary with or without fistula).

In comparison to other locations, isolated AVMs of the scalp and face give rise to two types of problems:
1. cosmetic (Figs. 10.8–10.10, 10.17)
2. technical (Figs. 10.11–10.13)

These lesions have a major psychological impact related to the magnitude of the cosmetic problem. The adverse psychological effects are aggravated by the fact that acute exacerbation occur during times of hormonal changes (premenstrual, last trimester of pregnancy or puberty). Management of these frequently invasive facial lesions, especially when they are lateral in location and involve the cutaneous musculature and the facial nerve, can be extremely challenging (Fig. 10.14).

Leikensohn reported 7 out of 8 patients in whom facial AVM where satisfactorily embolized and then operated upon either for bleeding or for

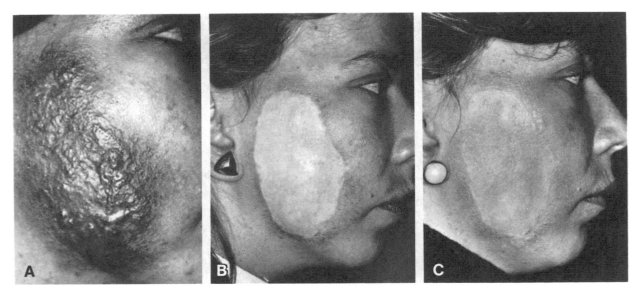

Fig. 10.11 A-C. 32 year old female presenting with a port wine stain and underlying capillary vascular malformation. The cheek became more tense discolored and pulsatile during her menstrual periods. A bruit and a thrill were noted clinically but no AVF was found at angiography. There was no previous history of trauma. She underwent microembolization with PVA followed by surgical resection. Split thickness skin grafting followed as combined treatment (By permission, from Berenstein, AJNR 2:261–267, 1981)

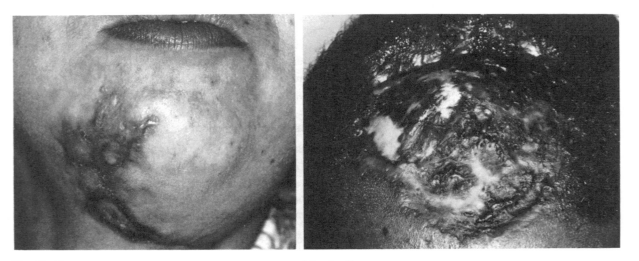

Fig. 10.12   **Fig. 10.13**

Fig. 10.12. Skin necrosis following IBCA injection through collateral circulation which developed after multiple ligations

Fig. 10.13. 32 year old black male with a vascular malformation of the forehead which was embolized with particles. Following an attempt to remove the lesion at surgery the patient was referred because of nonhealing of the infected incision. The area was treated by reembolization with microparticles (PVA) and reoperation with a full thickness graft from the thigh using vascular pedicles

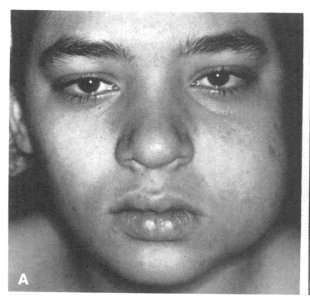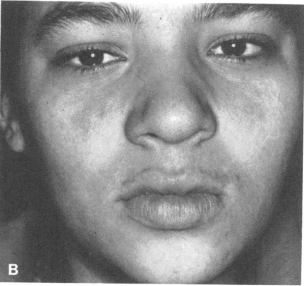

Fig. 10.14. High flow vascular malformation of the left cheek in a 19 year old female which became symptomatic at the time of puberty and was aggravated with menstruation **(A)**. After embolization with silicone fluid, the lesion could be removed entirely at surgery and has been stable over a 7 year follow up **(B)**. All branches of the VIIth nerve were preserved. (Same patient as Fig. 1.19)

mass effect with cosmetic problems. The remaining case illustrates disastrous effect of proximal embolization with silastic spheres (acting as a proximal ligation) and radiotherapy, which turned an easily reachable lesion into an almost unreachable one. To reach part of the nidus it was necessary at a later date to perform balloon manipulation in the intra-dural internal carotid artery and vertebral artery with IBCA embolization into the ophthalmic system resulting in blindness.

β) Bone Involvement in Face and Scalp AVMs. When planning the therapy of cutaneous scalp and facial AVMs, it is important to determine the presence or absence of associated bone involvement. One can determine that the bone is involved when bony arterial branches feed the AVM. Obviously cutaneous branches of bone arteries have to be identified carefully (inferior dental, medial mandibular, malar arteries) (Fig. 10.14). Nevertheless, CT images with bone windows are an important part of the pretherapeutic evaluation. In our experience, the bony changes are usually not related to the arterial nidus of the AVM, but to its venous drainage. Enlargement of vascular channels or grooves indicate increased flow in the vein or venous lakes (diploic) whereas hypertrophied bone may indicate only a constrainst or obstruction of the normal draining veins from the bone as occurs in Klippel Trenaunay syndrome of the legs with bone hypertrophy. In this latter situation, the AV shunts are always extraosseous (Figs. 10.11, 10.12). Similarly the bone hypertrophy observed in Struge Weber is thought to be related to a venular constraint as the associated leptomeningeal cutaneous malformations are of venous nature (see below). Other postulated causes for bone hypertrophy with subcutaneous-vascular malformation are increased temperature caused by hyperemia, and a

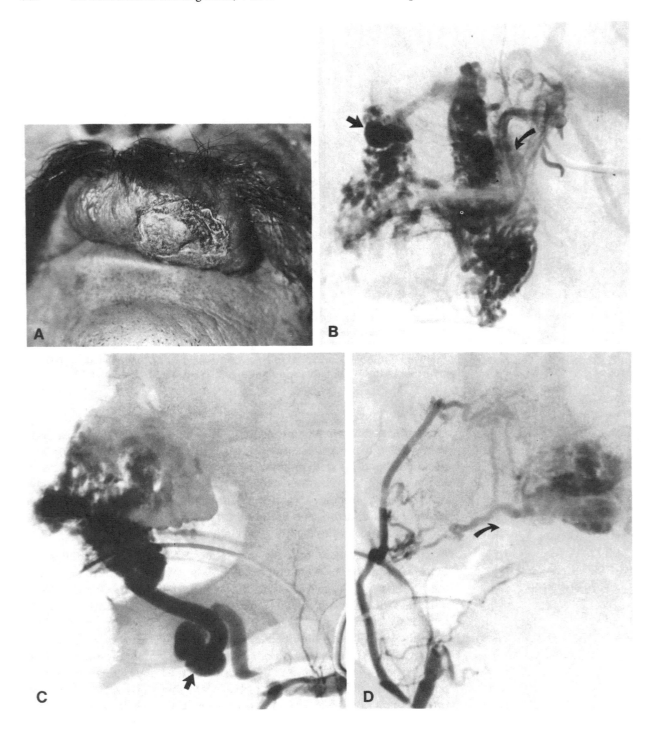

Fig. 10.15 A-F. 45 year old male presenting with a high flow vascular malformation of the upper lip and subjacent maxillar bone. **A** Close up view of a recently developed ischemic ulcer. **B** Distal internal maxillary artery injection demonstrating the supply to the bony component of the lesion *(curved arrow)* and intralesional vascular ectasia in the subcutaneous tissue *(solid arrow)*. **C** Ipsilateral facial artery injection demonstrating an aneurysm of the facial artery proximal to the vascular malformation. **D** Contralateral facial artery injection showing supply from unusual dysplastic vessels which join the most medial extension of the malformation *(curved arrow)*.

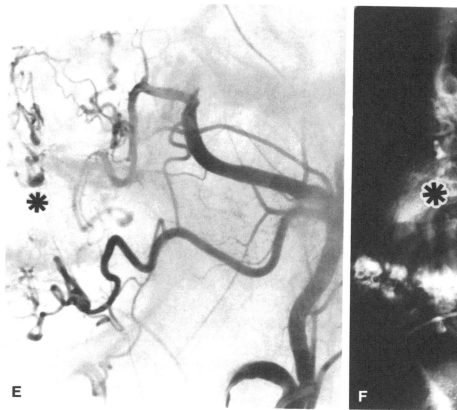
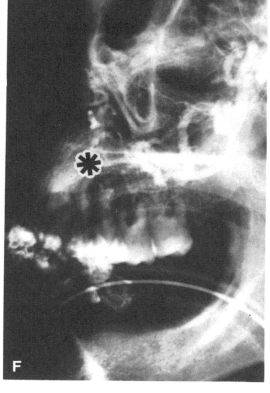

Fig. 10.15 E, F. Control angiograms after embolization with radiopaque IBCA. Since embolization the ischemic ulcer has healed and the lesion has been stable. No surgery was done in this case

generalized mesodermal dysplasia. Interesting is the usual absence of bone hypertrophy in scalp lesions in the parietotemporal or occipital region.

Although we have no satisfactory explanation to it, our impression is that the venous drainage of the bone can be directed towards different paths, so that no constraint is necessarily present to produce hypertrophy.

b) Ear AVMs

Vascular malformations in this territory are of the high flow type, often with direct arteriovenous fistulas. Trauma is frequently involved in their evolution. Ischemic ulceration can also be observed in these high flow lesions and is probably due more to venous obstruction than to acute arterial steal (Figs. 10.15–10.17). They classically produce frightening lesions with a higher risk of necrosis than AVMs of the tongue. To avoid this complication, embolization must be precise in delivery of the agent within the nidus exclusively. In general, we prefer IBCA to treat the subcutaneous and scalp AVMs even in the external ear location. PVA or other particles may reach normal territories since repetitive injections alter progressively the protective sump effect of the AVM. Since the goal of embolization is permanent stabilization (mass effect, bleed, bruit) without surgical correction, it is more likely that this will be achieved with IBCA (see Chapter 1).

c) Eyelid AVMs

Palpebral AVMs are potentially supplied by ophthalmic artery branches. This specific arterial disposition produces technical problems, and any

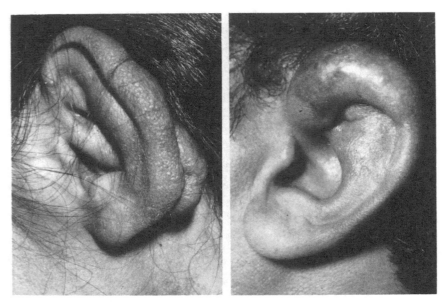

Fig. 10.16   **Fig. 10.17**

Fig. 10.16. Arterial vascular malformation of the ear with a post traumatic arteriovenous fistula on the medial surface of the helix

Fig. 10.17. Arterial vascular malformation of the ear with spontaneous (non traumatic) venous congestion

Fig. 10.18. High flow vascular malformation of the ear associated with a port wine stain and an ischemic ulcer of the helix **A** in a 15 year old female. This lesion required embolization for repeated hemorrhage. Note the high flow lesion with adjacent venous congestion seen on the **B** early and **C** late phases of the anterior auricular angiogram

▼

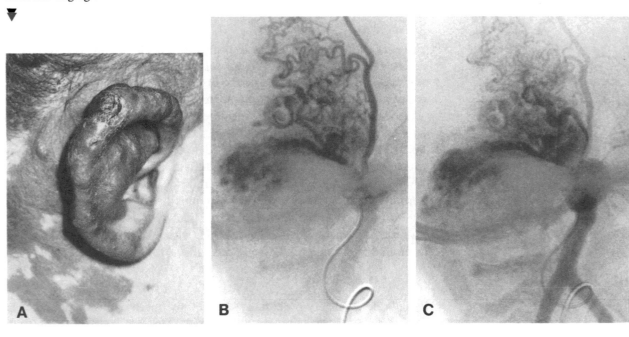

decision will therefore have to be carefully discussed if an attempt to reach the entire lesion either by embolization alone or combined approach is planned (Fig. 10.19).

If discoloration of the cutaneous covering of the ipsilateral frontal area or of the temporal area is present, careful search for an intracranial associated vascular anomaly must be achieved by contrast enhanced CT examination and proper selective injection during the pretherapeutic angiographic evaluation (Fig. 10.19).

d) Muscle AVMs (Fig. 10.20)

Intramuscular vascular malformations are usually of the arterial or capillary type. However, some of them will involve the capillary venous or venous channels. Intramuscular vascular malformations typically present in young adults although they can be seen at any age. They manifest as a rubbery pulsatile mass usually painful with periodic swelling during chewing. In the head and neck area, they concern mainly the masticatory muscles predominantly the masseteric muscle. Temporal and pterygoid muscles, are less frequently involved. Surgical correction in these deep locations is functionally more disabling. Malan in 1968 reported the Azzolini approach to the temporal and masseteric AVMs. Shklar and Meyer in 1965, recommended to wait at least until the age of 8 or 10 before undertaking surgery. They also deplore the use of any form of radiation in this type of lesions.

Fig. 10.19 A-I (see pp. 366 and 267). Vascular malformation of the eyelid in a 24 year old male. Spontaneous bleeding into the eyelid had led to occlusion of the eye.
A, B Axial CT image after contrast injection. Note the intraorbital extension of the malformation *(arrow)*. **C** Internal carotid angiogram which demonstrates the ophthalmic supply *(double arrow)*. **D** Anterior deep temporal artery injection shows that the orbital branch supplies the malformation *(broken arrow)*.
E Control immediately before IBCA deposition in oblique view. The catheter tip is in the orbital branch *(open arrow)* **(F)** following IBCA injection ("Sandwich" technique): the same 4 french catheter is still in place. The inferior portion of the lesion has been occluded and the upper compartment is now clearly seen *(arrowheads)*. Injection through this compartment produced reflux into the ophthalmic artery *(curved arrow)* better demonstrated in AP view **(G).** After determing by test injections of contrast material the necessary pressure to visualize the nidus without producing reflux into the ophthalmic system, the lesion was embolized through the same catheter in the same position with radiopaque IBCA.
H Control in the distal external carotid artery after the final IBCA deposition *(double arrow)*. **I** Immediate control angiogram of the internal carotid artery showing the disappearance of the lacrymal supply to the malformation.
The patient was operated upon without difficulty and the lesion was entirely removed. The cosmetic result was satisfactory and has been stable over a 3 years follow up. The dural lesion did not change and was embolized with IBCA 2 years later, because of concern about its drainage into the cortical venous system

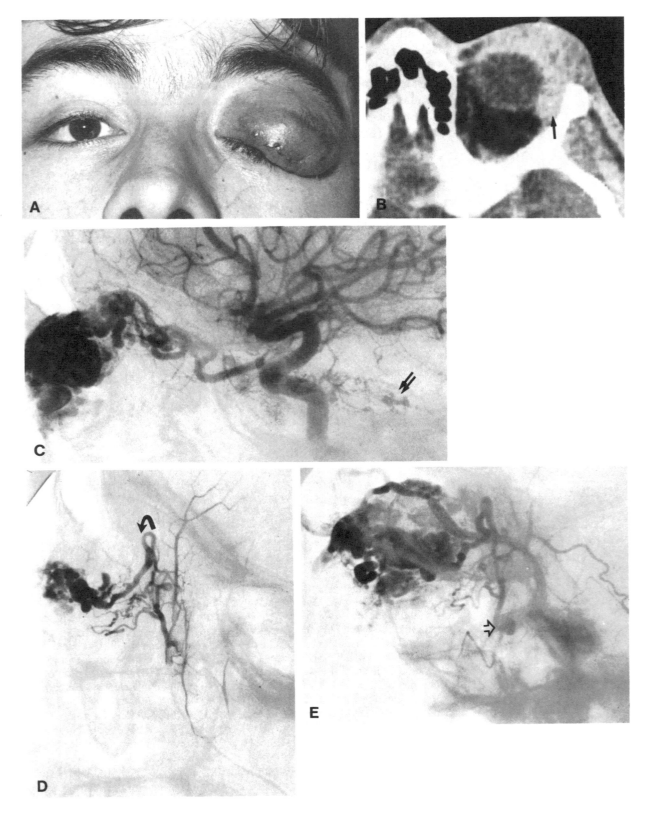

Fig. 10.19 A-E (legend see p. 365)

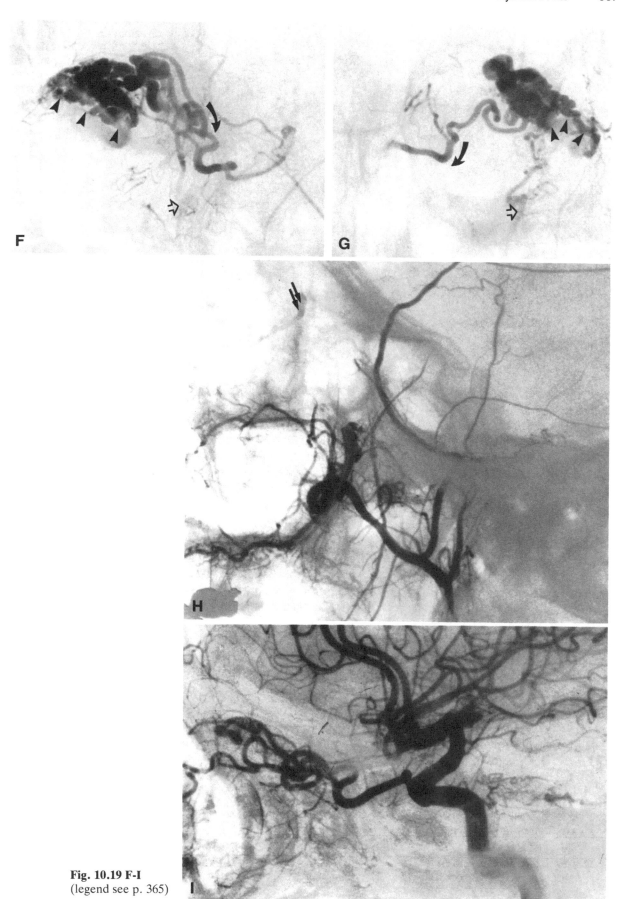

Fig. 10.19 F-I
(legend see p. 365)

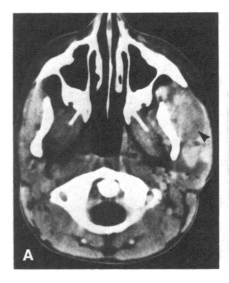
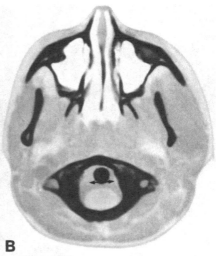

Fig. 10.20 A, B. Capillary vascular malformation *(arrowhead)* of the masseteric muscle **(A)** and **(B)**. Note the moderate displacement of the odontoid to compensate for the mandibular translation *(arrowhead)* **(B)**

3. Complex Vascular Malformations (Andre, 1974; Picard, 1968)

a) Cerebrofacial Vascular Malformations

Port wine stains represents localized dermal venular malformations, which can involve 0.3% of the population at birth (Jacobs 1976). Although they may occur anywhere, the face and neck represent the most frequent location (Knudsen 1979). The evolution of these skin lesions is not clear. They usually remain stable. These discolorations have to be individualized within birthmarks which have a high incidence (30% of the newborns) and from skin discoloration of subcutaneous hemangiomas. The latter usually regress spontaneously usually without sequelae (Figs. 9.6, 9.12).

From Wisnicki, 1 to 2% of port wine strains carry the diagnosis of Sturge Weber syndrome (Stevenson 1974) (Figs. 10.21–10.23). This encephalotrigeminal angiomatosis is a nonfamilial disease with a skin discoloration (port wine) in the V_1 territory associated to a calcified leptomeningeal venous malformation of the ipsilateral supratentorial hemisphere. Symptoms appear before the second year of age and include the cosmetic problems, neurological problems, related to subjacent cerebral atrophy leading to epilepsy, deficits, mental retardation (Figs. 10.21–10.23).

The lesions do not bleed except for extensive associated AVM of the cavum or pharynx which have to be differenciated from the gingivorrhagia related to some antiepilectic medications. Glaucoma occurs in one third of patients with Sturge-Weber syndrome due to the presence of a retinal vascular malformation probably of the venous type. This angiomatosis is usually unilateral, but it can involve the midline and is reported to extend to the chest, trunk and limbs in some cases.

From our experience, we have tried to individualize a full syndrome that we both have encountered in 8 instances:
- Port wine stains in the trigeminal territory (either V_1, V_2 or V_3).
- Lymphangiomatous malformation of the cheek area (Fig. 10.21).
- Maxillofacial (malar, frontal or maxilla) bone hypertrophy (Fig. 10.24).
- Pial vascular malformation supra or infratentorial.

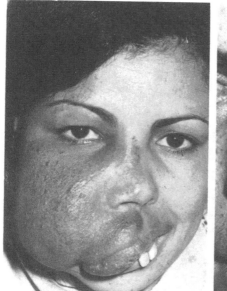 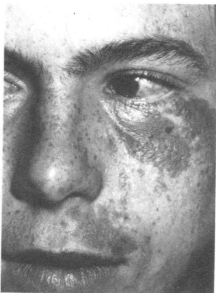

Fig. 10.21   **Fig. 10.22**

Fig. 10.21. Typical aspect of a complete encephalotrigeminal vascular malformation complex (Sturge-Weber syndrome) with at the maxillofacial level a lymphangioma of the cheek, port wine stain and bone hypertrophy

Fig. 10.22. Minimal expression of the Sturge-Weber syndrome, limited to a port wine stain. Conjunctival hyperemia was not associated with visual impairment

Although this form can be encountered, incomplete ones corresponding to the same neural crest disorder, are more frequent. In that regard, cheek lymphangioma with V_2 territory port wine stain and maxilla hypertrophy are not a rare association.

Using Couly's approach to regroup the neural tube and neural crest derivatives, one can appreciate the association between certain maxillofacial and central nervous system malformations. However, the pharynx, the floor of the mouth and tongue including inferior lip and chin, differ in that they are probably related developmentally to another organ system (pharyngeal digestive tract) and therefore are not involved in these malformations (Fig. 10.25).

Using CT, one should look for maxillofacial bone changes, brain atrophy, supra or infratentorial lesion, cortical calcification, and subarachnoidal cysts (Fig. 10.24).

In fact, the Sturge-Weber syndrome appears to involve metameric vascular malformation in the head and neck area as the Cobb syndrome at the spinal level. It can in some patients involve two or three consecutive metamers and be more or less complete in all the tissues derived at a given level.

Other combined maxillofacial central nervous system anomalies illustrates either the direct relationships between the neural tissue and the neural crest at the specific level, or the gap that may exist betwen two consecutive levels. Tessier (1976) in his classifications found 14 meridians to represent the most critical area in the upper and lower frontomaxillary region. We have already mentioned that some vascular malformations of the face may behave like clefts and receive unusual blood supply from rare

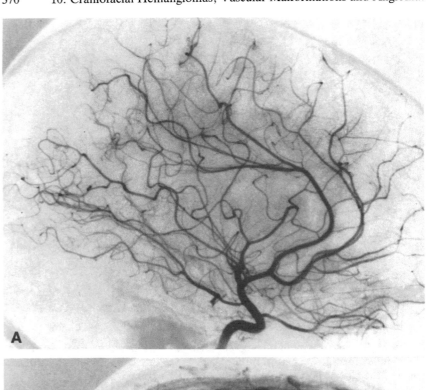

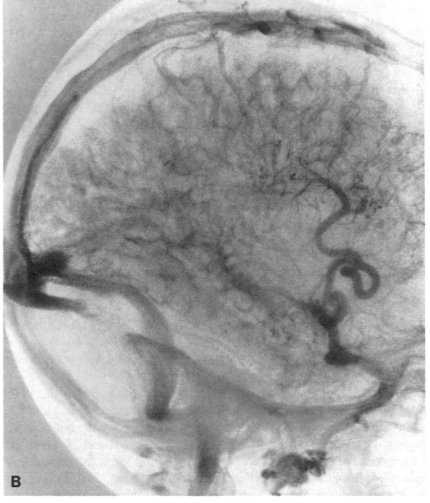

Fig. 10.23. Typical angiographic findings of a Sturge-Weber syndrome (A), early and (B) late phase of the internal carotid angiogram. Note the absence of arterial or capillary lesions. The venous system is abnormal and the drainage occurs late during the series.

Fig. 10.23. C Early and **D** late phase of the vertebral artery angiogram in the same patient. Note the similarity of the venous alterations in the right cerebellar hemisphere

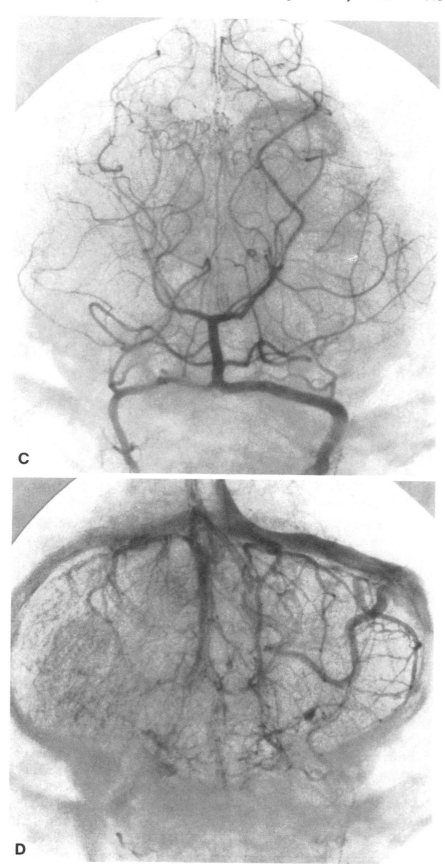

C

D

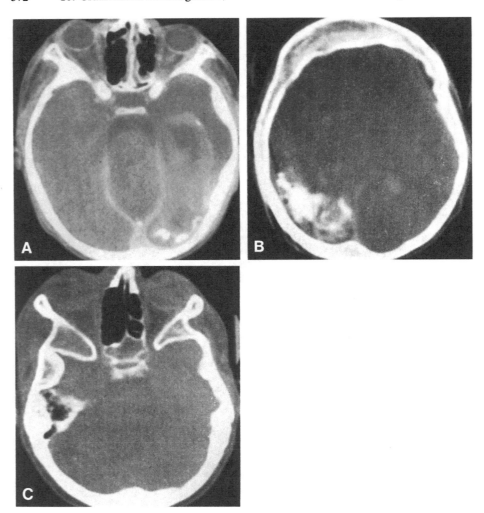

Fig. 10.24. Bony and cerebral changes in a complete form of encephalotrigeminal vascular malformation **(A)**. Note the short anterior floor on the cranial base and the atrophy and calcification of the righ temporal lobe. **B** Same patient, the higher section demonstrates the significant frontal bone hypertrophy and calcification of the left occipital pole. **C** Same patient, note the sphenoid bone hypertrophy and the asymmetry of the pneumatization of the ethmoid bone

arterial variations (see Vol. 1) (Fig. 10.26). Cleft margins are known to be highly vascularized (pre malformative or hemangiomatous state). In one of our cases, the cleft was associated with another midline vascular lesion confirmed at surgery (Fig. 10.27). Recently, Reid (1985) reported one case of facial port wine stain associated with an intracranial aneurysm treated by balloon trapping. Obviously not every vascular lesion of the face should undergo a complete angiographic study. However, when evaluating a vascular malformation on the face, one should consider it as part of a more generalized malformation until proven otherwise. Careful clinical examination and CT performed with an understanding of the CNS-neutral crest correspondance are usually adequate to exclude the complex diseases anomalies (Fig. 10.28).

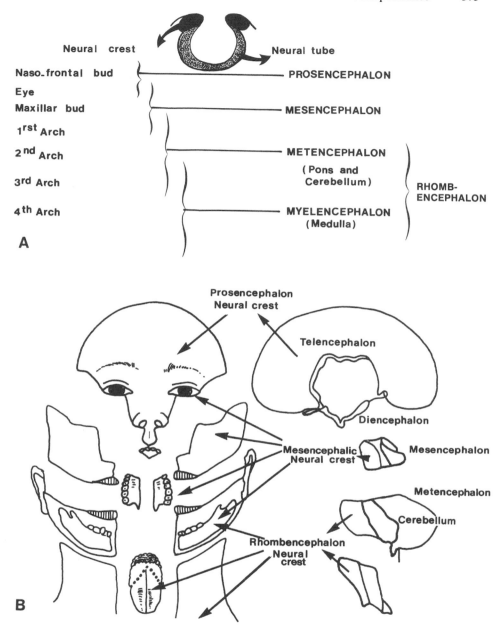

Fig. 10.25 A, B. Schematic representation of the maxillofacial correspondance to the cerebral nervous system. **A** Embryonic stage. **B** Final stage (From G. Couly with permission)

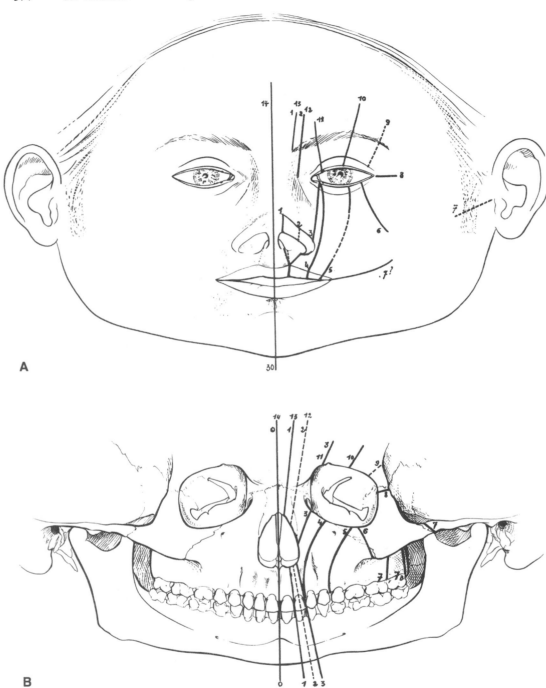

Fig. 10.26 A, B. Schematic representation of facial, craniofacial and laterofacial clefts. **A** and **B** demonstrate the localization in the soft tissue **(A)** and skeleton **(B)**. Dotted lines indicate either uncertain localization or uncertain clefts (From Tessier with permission)

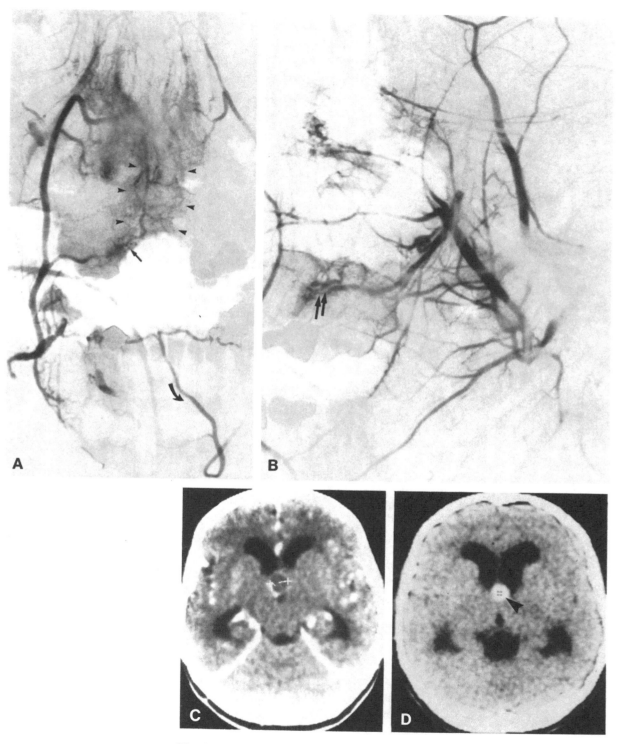

Fig. 10.27 A-F. 26 year old patient who presented with a chiasmatic syndrome and a cleft palate. **A** Selective injection of the ipsilateral facial artery. Note the hyperhemic cleft margins *(arrowheads)*. The upper lip also has hyperemic zone *(arrow)*. Note the medial branch to the inferior labial arcade *(curved arrow)*. **B** Internal maxillary artery injection in the same patient. Note the interruption of the greater palatine artery corresponding to the margin of the cleft. Axial CT without **(C)** and with **(D)** contrast injection. Note the contrast enhancing lesion of the area of the anterior commissure.

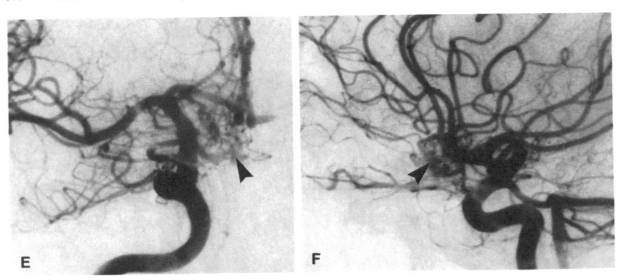

Fig. 10.27. E right and **F** left internal carotid arteries angiograms demonstrate a vascular lesion of an arteriolocapillary type corresponding to the CT images *(arrowhead)*. At the surgery, the lesion was found to be a vascular malformation

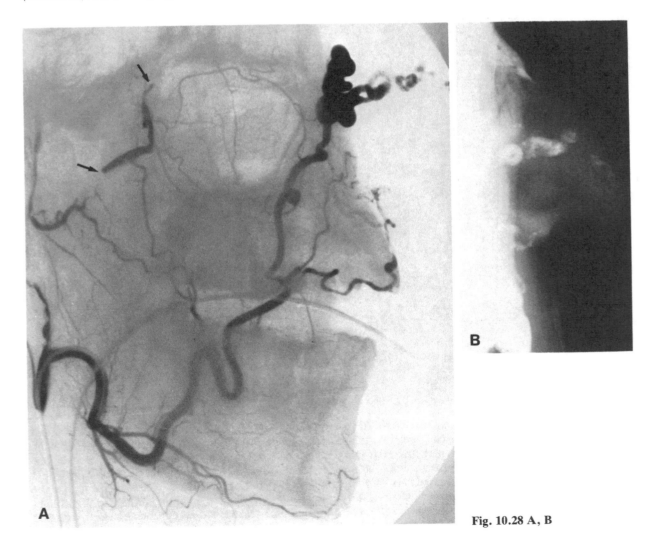

Fig. 10.28 A, B

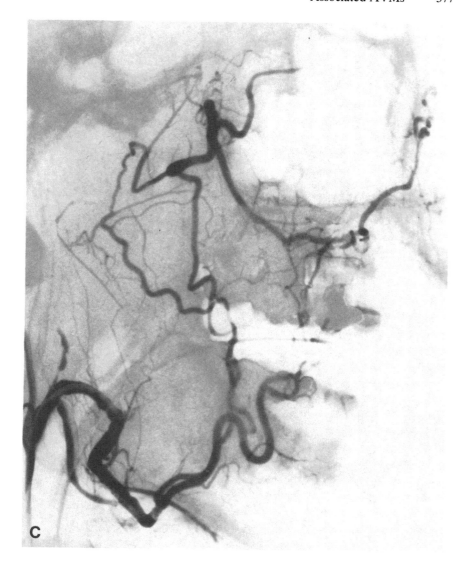

Fig. 10.28 A-E. 47 year old male presenting with a vascular malformation of the nose. **A** Facial artery injection following embolization of the internal maxillary artery with particles to redirect the flow *(arrows)*. **B** IBCA deposition into malformation. **C** Control angiogram one year after the embolization of the facial artery.

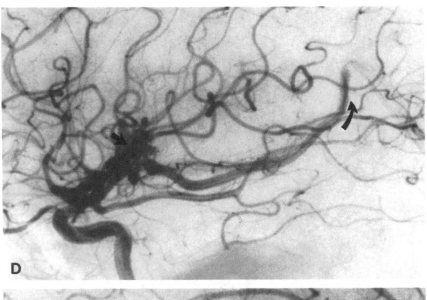

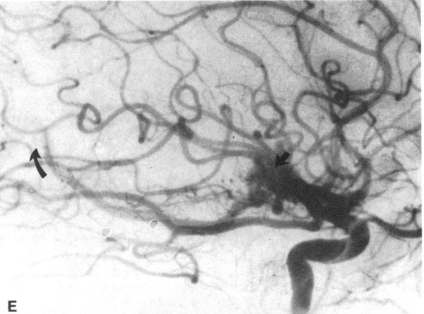

Fig. 10.28. D and **E** Discovery of a vascular malformation at the level of the mamillary body *(solid arrow)* draining into the basal vein of Rosenthal on the left side *(curved arrow)*

In our experience, angiography failed to demonstrate hypervasculariza-tion in these lesions. Bone hypertrophy as mentioned above, should be related to the venular type of malformation which is already responsible for the leptomeningeal lesion and port wine stain. As already mentioned in the high flow lesions of the oral cavity and known for a long time in Klippel Trenaunay disease, the venous anomalies at the venular level are likely to be responsible for this bone hypertrophy. Therefore, all the lesions observed seem linked to the same embryonic stage of maturation of the vascular system in which venous and lymphatic malformation are formed.

Therapeutic angiography in these cases have been carried out when facial reconstruction for cosmetic purposes was indicated. Usually, the maxilla and cheek deformities will induce so many disturbances in the maxillo-facial growth that the plastic and reconstructive surgeon may feel obliged to perform osteotomies and debulking surgery on the cheek masses. Presurgical angiography and embolization with a large particle will avoid the surprise of some high flow lesions which can be associated to this disease and will devascularize the operative field reducing the peri operative blood loss in this difficult bony reconstructions.

b) *Rendu-Osler-Weber Disease* (Picard, 1974)

The hemorrhagic hereditary telangiectasia of Rendu-Osler-Weber (ROW) is a rare autosomic dominant disease with a variable expressivity. Only the heterozygous form seems viable. The disease evolves through 4 stages: latency, hemorrhages, telangiectasias and anemic. Although telangiectasias of the skin are exposed to repeated trauma, mucous membrane hemorrhages are usually the bleeding localizations of the disease. The distribution of the telangiectasias in the symptomatic states (second or third) are listed in Table 10.4 (Fig. 10.29).

The hemorrhagic manifestations in ROW have the following distribution: 85% epistaxis, 20% oral, 20% digestive, 10% genitourinary, 17% lungs (Golding and Wood). Epistaxis is the major cause of death 4 to 27% depending on the series. Pathologically, there are no specific findings related to this disease, although Patterson in his comment on Harrison's (1982) paper, pointed out the similitaries of the pathological pictures of ROW with that of juvenile angiofibromas. The diagnosis of the disease is exclusively clinical and can be made from the hemorrhagic symptoms, usually epistaxis, the family history and the telangiectasias. However, the telangiectasias may occasionally be found only if searched for carefully. They often occur under the nails or on the tip of the fingers and toes. The family history may be poor since the penetrance is variable: some generations may not present any type of hemorrhagic symptoms but will transmit the disease (see Fig. 10.29). Finally confronted with the first epistaxis in an adult, the diagnosis of Rendu-Osler-Weber disease has in our experience always been possible even with no family history nor obvious telangiectasias. In our review of 25 cases, 100% of the patients presenting epistaxis had liver telangiectasias although they did not present with any digestive symptoms. In the investigation of patients referred for embolization for epistaxis it is now our protocol to perform hepatic angiography, if there is a suspicion of Rendu-Osler-Weber disease (Fig. 10.30).

In our cases presenting epistaxis, we have never been confronted with a hemorrhagic complication in another area which required therapeutic angiography aside from the nasal cavities.

Table 10.4. Row distribution of telangiectasis

	%		%
Face	40	Hand	40
Lips	65	Digestive system 15	30
Nose	65	Lungs and chest 15	20
Liver	30–70	Feet	20
Tongue	45	Genito-urinary	5
Ear	40	Spinal cord	4
		Brain	2,5

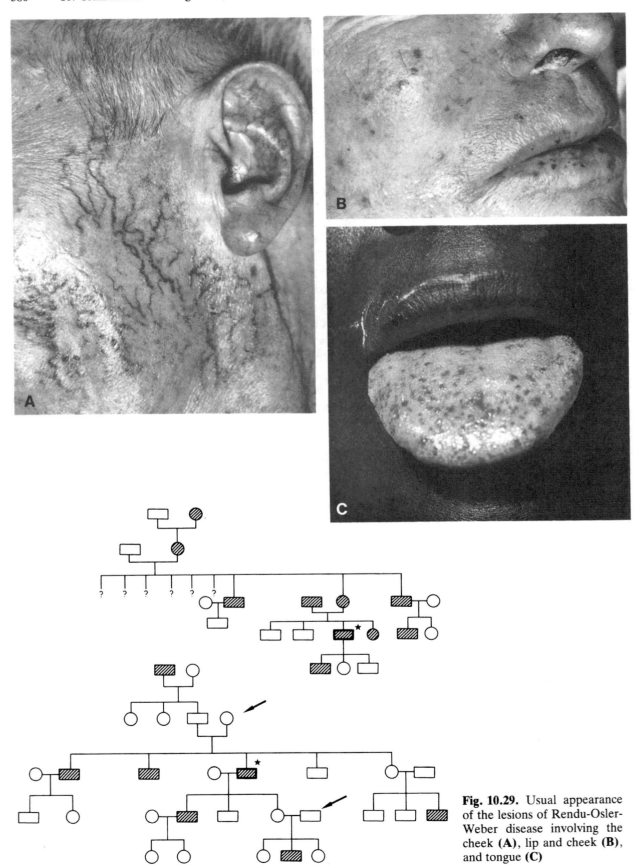

Fig. 10.29. Usual appearance of the lesions of Rendu-Osler-Weber disease involving the cheek (**A**), lip and cheek (**B**), and tongue (**C**)

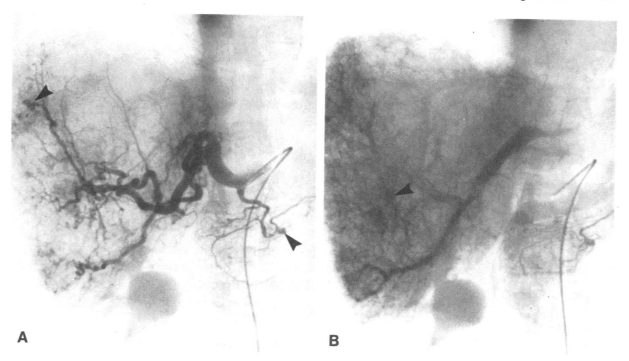

A   B

Fig. 10.30. Hepatic artery injection in a patient with Rendu-Osler-Weber disease. Note the multiple angioectasias *(arrowhead)* during early (**A**) and late (**B**) phase

The central nervous system is rarely involved and when involved, it frequently is not symptomatic. In his very complete review, Merland emphasized the role played by the pulmonary fistulas in the neurological symptoms. They can produce multiple CNS manifestations (Roman, 1978), septic or even air emboli. When CNS manifestations are seen in patients with ROW, search for arteriovenous fistulas and their obliteration should be done; when this type of secondary clinical manifestation is encountered with brain AVMs it should not lead to local treatment but to the search of pulmonary AVF first. Intracranial bleeding is rare in the lesions of the brain or dura but it may occur. Among 25 patients, seen at Bicetre, 4 presented with brain AVMs (1 capillary, 1 multiple capillary, 2 arterial with shunts) but only 1 presented with symptoms which could be related to the central nervous system lesion (epilepsy). Three of the 25 had a pulmonary arteriovenous fistula, only one had both, none was symptomatic.

Pretherapeutic evaluation should be limited to the symptomatic area. Brain CT will demonstrate the intracranial lesion if present, however a normal DIVA should not be considered a satisfactory procedure to rule out AVMs. Additional medical assessment of the various complications of repeated blood transfusions is necessary.

Appreciation of the evolution of the disease is extremely difficult but of paramount importance in selection of the most appropriate treatment. Complete cure is not possible in this systemic disease; no drugs can satisfactorily stabilize the evolution of the telangiectasias. Our only objective is the stabilization of the bleeding which in itself constitutes and ambitious goal. In our review, a few clinical features appeared to be of some significance in prognosis: the high familial expression of the disease and extensive involvement with telangiectasias seem to be the most predictive signs. Presentation of hemorrhagic episodes at an early or late age does not modify the response for treatment (Lasjaunias, 1983). Several types of

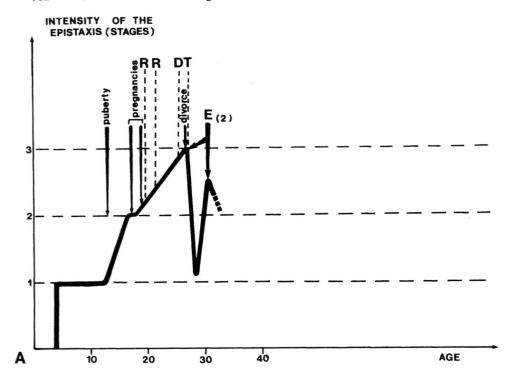

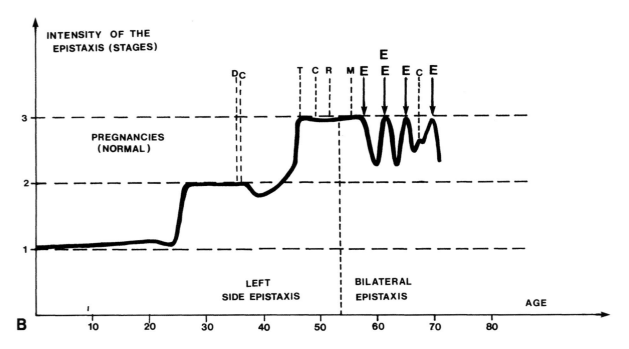

Fig. 10.31. **A** Diagrammatic representation of the evolution of the Rendu-Osler-Weber disease in a given patient which shows the acute changes observed following hormonal events. Two embolizations were needed to bring this patient from stage 3 to stage 2. **B** Diagrammatic representation in a patient with Rendu-Osler-Weber disease in whom evolution has been slowly progressive without evidence of hormonal dependence. After failure of several types of treatments, five embolizations were carried out in a ten years period to maintain the patient at stage 2, allowing satisfactory quality of life. *M* packing, *R* radiation, *C* electrocoagulation, *T* transfusion, *D* dermoplasty, *E* embolization

evolutive patterns demonstrate either the slowly evolutive course of the disease or the course characterized by marked sensitivity to hormonal changes (Fig. 10.31).

In an attempt to appreciate the effect of the disease on the life style of the patient, we suggested three stages: 1. episodic but spontaneously resolutive bleeding requiring no specific treatment and often ignored by the patient, 2. periodic bleeding sometimes following mechanical trauma (sneezing, blowing nose) requiring no more than one hospitalization and one transfusion per year, permitting normal professional activity, 3. frequent spontaneous bleeding requiring multiple hospitalization per year with incapacitation.

Considering the available treatments (Fig. 10.31), it seems reasonable to progressively increase the agressiveness of the therapeutic approach knowing that some treatments carry more hazards than others. Patients in stage I usually do not require treatment. Stage II should be treated whenever blood transfusion is necessary. Local therapy should be attempted first, arterial ligation should be avoided at all cost and radiation therapy should be delayed unless embolization is not available.

Further evolution of the disease should be treated by an endovascular approach unless the lesions are inaccessible due to unreachable collateral circulation from the ethmoidal arteries. There is some controversy as to whether or not orbital clipping of the ethmoidal arteries should be carried out prior to distal internal maxillary embolization. However, there is no evidence that further stabilization is better following either strategy.

The inability to stabilize the patient with embolization at stage II or to convert him from stage III to stage II should lead to more aggressive treatment. Radiation therapy has proven to be effective but makes subsequent endovascular therapy more difficult. Estrogen therapy was used in 118 patients over 25 years by Harrison, who claimed excellent results but with some side effects and complications.

In our experience, dihydrostybestrol has proven to be effective in the treatment of the epistaxis in this disease. The rationale lies in the specific nature of the nasal mucosa which has been described in Chapter 3. The doses employed vary from 1 mg to 2 mg per day. Careful gynecological and biological monitoring and the addition of testosterone may be necessary to prevent side effects or complications of the treatment: alteration of sexual characteristics, and libido, phlebothrombosis, gynecomastia in males, cancer of the endometrium etc.

In general, embolization with particles in Rendu-Osler-Weber disease gives a satisfactory immediate hemostasis which usually lasts from 2 month to 2 years. Bilateral embolization of the internal maxillary and facial arteries has to be done to insure adequate control of the hemorrhage. Embolization should be tried each time it is necessary and possible. Nonsymptomatic telangiectasias should not be treated; the treatment of asymptomatic pulmonary AV fistula is controversial because of the potential for brain complications. Preloaded microcapsules with estrogens may represent a possible useful treatment in the near future.

c) Other Epistaxis

Epistaxis may be the presenting symptom of other diseases and may create specific complications related to the particular conditions of the patient (see Vol. 1, Fig. 14.6).

Coagulopathy. Epistaxis is a frequent complication of coagulopathies in children. If needed, they can be controlled and stabilized by particle embolization in addition to the general treatment of the primary disease. Angiography usually shows a normal appearance of the nasal mucosa. The goal is therefore only local desarterialization with careful avoidance of the orbital anastomosis which are usually widely patent in children (see Vol. 1).

Spontaneous Epistaxis. They usually occur in the fifth decade. Usually when associated with hypertension or hepatic insufficiency, epistaxis resolves after packing and usually does not reccur. However, in some patients, the intensity or repetition of hemorrhages in a short period of time may be an indication for more invasive treatment. In this situation, embolization is preferred to ligation since it conforms to any atomic variation and results in the hemostasis allowing removal of the packing in the angio room. Treatment of the hypertension or the liver disease must obviously be adressed simultaneously (see Vol. 1).

Tumoral Epistaxis. They may form part of the presenting symptoms with lesions such as juvenile angiofibroma, capillary hemangiomas of the nasal fossa or malignant tumors. Although embolization may allow removal of the packing, a strategy attempting to treat the primary disease as well as its hemorrhagic complication should be considered simultaneously. Therefore, patients presenting with spontaneous epistaxis in the fifth decade should initially undergo CT examination to rule out the possible nasal tumor or a sphenoid lesion (see Chapter 5, II).

Biopsy. Diffuse epistaxis may follow biopsy of an unexpectedly highly vascular lesion. Embolization will again provide hemostasis if it cannot be obtained by conventional packing. Endovascular desarterialization of the area of the base of the skull or the nasal fossa prior to biopsy in a highly vascularized lesion (Fig. 10.32) most of the time does not alter, the pathological diagnosis if the embolization is performed with particles. On the other hand, since misinterpretation of the histologic findings due to local tumoral necrosis may occur, fluid embolization should not be used in this situations if possible.

Traumatic Epistaxis. These events illustrate the most rewarding aspect of embolization when one considers the efficiency of minimal endovascular treatment required to help a normal vasculature to produce hemostasis. Internal carotid artery angiography should be carried out first to rule out bleeding from this vessel into the sphenoid sinus (see Chapter 7). Attention should be paid to the ethmoidal arteries as a possible source of bleeding. Then the protocol of embolization can be carried on and the packing removed at the end of the procedure prior to with drawal of the angiographic catheters. In general, embolization is indicated when anterior and posterior packing is not effective, when the epistaxis recurs after removal of the packing, or when septic complications develop in patients with fractures of the paranasal sinuses (Fig. 10.33).

As a general principle we feel that every patient with epistaxis should initially receive traditional treatment with nasal packing; embolization which almost always produces hemostasis should be prefered over vascular ligation. Angiography will not demonstrate extravasation if the packing is

Fig. 10.32. Acute hemorrhage occurring after biopsy in a patient with a vascular malformation of the nasal fossa. Note the forceps *(arrowhead)* necessary to ensure hemostasis. In this case, the nasal branch of the ophthalmic artery represents the major supply to the lesion. The other feeders from the internal maxillary and facial arteries have been embolized. Manual compression on the medial canthus after the external carotid embolization allowed satisfactory control of the bleeding

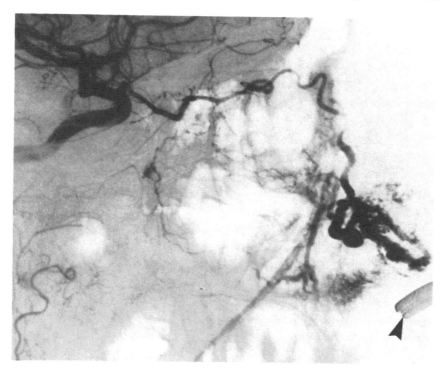

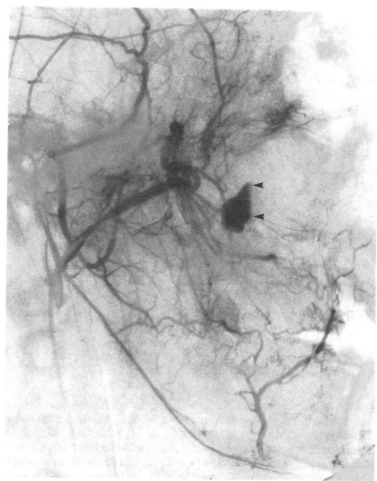

Fig. 10.33. Intrasinusal extravasation of contrast *(arrowheads)* following maxillofacial trauma

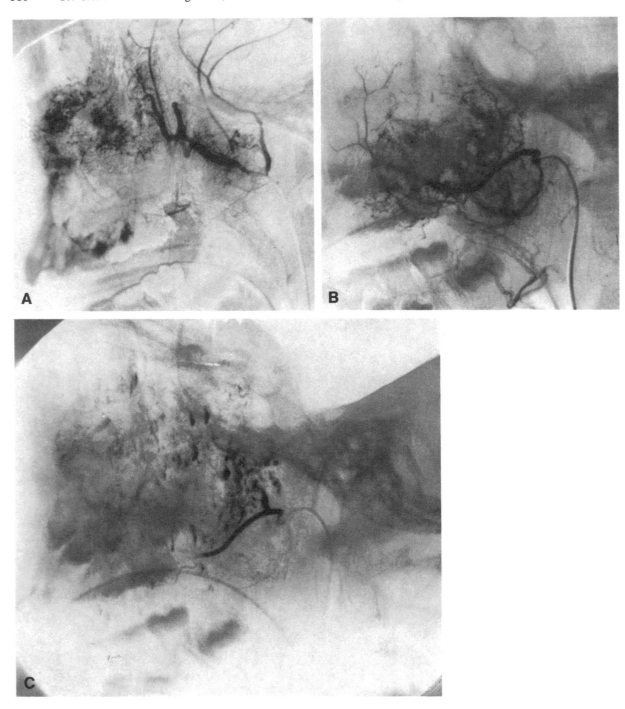

Fig. 10.34 A-E. 9 year old black boy presenting with a capillary venous malformation. **A** Internal maxillary artery injection showing the late arterial phase blush, also demonstrated during the transverse facial injection **(B)**. **C** Late phase of the transverse facial artery shows ectatic venules with fluid levels. **D** Control angiogram post embolization with PVA microparticles. The proximal transverse facial artery *(arrows)* is patent. **E** Direct injection in the lesion in the cheek demonstrates the deep extension towards the pterygoid area

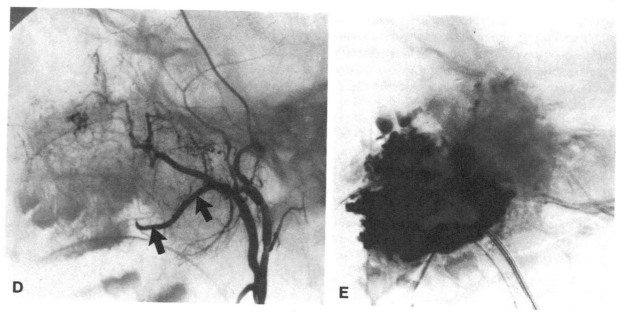

Fig. 10.34 D, E

effective enough to transiently produce the necessary hemostasis. Surgical clipping of the ethmoidal arteries is indicated when there is angiographic evidence of their involvement.

4. Capillary Venous Malformations

Capillary venous malformations develop on the capillary venous side of the vascular tree. They are slow flow lesions presenting vascular lakes of small size visualized in the late capillary venous phase of the angiograms. They eventually drain into normal venous system through normal venous channels. The triggering factors leading to angioectatic activity are unclear. They are nonproliferative lesions and therefore noninvolutive. They present clinical and anatomical similarities to hemolymphangiomas and present the same type of therapeutic problems.

a) Clinical Presentation and Natural History

Capillary venous malformations seem to have specific clinical and angiographic appearance (Berenstein, 1983; Riche, 1983). They usually present in young patients where they produce facial asymetry in relation to mass effect without bony involvement. The skin or mucous membranes are usually not involved. No abnormal pulsations, thrills or bruits can be palpated or auscultated. The lesion may increase in size or tension with dependent position, valsalva or other maneuvers that increase venous pressure. They are rubbery in consistancy and cannot be easily emptied on manual or carotid compression.

The lesions may fluctuate with periods of increased swelling usually associated with pain or tenderness; they occasionally have minor bleedings with or without trauma that stop spontaneously or after manual compression at which time they decompress with relief of tension and discomfort.

With time the lesion has little tendency to grow and usually remains stable and grows commensurately with the child (Mulliken, 1983). However, when present in the growing face or mouth, due to their mass effect, they may interfere with normal growth of the maxillofacial area. They may induce secondary functional impairments and dysmorphism (see Chapter 10, II 1).

b) Pretherapeutic Evaluation and Therapeutic Goals

Indications of treatment are primarily related to complications (major functional disturbances, bleeding, psychological problems). Therefore, if no treatment is contemplated, conservative follow up should include documentation of the initial presentation by photography and measurements of the mass in relationship to surrounding structures and yearly follow up. If treatment is indicated, CT scanning before and after the intravenous administration of contrast material will show the mass effect and its relationships with the airways adjacent bone overlying skin and muscles (Fig. 10.35).

Bony overgrowth is rare in this type of lesion and bony changes when present have to be related to an important capillary component. Phleboliths are not present in any of our patients with this type of capillary venous malformation. Enhanced CT may appear inhomogeneous, suggesting puddling within the lesion. Less frequently, cystic, low attenuation areas can be recognized (Fig. 10.34).

At the pretherapeutic stage, the arterial capillary component of the capillary venous malformation must be evaluated. As in other situations, the same topographic angiographic protocol is followed for the analysis of the vascular architecture, topographic extent of the lesion and the hemodynamic characteristics, the venous outflow and the adjacent territories. Nonselective angiography in these patients is not only useless but also carries the dangers of false impression of an avascular mass. Superselective angiography demonstrates the feeding arteries of normal caliber, displacement and hypervascularity in the mid and late capillary phase (Fig. 10.33). A dense blush is seen when the patient is in the supine position at the declive position of the malformation (Figs. 10.33, 10.34). Venous puddling or lakes with relatively slow flow will be seen in later phase.

The limitation of arterial studies is in its ability to fully visualize the lesion itself. Direct percutaneous contrast injection demonstrates the entire architecture. However, direct percutaneous and in situ catheterization should be done after the arterial side is embolized with microparticles. Multicompartmental capillary venous malformations would require multiple puncture to be studied thoroughly. This constitutes an important difference between management of capillary venous and purely venous malformation, where neither angiography nor arterial embolization are required.

c) Treatment

An arterial microembolization with flow control can decrease some of the mass effect that is altering normal maxillofacial growth. If arterial microembolization fails, one may then entertain surgery or one may attempt direct ethanol in situ injection. However, this latter technique has not produced

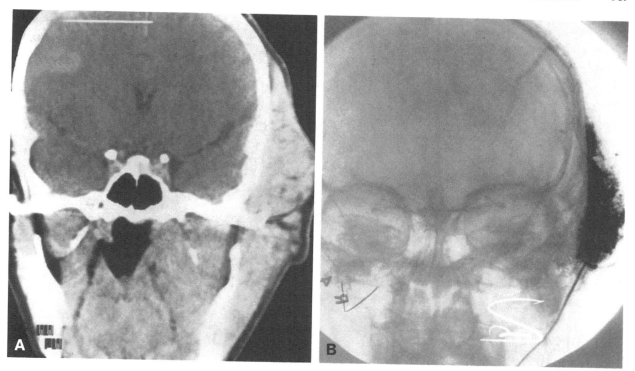

Fig. 10.35. Capillary venous malformation of the temporal muscle **(A)**. The coronal enhanced CT image demonstrates the extension of the lesion to the masseteric muscle. **B** Selective injection of the middle deep temporal artery shows the late arteriolocapillary phase blush with no demonstrable arteriovenous shunting

the same result as in purely venous lesions (see below). Combined endovascular and surgical approach may facilitate removal and prevent excessive bleeding with better possibilities of preserving important structures and nerves. Surgery for these lesions, primarily preceded by embolization is usually successful. However, as in other malformations it is important that venous outflow is respected emphasizing the link between these lesions and the arterial capillary system. In patients referred after partial removal of capillary venous malformation, the main therapeutic problem has been excessive swelling and edema that may even compromise the airway and/or alimentary passages. Arterial ligations have no lasting effect. They take away the opportunity to reach the lesion leading to use unfavorable and dangerous routes to reach the capillary level (collateral circulation to a slow flow lesion).

5. Venous Vascular Malformations

Purely venous vascular malformations develop on the venous side of the vascular tree. They do not have any connection with the arterial capillary system and cannot be visualized through it by conventional angiography. They are constituted by large communicating or septated venous spaces. They are nonproliferative and therefore not involutive.

Pure venous malformations may present as part of a combined port wine stain in the skin surface with a deep venous component. Although the port

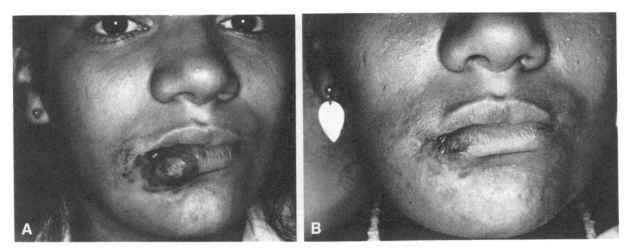

Fig. 10.36. Clinical results of direct alcohol injection in a venous vascular malformation of the lip in a young female **(A)** before and **(B)** after four alcohol injections.

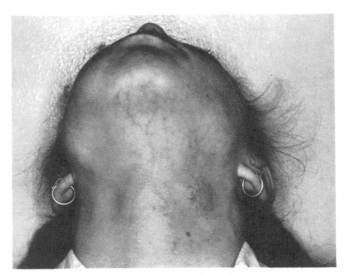

Fig. 10.37. 9 year old female presenting with a venous vascular malformation on both side of the face more marked on the right. The clinical photograph demonstrates the dominant mass effect in the right mandibular region, the dilatation of the small veins of the skin of the neck. The lesion was multi-compartmental and the patient complained of episodes acute pain which were followed by formation of radiopaque phleboliths

wine portion may remain of the same size, simulating involution, the deep seated venous malformation usually presents a little tendency to expand and grow with the child (Figs. 10.36, 10.37).

In the head and neck, the lesions are present usually since birth, although they may become apparent some weeks or even years after birth. They may have bluish discoloration at apparently distal areas. When seen at a later stage, parts of the lesion might have regressed clinically but during vascular studies, the contrast will reach the nonapparent or "dormant" areas. In

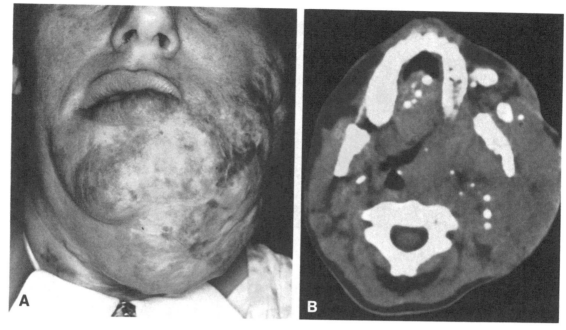

Fig. 10.38. A Extensive venous vascular malformation of the floor of the mouth extending to the larynx. **B** The phlebolithes are clearly seen on CT examination and confirm the venous nature of the lesion, and the airway and oesophagus impairment

venous vascular malformations, the apparent triggering factor for angioectatic activity seems to be in relation with any venous type of hyperpressure.

Direct venous sampling of the lesion has demonstrated a uniform fibrinolytic depletion as compared to peripheral blood and slightly elevated P_aO_2. In all these patients the cellular element of blood including platelets in the systemic circulation were normal. With the available information, one question remains: is the fibrin splitting factor consumption responsible for maintaining the permeability of the abnormal pouches or is the partial thrombosis followed by clot lysis responsible for the coagulation factor consumption?

a) Clinical Presentation

Venous vascular malformations are more frequent in females (2/1) than males; they do not usually fluctuate with hormonal changes. Uniquely there is a bluish discoloration of the skin and/or mucous membrane and may be quite disfiguring (Fig. 10.38). The skin temperature is normal and no abnormal pulsations, thrill or bruit can be found. Spontaneous bleeding is rare. We have seen it only once with a nasal venous malformation in over 50 patients. The patient presented as sporadic small epistaxis for which she never required blood transfusion.

The lesion can increase in size by maneuvers that increase venous pressure such as dependent position or valsalva maneuver. The malformations are usually larger in the morning, and as the patient ambulates and improves venous drainage by gravity, the lesion becomes softer and smaller. The lesions are soft and easily compressible. One can empty the pouches by manual compression; refilling occurs in seconds. On palpation

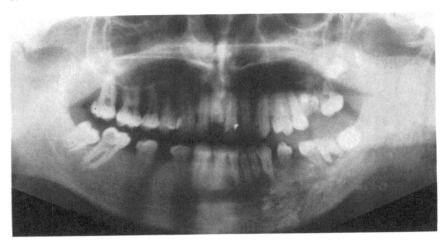

Fig. 10.39. Phlebolithes can be seen on plain panoramic films as demonstrated in this case of left lower cheek and floor of the mouth venous vascular malformation

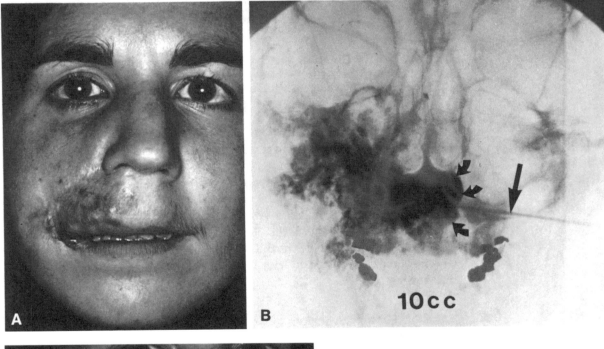

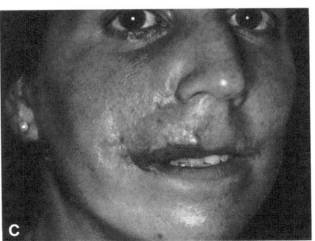

Fig. 10.40. A Venous vascular malformation of the upper lip. **B** Direct puncture from the opposite side, allows after injection of 10 CC of contrast a satisfactory filling of the venous compartment. Note the typical convex outwards configuration observed following full opacification of the compartment *(small arrows)*. **C** Clinical aspect after two sessions of alcohol injection into the lesion

phleboliths are usually found. During acute episodes of phlebothrombosis, there is tenderness and a more rubbery consistency although this occurs only in portions of the lesion. Functional disturbances in arway and/or alimentary passage can be significant and necessitate intervention such as tracheostomy or nasogastric intubation. Due to the phleboectasia chronic localized pain may also occur in the anomalous vein. Edema, ectasias, dermatitis and ulcerations are late stage problems and usually seen when the extremities are involved.

b) Pretherapeutic Evaluation

From a purely clinical assessment, the diagnosis can be made and the decision as to conservative observation or therapeutic intervention easily taken. If observation is indicated, one can postpone further studies and document the extent of the lesion by photography and measurements as usual in vascular lesions. If treatment is indicated, biological (complete coagulation profile) and morphological studies should be obtained.

CT scanning before and after the intravenous administration of contrast material demonstrates the extent of the lesion; phleboliths are constantly found (Figs. 10.37–10.39). Bony displacement but with no hypertrophy or direct involvement is seen. In lesion that have a deep extension, special attention has to be paid to the airway and alimentary passages.

Arterial studies are not needed in patients in which the clinical diagnosis of a purely venous malformation is evident. The late capillary phase blushes sometimes mentioned in this type of lesion following high volume contrast injection (Riche, 1983) correspond either to a venular compartment to the lesion or to a chronic inflammatory appearance of the adjacent tissue.

For best visualization of their extent and anatomy, direct (Fig. 10.40) percutaneous puncture of vascular malformations is indicated. The procedure can be divided into a diagnostic evaluation and therapeutic one (in situ alcohol infusion). At the beginning of our experience, we performed each procedure at different stages. At present, both parts are carried out in the same sitting.

The full extent of the lesion may not be appreciated nor treated through one single puncture site. Depending on the preliminary clinical and CT determination of the potential extent of involvement, various puncture sites may be needed. Multicompartments can be found either because of previous areas of partial thrombosis or from previous incomplete surgical or other types of treatments.

Vascular malformations of the tongue (Fig. 10.35) are present in many patients, and compared to other vascular malformations, this localization is rarely symptomatic. This may be due to the soft nature of the mass which produces less growth deformity. Rarely tongue enlargement produces airway obstruction or difficulty in closing the mouth. Lesions with bilateral involvement may be opacified or reached from only one side if gravity is used. The venous drainage can further be compromised when patients have had some types of surgery. Although Riche (1983) recommended arterial embolization prior to direct percutaneous puncture of the lesion, in our experience of purely venous malformations, no arterial embolization appears to be needed if clinical examination has excluded a capillary venous malformation.

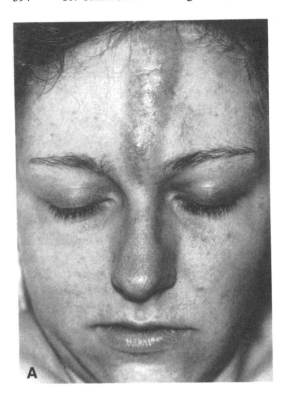

Fig. 10.41 A-C. 28 year old female complaining with cosmetic problems related to a subcutaneous midline varix of the forehead. The plastic surgeon prior to surgery requested an angiogram

c) Embolization

Multiple reports of sclerosing agents such as hypertonic saline or glucose or sodium murrhate were found to produce at least some benefit. Unfortunately, none of these treatments have gained acceptance due to the high incidence or recurrence. The use of Ethibloc in the cases reported by Riche and Merland (1983) required surgical resection. The agent they used has a 60% alcohol content and takes 10–20 minutes to harden; some types of compression is suggested by the author which can be easily done in an extremity, but is more difficult in the head and neck.

Attention should also be paid to intracranial or spinal venous drainage or communications (Figs. 10.40–10.43).

Over 50 patients were treated with in situ 95% ethanol (see Chapter 1). 4 had surgical removal of the vascular malformation after 1–4 alcohol injections with excellent cosmetic and/or functional results. Except for a surgically removed lesion, there has not been complete disappearance of the malformation. However, all patients have been improved by the treatment (Figs. 10.35, 10.39–10.43).

Alcohol levels taken in our patients failed to reach toxic level. A blister was noted within 12 hours after the alcohol injection on four occasions. These resulted in an ulceration at that point which healed by granulation in all cases without sequelae.

Venous lesions of the mucosa can sometimes respond in a dramatic fashion (Fig. 10.44); however diffuse malformations in the maxillofacial area will be difficult to approach, particularly when different channels (veins, lymphatics) and lesionnal architecture (venous or lymphatic pouches or cysts) will be encountered (Fig. 10.45).

Fig. 10.41. B, C Left and right venous phases of the respective internal carotid angiograms demonstrate complex nonmalformative venous anomalies. The varix could be identified as a sinus pericranii draining part of the right cerebral hemisphere. Treatment of this varix was not and should not be undertaken

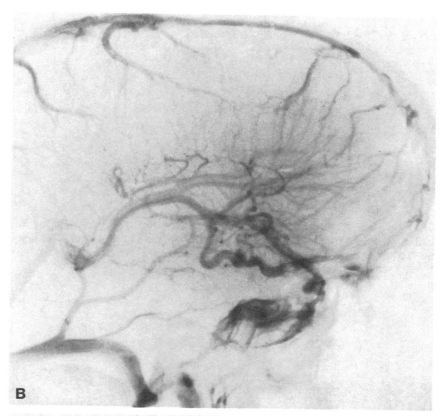

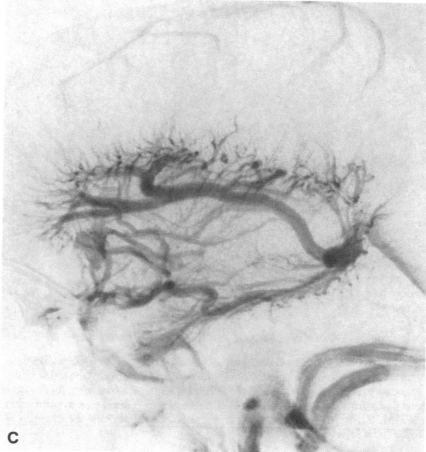

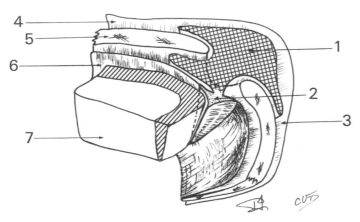

Fig. 10.42. Schematic representation of a nuchal venous vascular malformation with transosseous communication with a median occipital venous sinus. 1 cutaneous and epidural venous pouch, 2 dural sinus, 3 subcutaneous region, 4 cutaneous cover, 5 occipital bone, 6 dura, 7 cerebellar hemisphere

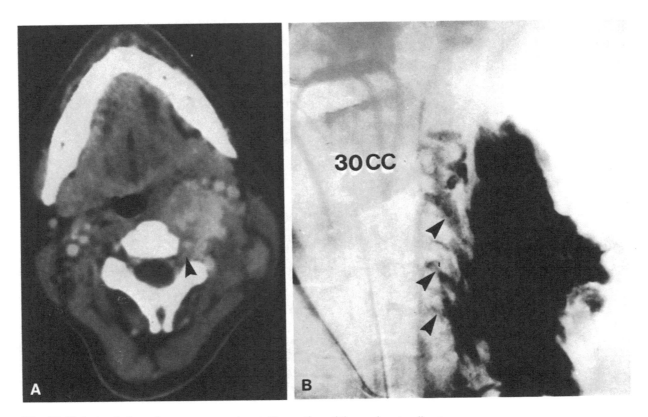

Fig. 10.43. Lateral view of a venous vascular malformation of the neck extending to the base of the skull. CT demonstrates the anatomic relationships of the lesion to the upper cervical spine *(arrowhead)* at the level of the foramen transversarium. After direct puncture and injection of 30 CC of contrast, the epidural venous plexus was opacified; this represented the significant end point to determine the quantity of alcohol to be injected

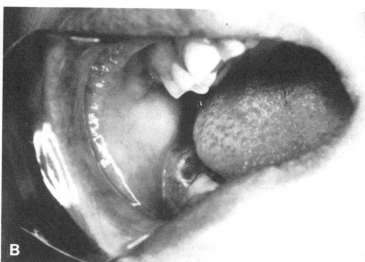

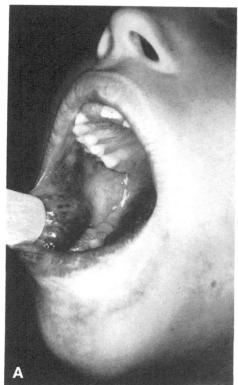

▲
Fig. 10.44 A, B. 13 year old female presenting with a venous vascular malformation of the cheek. **A** Note the submucosal discoloration of the cheek. **B** Appearance of the same region one month after the third alcohol injection

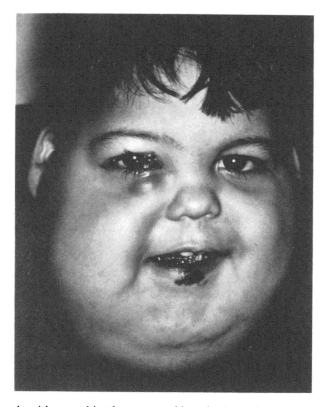

Fig. 10.45. 4 year old male with a combined venous and lymphatic malformation. Two venous pouches could be demonstrated in the lower lip and the lower eyelid. Puncture of the neck area yielded yellow fluid which led to the diagnosis of associated cystic hygroma

References

Abele J (1978) Balloon catheters: What is available, how they are made and how they are used. MediTech Division

Adams JE, Dams PH, Mamtora H, Isherwood I (1981) Computed tomography and the localisation of parathyroid tumors. Clin Radiol 32:251–254

Agarwal MK, Gupia OP, Smamant HO, Gupia S (1980) Neurilemmoma of the maxillary sinus. J Oral Surg 38:698–699

Ahn HS, Kerber CW (1983) Therapeutic embolization of external carotid cavernous fistula in infancy. J Neuroradiology 10:261–264

Akerson HA, Allen GW, Solomson (1981) Ossifying angioma: an unusual mandibular lesion in an infant. J Oral Surgery 39:954–957

Albores-Saavedra J, Espino-Duran M (1968) Thyroid carcinoma and chemodectoma. Am J Surgery 116:887–890

Albrecht R (1959) Die Wasenchentumoren und ihre Behandlung. Arch Ohr 8: 175:1–68

Albright AL, Latchaw RE, Price RA (1983) Posterior dural arteriovenous malformation in the infancy. Neurosurgery 13:129–135

Alexander E, Wigser SM, Savis SM, Davis CH (1966) Bilateral extracranial aneurysms of the internal carotid artery. Case report. J Neurosurg 25:437–442

Alford BR, Guilford FR (1962) A comprehensive study of tumors of the glomus jugulare. Laryngoscope 72:765–805

Ali S, Jones WI (1982) Clinical records: extranasopharyngeal angiofibromas (sex incidence and age distribution). J Laryng Otol 96:559–565

Ali S, Aird W, Bihari J (1983) Pain inducing laryngeal paragangliomas (nonchromaffin). J Laryng Otol 97:181–188

Aminoff MJ (1973) Vascular anomalies in the intracranial dura mater. Brain 96:601–612

Aminoff MJ, Kendall BE (1973) Asymptomatic dural vascular anomalies. Br J Radiol 46:662–667

Anderson JH, Grisius RJ, McKean TW (1981) Arteriovenous malformation of the mandible. J Oral Surg 52:118–125

Andre JM (1973) Les dysplasies vasculaires systématisées. L'expansion scientifique française, 58–87

Angervall L, Kindblom L-G, Nielsen JM, et al. (1978) Hemangiopericytoma: a clinicopathological, angiographic and microangiographic study. Cancer 42:2412–2427

Apfelberg DB (1983) Argon laser treatment of port-wine hemangiomas: summary of 10 years' experience. In: Williams HB (ed) Symposium of vascular malformations and melanotic lesions, Mosby. St-Louis pp 95–100

Apostol JV, Frazell EL (1965) Juvenile nasopharyngeal angiofibroma: a clinical study. Cancer 18:869–878

Armstrong EA, McLennan JE, Benton C, Chambers AA, Perlman AW, Conners JW (1981) Maffucci's syndrome complicated by an intracranial chondrosarcoma and a carotid body tumor. Case report. J Neurosurg 55:479–483

Arutinov A, Burlutsky AP (1984) (New modification of Brooks operation) in Material k ob'einenoy conferencii neurichirurgov. Leningrad, p 67–69

Askenazy HM, Behmoaram AD (1960) Subarachnoid hemorrhage in meningiomas of the lateral ventricle. Neurology (Minneapolis) 10:484–489

Aubin A (1933) Récidive de polype nasopharyngien: extirpation totale par voie palatine. Ann Oto-laryngol 8:974–976

Aufdemorte TB (1981) Hemangiopericytoma-like tumor of the nasal cavity. Arch Otolaryngol 107:172–174

Auriol M, Coutant A, Crinets V, et al. (1985) Sensibilité proprioceptive et fonctions oro faciales. Rev Stomatol Chir Maxillofac 86:137–146

Awbrey BJ, Hoak JC, Owep WG (1979) Binding of human thrombin to cultured human endothelial cells. J Biol Chem 254:4092–4095

Awe AC, Roberts W, Braunwald NS (1967) Rapidly polymerizing adhesive as a hemostatic agent: Study of tissue response and bacteriological properties. Surgery 54:322–328

Azzolini A, Bertani A, Riberti C (1982) Superselective embolization and immediate surgical treatment. Our present approach to treatment of large vascular hemangiomas of the face. Ann Plastic Surg 9:43–60

Bahar F, Chiras JP, et al. (1984) Spontaneous vertebral-arteriovenous fistula associated with fibromuscular dysplasia. Neuroradiology 26:45–49

Bailey OT, Ingraham FD, Weadon PS et al. (1952) Tissue reactions to powdered tantalum in the central nervous system. J Neurosurg 9:83–92

Barbin JY, Lebatard-Sartre R, Menegalli D, Lajat Y (1981) Tumeurs du glomus carotidien: reflexion à propos de 4 cas dont 2 bilatéraux survenus dans une même famille. Chirurgie 107:577–584

Bardach J, Panje W (1981) Surgical management of the large cavernous hemangioma. Otolaryngol Head Neck Surg 89:792–796

Barker WF (1954) Mycotic aneurysms. Ann Surg 139:84–98

Barker WF, Stern WE, Krayenbuhl H, et al. (1968) Carotid endarteriectomy complicated by carotid cavernous fistula. Ann Surg 167:572

Barnett HJM (1979) Delayed cerebral ischemic episodes distal to occlusion of major cerebral arteries. Neurology (NY) 28:769–774

Barnett HJM, Peerless SJ, Kaufmann JCE (1978) "Stump" of internal carotid artery: a source of further cerebral embolic ischemia. Stroke 9:448–456

Barr HWK, Blackwood W, Meadows SZ (1971) Intracavernous carotid aneurysm: a clinical pathological report. Brain 94:607–622

Barrett JH, Lawrence VL (1960) Aneurysm of internal carotid artery as complication of mastoidectomy. AMA Arch Otolaryng 72:366–368

Barth KH, Strandemberg JD, White RI (1977) Long term follow-up of transcatheter emboli with autologous clot, oxysele and gelfoam in domestic swine. Invest Radiol 12:273–280

Barth KH, White RI Jr, Kaufmann SL, et al. (1979) Metrizamide, the ideal radiopaque filling material for detachable silicone balloon embolization. Invest Radiol 14:35–40

Bartol AD, Levy M (1972) Excision of congenital suboccipital vertebral arteriovenous fistula. J Neurosurg 37:452–456

Batsakis JG (1979) Tumor of the head and neck, clinical and pathological considerations. Williams & Wilkins, 2nd edition, 296–301

Batsakis JG, Klopp CT, Newman W (1955) Fibrosarcoma arising in a "juvenile" nasopharyngeal angiofibroma following extensive radiation therapy. Am J Surg 21, 786

Batsakis JG, Jacobs JB, Templeton AC (1983) Hemangiopericytoma of the nasal cavity: electron-optic study and clinical correlations. J Laryng Otol 97: 361–368

Batzdorf V, Bentson JR, Marchleder H (1979) Blunt trauma to the high cervical carotid artery. Neurosurgery 5:195–210

Beall AC Jr, Crawford ES, Cooley SA, DeBakey ME (1962) Extracranial aneurysms of carotid artery: report of 7 cases. Postgrad Med 32:102–104

Beall AC, Shirkey AL, DeBakey ME (1983) Penetrating wounds of the carotid arteries. J Trauma 2:276–287

Bean WJ (1981) Renal cyst: treatment with alcohol. Radiology 138:329–331

Beatty RA (1977) Dissecting hematoma of the internal carotid artery following chiropractic manipulations. J Trauma 17:248–249

Belsheim MR, Sullivan SN (1982) Blue rubber bleb nevus syndrome. Can J Surg 23:146

Benedict WF, Porter IH, Brown CD, et al. (1970) Cytogenetic diagnosis of malignancy in recurrent meningiomas. Lancet 1:971–973

Bentson JR, Crandall PH (1972) Use of the Fogarty catheter in arteriovenous malformations of the spinal cord. Radiology 105:65–68

Benvenuto R, Despres JP, Pribram HFW, Callaghan JC (1961) Excision of extracranial aneurysm of internal carotid artery employing hypothermia. J Cardiovasc Surg 2:165–167

Berenstein A (1980) Flow controlled silicone fluid embolization. AJNR 1:162–166

Berenstein A (1983 a) Brachiocephalic vessel: Selective and superselective catheterization. Radiology 148:437–441

Berenstein A (1983 b) Discussion on the treatment of capillary venous malformation using a new fibrosing agent by MC Riche, E Hadjaen, T Tran-Ba-Huy and JJ Merland. Plastic Reconstruct Surg 71:613–614

Berenstein A, Graeb D (1982) Convenient preparation of ready-to-use polyvinyl alcohol foam suspension for embolization. Radiology 145(3):846–850

Berenstein A, Kricheff II (1979 a) Catheter and material selection for transarterial embolization: technical considerations, I. Catheters. Radiology 132(3):619–632

Berenstein A, Kricheff II (1979 b) Catheter and material selection for transarterial embolization: technical considerations. II. Materials. Radiology 132(3):631–639

Berenstein A, Kricheff II (1979 c) Balloon catheters of the investigating of carotid cavernous fistulas. Radiology 132(3):762–764

Berenstein A, Kricheff II (1979 d) A new balloon catheter for coaxial embolization. Neuroradiology 18:239–241

Berenstein A, Kricheff II (1980) Treatment of vascular abnormalities of the vertebral artery with detachable balloons. AJNR 1:358

Berenstein A, Kricheff II (1981 a) Neuroradiologic interventional procedures. Seminars Roentgenol 16(2):79–94

Berenstein A, Kricheff II (1981 b) Microembolization techniques of vascular occlusion: Radiologic, pathologic and clinical correlation. AJNR 2:261–267

Berenstein A, Kricheff II, Ransohoff J (1980) Carotid-cavernous fistulas: intra-arterial treatment. AJNR 1:449–457

Berenstein A, Ransohoff J, Kupersmith M, Flamm E, Graeb D (1984 a) Transvascular treatment of giant aneurysm of the cavernous carotid and vertebral arteries. Functional investigation and embolization. Surg Neurol 21:3–12

Berenstein A, Wisey, Ransohoff J, Benjamin V, Merkin S (1984 b) Somatosensory evoked potentials during spinal angiography and therapeutic transvascular embolization. J Neurosurg 60:777–785

Berg NO (1950) Tumors arising from the tympanic gland (glomus jugularis) and their differential diagnosis. Acta Pathol Microbiol Scand 27:194–221

Bergquist E, Bergstrom K, Hugosson R, et al. (1971) Complicated arteriovenous fistula after vertebral angiography. Neuroradiology 2:170–175

Bernini FP, Cioffi FA, Muras I (1982) Arteriovenous shunts between dural branches of the carotid artery and the cavernous sinus. Surg Neurol 18:102–107

Besznyak I, Markos G (1961) Chemodectoma malignum. Zentralbl Allg Pathol 102:298–305

Bickerstaff ER (1964) Etiology of acute hemiplegia in childhood. Br J Med II:82–87

Bickerstaff ER, Howells JS (1953) The neurological importance of tumors of the glomus jugulare. Brain 76:576–593

Bickerstaff ER, Small JM, Guest IA (1958) The relapsing course of certain meningiomas in relation to pregnancy and menstruation. J Neurol Neurosurg Psychiat 21:89–91

Biller HF, Sessions DG, Ogura JH (1974) Angiofibromas: a treatment approach. Laryngoscope 84:171–176

Bingham HG (1979) Predicting the course of a congenital hemangioma. Plast Reconstr Surg 63:161

Binkley W, Vakili ST, Worth R (1982) Paraganglioma of the cauda equina. J Neurosurg 56:275–279

Bismuth A, Bergue A, Frija G, Baviera E, Blery N, Gaux JC (1975) Etude anatomoradiologique des artères thyroidiennes inférieure. Interêt pour le diagnostic des adénomes parathyroidiens. J Radiol 56:453–458

Bitoh S, Hasegawa H, Fujiwara M, Nakata M (1980) Traumatic arteriovenous fistula between the middle meningeal artery and cortical vein. Surg Neurol 14:355–358

Bitoh S, Hasegawa H, Fujiwara M, Sakurai M (1982 a) Angiographically occult vascular malformations causing intracranial hemorrhage. Surg Neurol 17:35–42

Bitoh S, Hasegawa H, Fujiwara M, Nakao K (1982 b) Irradiation of spontaneous carotid-cavernous fistulas. Surg Neurol 17:282–286

Blackfield HM, Morris FA, Torrey FA (1957) Visible hemangiomas. A preliminary statistical report of a 10-year study. Plast Reconstr Surg 26:313

Blix A, Aas K (1961) Giant hemangioma, thrombocytopenia, fibrinogenopenia, and fibrinolytic activity. Acta Med Scand 169:63–70

Blumenkopf B, Boekelheide K (1982) Neck paraganglioma with a pituitary adenoma. Case report. J Neurosurg 57:426–429

Boatmann KK, Bradford VA (1958) Excision of internal carotid artery aneurysm during pregnancy employing hypothermia and vascular shunt. Ann Surg 148:271–275

Boldrey E, Maas L, Miller E (1957) Role of atlantoid compression in etiology of internal carotid thrombosis. J Neurosurg 13:127–139

Bostrom K, Lliequist B (1967) Primary dissecting aneurysm of the extracranial part of the internal carotid and vertebral arteries. Neurology 17:179–186

Bowers RE, Graham EA, Tomlinson KM (1980) The natural history of strawberry nevi. Arch Dermatol 82:667

Braine J, Funck-Brentano P (1934) Les variations des artères du corps thryoide. Ann Anat Pathol 11:125–155

Brainin M, Samec P (1983) Venous hemodynamics of arteriovenous meningeal fistulas in the posterior cranial fossa. Neuroradiology 25:161–169

Bratt GW (1979) Glomus tumor of the middle ear: origin, symptomatology, and treatment. J Speech Hear Dis 44:121–135

Braun IF, Levy S, Hoffman JC (1985) The use of transarterial microembolization in the management of hemangiomas of the perioral region. J Oral Maxillofac Surg 43:239–248

Brem S (1976) The role of vascular proliferation in the growth of brain tumors. Clin Neurosurg 33:440–453

Brice JG, Dowsett DJ, Lowe RD (1974) Hemodynamic effects of carotid artery stenosis. Br Med J 2:1363

Bridger MWM (1976) Haemangioma of the nasal bones. J Laryngol 90:191

Brismar J, Brismar G (1976) Phlebographic appearance and relation to thrombosis. Acta Radiol Diagnosis 17:180–192

Brismar J, Lasjaunias P (1978) Arterial supply of carotid-cavernous fistulas. Acta Radiol Diagnosis 19:897–904

Brooks B (1931) Discussion, Noland L, and Taylor AS. Trans South Surg Ann 43:176–177

Browder JD, Browder A, Kaplanha (1972) Benign tumors of the cerebral dural sinuses. J Neurosurg 37:576–579

Brown J (1947) Surgical treatment of nasopharyngeal fibroma. Ann Otol Rhinol Laryngol 56:294–297

Browns SH, Neerhout RC, Fonkalsrud EW (1972) Prednisone therapy in the management of large hemangiomas in infants and children. Surg 71:168–173

Bryan RN, Sessions RB, Horowitz BL (1981) Radiographic management of juvenile angiofibromas. AJNR 2:157–166

Buchta K, Sands J, Rosenkrantz H, Roche WD (1982) Early mechanism of action of arterially infused alcohol in renal devitalization. Radiology 145:45–48

Buckingham RA, Aimi K, Perrelli SC (1959) Multicentric origin of glomus jugulare tumors. Arch Otolaryngol 70:94–97

Buckwalter JA, Sasaki CT, Virapongse C, Kier EL, Bauman N (1983) Pulsatile tinnitus arising from jugular megabulb deformity: a treatment rationale. Laryngoscope 93:1534–1539

Burns JC, Julian J, Alexander J (1985) Arteriovenous malformation of the submandibular gland. J Oral Maxillofac Surg 43:294–296

Burrows PE, Mulliken JB, Fellows KE (1983) Childhood hemangiomas and vascular malformations: angiographic differentiation. AJR 141:483–488

Buxton JT Jr, Stevenson TB, Stallworth JM (1964) Arteriosclerotic aneurysm of extracranial internal carotid artery treated by excision and primary reanastomosis under controlled hypertension. Ann Surg 159:222–226

Calbucci F, Scialfa C (1977) Congenital arteriovenous malformation of the cervical region. J Neurosurg Sciences 21:211–220

Calcaterra TC, Rich R, Ward PW (1980) "Neurilemmona of the sphenoid sinus" Arch Otolaryng 100:385–386

Campiche R, Oberson R (1972) Syndrome d'emaciation provoque par un meningiome du tubercule sellaire. Oto-Neuro-Ophthalmol 44:353–358

Cantrell RW, Chew JY, Morika WT (1968) Hemangiopericytoma of the nasopharynx. J Laryngol Otol 82:839–844

Carella RJ, Ransohoff J, Newall J (1982) Role of Radiation Therapy in the management of meningioma. Neurosurg 10(3):332–338

Cares HL, Roberson GH, Grand W, et al. (1978) A safe technique for the precise localization of carotid-cavernous fistula during balloon obliteration. J Neurosurg 49:146–149

Carmody RF, Seeger J, Horsly WW, Smith JR, Miller RW (1983) Digital subtraction angiography of glomus tympanicum and jugulare tumors. AJNR 4:263–265

Castaigne P, Bories J, Brunet P, Merland JJ, Meininger V (1976) Les fistules artérioveineuses méningés pures à drainage veineux cortical. Rev Neurol 132:169–181

Chambers EF, Norman D, Dedo HH, Ferrel LD (1982) Case report: primary nasopharyngeal chemodectoma. Neuroradiology 23:285–288

Chang SC, Schi YM (1984) Neurilemmoma of the vagus nerve. A case report and brief literature review. Laryngoscope 94:946–949

Chasmar LR, Robertson DC, Former AW (1957) Irradiation fibrosarcoma. Plast Reconstr Surg 20:55

Chaudhary MY, Sachved VP, Cho SH, Weitzner I, Puljic S, Huang YP (1982) Dural arteriovenous malformation of the major venous sinuses: an acquired lesion. AJNR 3:3–19

Chiras J, Bories J, Leger JM, Gaston A, Launay M (1982) CT scan of dural arteriovenous fistulas. Neuroradiology 23:185–194

Choi NW, Schuman LM, Gullen WH (1970) Epidemiology of primary central nervous system neoplasms in Minnesota. Am J Epidemiol 91:238–259

Chou SN, French LA (1964) Arteriovenous fistula of vertebral vessels in the neck. J Neurosurg 22:77–80

Chou SN, Story JL, Seljeskog E, French LA (1967) Further experience with arteriovenous fistula of the vertebral artery in the neck. Surgery 62:779–788

Christiansen TA, Duvall AJ, Rosenberg Z (1974) Juvenile nasopharyngeal angiofibromas. Otolaryngol 78:140–147

Chunn GMH, Ellestad MH (1971) Perforation of the pulmonary artery by a Swan-Ganz Catheter. N Engl J Med 284:1041–1042

Cifarelli F, Sadiq S (1971) Bilateral cervical carotid aneurysms treated by resection and replacement grafts. Report of a case. Arch Surg 102:74–75

Clemis JD, Briggs DR, Changus GW (1975) Intramuscular hemangioma in the head and neck. Canadian J Otolarygol 4:339–347

Cole IE (1982) Haemangioendothelioma of the head and neck. J Laryng Otol 96:545–558

Collins JA, Pani KC, Lehmann RA (1966) Biological substrates and cure rates of cyanoacrylate tissue adhesives. Arch Surg 93:428–432

Compagno J, Hyams VJ (1976) Hemangiopericytoma like intranasal tumors: a clinicopathologic study of 23 cases. Am J Clin Pathol 65:672–683

Conley JW (1968) Nasopharyngeal angiofibroma in the juvenile. Surg Gynec Obst 126:825–837

Conley JJ, Clairmont AA (1977) Intramuscular hemangioma of the masseter muscle. Case report. Plast Reconstr Surg 60:121–125

Cophignon J, Djindjian R, Rey A (1974) Treatment of carotid cavernous fistulae. Ann Radiol 17:275–277

Cosmann B (1980) Experience in the argon laser therapy of port wine stains. Plast Reconstr Surg 65:119

Couly G, Lelievre Ayer C (1983) Malformations latéro-faciales (neurocristopathies maxillo mandibulaires) associées à des anomalies du tronc cérébral et des nerfs craniens. Rev Stomatol Chir Maxillofac 84:254–263

Couly G, Monteil J (1982) Classification neurocristopathique des anomalies dentaires. Rev Stomatol Chir Maxillofac 83:293–298

Cox GG, Lee KR, Price HI, Gunter KI, Noble MJ, Mebust WK (1982) Colonic infarction following ethanol embolization of renal-cell carcinoma. Radiology 145:343–345

Cox RH, Fisher GM (1978) Effects of sex hormones on the passive mechanical properties of rat carotid artery. Blood vessels 15:266–276

Cragg AH, Galliani CA, et al. (1982) Endovascular diathermic vessel occlusion. Radiology 144:303

Cromwell LD, Kerber CW (1979) Modification of cyanoacrylate for therapeutic embolization: preliminary experience. Am J Roentgenol 132:799–801

Crouse SK, Berg BO (1972) Intracranial meningiomas in childhood adolescence. Neurology (Minneapolis) 22:135–141

Cummings BJ (1980) Relative risk factors in the treatment of juvenile nasopharyngeal angiofibroma. Head Neck Surg 3:21–26

Cummings BJ, Blend R, Fitzpatrick P, Clark R, Harwood A, Keane T, Beale F, Garrett P, Payne D, Rider W (1984) Primary radiation therapy for juvenile nasopharyngeal angiofibroma. Laryngoscope 94:1599–1605

Curtis GM (1930) The blood supply of the human parathyroids. Surg Gynecol Obstet 315:805–809

Cushing H, Eisenhardt L (1929) Meningiomas arising from the tuberculum sellae with the syndrome of primary optic atrophy and bitemporal field defects combined with a normal sella turcica in a middle-aged person. Arch Ophthalmol (Chic) 1:1–41, 166–205

Cushing H, Eisenhardt L (1938) Meningiomas; their classification, regional behaviour, life history and surgical end results. Charles C. Thomas, Springfield, III, pp. 71–73

Dandy WE (1946) Arteriovenous aneurysms of the scalp and face. Arch Surg 51:1–32

Dandy WE (1982) Arteriovenous aneurysm of the brain. Arch Surg 17:190–243

Dane WH (1954) Juvenile nasopharyngeal fibroma in state of regression. Ann Otol Rhin Laryngol 63:997–1014

Davies D (1964) Cavernous hemangioma of the mandible. Plast Reconst Surg 33:457

Davis JM, Zimmerman RA (1983) Injury of the carotid and vertebral arteries. Neuroradiology 25:55–69

Day AL, Rhoton AL (1982) Aneurysms and arteriovenous fistulae of the intracavernous carotid artery and its branches. In: Youmans JR (ed) Neurological Surgery, Saunders, Philadelphia, p. 1774

Deans WR, Block S, Leibrock L, et al. (1982) Arteriovenous fistula in patients with neurofibromatosis. Radiology 144:103–107

Debrun G, Chartres A (1972) Infra and supratentorial arteriovenous malformations: a general review about two cases of spontaneous supratentorial arteriovenous malformations of the dura. Neuroradiology 3:184–192

Debrun G, Lacour P, Caron JP, et al. (1975 a) Inflatable and released balloon technique. Experimental in Dog-application in men. Neuroradiology 9:267–271

Debrun G, Lacour P, Caron JP, Hurth M, et al (1975 b) Traitement des fistules arterioveineuses et d'anevrysmes par balloon gonflable et largable. Nouv Press Med 2315–8

Debrun G, Lacour P, Caron JP, et al. (1978) Detachable balloon and calibrated leak balloon technique in the treatment of cerebral vascular lesions. J Neurosurg 49:635–649

Debrun G, Legre J, Kasbarian M, et al (1979) Endovascular occlusion of vertebral fistulas by detachable balloons with conservation of the vertebral blood flow. Radiology 13:141–147

Debrun G, Lacour P, Viñuela F, et al. (1981) Treatment of 54 traumatic carotid-cavernous fistulas. J Neurosurg 55:678–692

Debrun G, Viñuela FV, Fox AJ, et al. (1982) Two different calibrated leak balloons: Experimental work and application in humans. AJNR 3:407

De Campos JM, Lopez Ferro MO, Burcazo JA, Boixados JR (1982) Spontaneous carotid-cavernous fistula in ostegenesis imperfecta. J Neurosurg 56:590–593

Deen HG, Scheithauer BW, Ebersold MJ (1982) Clinical and pathological study of meningiomas in the first two decades of life. J Neurosurg 56:317–322

Delarue J, Paillas J, Payen J, Burgeat M (1956) Les fibromes naso-pharyngiens; étude anatomopathologique. Semaine Hop 32:3801–3809

Deterling RA Jr (1952) Tortuous right common carotid artery simulating aneurysm. Angiology 3:483–492

Devlamynck S, Rossazza C, Jan M, et al. (1978) Ocular complications sustained after the occlusion of a carotid cavernous fistula with a Fogarty balloon catheter. Rev Otoneuroophthalmol 50:409–412

Deysine M, Aidiga R, Wilder JR (1969) Traumatic false aneurysm of the cervical internal carotid artery. Surgery 66:1004–1007

Dickens WJ, Million RR, Cassisi NJ, Singleton GT (1982) Chemodectomas arising in temporal bone structures. Laryngoscope 92:188–191

Di Stefano JF, et al. (1979) False aneurysms of the lingual artery. J. Oral Surg 35:918–920

Di Tullio MV, Rand RE, Frisch E (1976) Development of a detachable vascular balloon catheter. A preliminary report. Bull Los Angeles Neurol Soc 41:2–5

Di Tullio MV, Rand RE, Frisch E (1978) Detachable balloon catheter. Its application in experimental arteriovenous fistulae. J Neurosurg 48:717–723

Dixon JM (1954) Angloid streaks and pseudoxanthomal elasticum with aneurysm of internal carotid artery. Amer J Ophthal 34:1322–1323

Djindjian R, Houdart R (1975) Arteriographie superselective de la carotide interne et embolization. Rev Neurol (Paris) 131:829–846

Djindjian R, Merland JJ (1978) Superselective arteriography of the external carotid artery. Springer, Berlin Heidelberg New York

Djindjian R, Cophignon J, Comoy J, Rey J, Houdart R (1968) Polymorphisme neuroradiologique des fistules carotido-caverneuses. Neurochirurgie 14:881–890

Djindjian R, Manelfe C, Picard L (1973 a) Fistules arterioveineuses carotide externe-vinus caverneux; étude angiographique à propos de 6 observations et revue de la littérature. Neurochirurgie 19:91–110

Djindjian R, Cophignon J, Theron J, et al. (1973 b) Embolization by superselective arteriography from the femoral route in neuroradiology. Review of 60 cases. Neuroradiology 6:20–26

Dohrmann PJ, Hunt BH, Samson D, Suss R (1985) Recurrent subarachnoid hemorrhage complicating a traumatic carotid cavernous fistula. Neurosurgery 17(3):480–483

Donnell MW, Meyer GA, Donegan WI (1979) Estrogen-receptor protein in intracranial meningiomas. J Neurosurg 50:499–502

Doppman JL (1980 a) The treatment of hyperparathyroidism by transcatheter techniques. Cardiovasc Intervent Radiol 3:268–281

Doppman JL (1980 b) The localization and treatment of parathyroid adenomas by angiographic techniques. Ann Radiol 23:253–258

Doppman JL, Zapol W, Pierce J (1971) Transcatheter embolization with a silicone rubber preparation. Experimental observations. Investigative Radiology 304–309

Doppman JL, Marx S, Speigel AM, et al. (1975) Treatment of hyperparathyroidism by percutaneous embolization of a mediastinal adenoma. Radiology 115:37–42

Dora F, Zileli T (1980) Common variations of the lateral and occipital sinuses at the confluence sinuum. Neuroradiology 20:23–27

Dorfman HD, Steiner GC, Jaffer HL (1971) Vascular tumors of bone. Hum Pathol 2:349

Dotter CT, Goldman ML, Rosch J (1975) Instant selective arterial occlusion with isobutyl-2-cyanoacrylate. Radiology 144:227–230

Doyon D, Metzger J (1973) Malformations vasculaires duremeriennes sustentorielles. Acta Radiol 13:792–800

Doyon D, Meyer B, Lasjaunias P, Quillard J, Josset P (1980) A case of an intratympanic meningioma. J Neuroradiology 7:209–214

Drake CG (1979) Giant intracranial aneurysms: Experience with surgical treatment in 174 patients. Clin Neurosurg 26:12–95

Drouet L (1980) Oestrogènes androgènes et vaisseaux. Quot Med Suppl 2150–2, 16–31

Du Boulay G, Darling M (1975) Autoregulation in external carotid artery branches in the baboon. Neuroradiology 9:129–132

Dunlop DAB, Papapoulos SE, Lodge RW, Fulton AJ, Kendall BE, O'Riordan JLH (1980) Parathyroid venous sampling: anatomic considerations and results in 95 patients with primary hyperparathyroidism. Brit J of Radiol 53:183–1191

Duplay J, Cossa P, Marchal E (1957) Anevrismes multiples de la carotide interne dans son segment exocranien et dans son segment endocranien. Presse Med 65:143–144

Dutton J, Isherwood I (1970) Iatrogenic vertebral arteriovenous fistulae Neurochirurgia 13:49–60

Duvall E, Johnston A, McLay K, Piris J (1980) Carcinoid tumor of the larynx. A report of two cases. J Laryng and Otol 97:1073–1080

Earle KM, Richany SF (1969) Meningiomas. Med Ann D C 38:353–358

Edgerton MT (1976) The treatment of hemangiomas with special reference to the role of steroid therapy. Annals of Surgery 183:517–532

Edwards MS, Connoly RS (1977) Cavernous sinus syndrome produced by communication between the external carotid artery and the cavernous sinus. J Neurosurg 46:92–95

Ehni G, Barrett JH (1960) Hemorrhage from ear due to aneurysm of internal carotid artery. N Engl J Med 262:1323–1325

Ehrenfeld WK, Hays RJ (1972) False aneurysms after carotid endarterectomy. Arch Surg 104:288–291

Ehrenfeld WK, Wylie EJ (1974) Fibromuscular dysplasia of the internal carotid artery. Surgical management. Arch Surg 109:676–681

Ekelund L, Jonsson N, Treugut H (1981) Transcatheter obliteration of the renal artery by ethanol injection: experimental results. Cardiovasc Intervent Radiol 4:1–17

Elders RA (cited by Zak) (1962) Paraganglioma. Een overzicht en een besspreking van 92 Nederlandse patienten. Thesis, University of Groningen. 333 p

El Gindi S, Andrew J (1966) Successful closure of carotid cavernous fistulas by the use of acrylic. J Neurosurg 153–156

Ellman BA, Green CE, Eigenbrodt E, et al. (1980) Renal infarction with absolute ethanol. Investigat Radiol 15:318–322

Ellman BA, Parkhill BJ, Curry III TS, Marcus PB, Peters PC (1981) Ablation of renal tumors with absolute ethanol: a new technique. Radiology 141:619–626

Ellman BA, Parkhill BJ, Marcus PB (1984) Renal ablation with absolute ethanol. Mechanism of action. Investigat Radiol 19:416–422

Enker SH (1979) Progression of a dural arterio-venous malformation resulting in an intra cerebral hematoma. Angiology 30:198–204

Enzinger FM, Smith BH (1976) Hemangiopericytoma. An analysis of 106 cases. Human Pathol 7:61–82

Evans CE (1984) Internal carotid artery aneurysm: a singular anomaly. Head Neck Surg 6:1043–1050

Ewing JA, Shively EH (1981) Angiofibroma: a rare case in an eldery female. Otolaryngol Head Neck Surg 89:602–603

Fabiani JN, Mercier JN, Ribierre M (1979) Traitement par embolisation d'une fistule arterio-veineuse vertebrale congenitale. Arch Franc Pediat 36:34–39

Farr HW, Gray GF, Vrana M, Panio M (1973) Extracranial meningioma. J Surg Oncol 5:411–420

Farrior JB, Hyams VJ, Benke RH (1980) Carcinoid apudoma arising in a glomus jugulare tumor: review of endocrine activity in glomus jugulare tumors. Laryngoscope 90:110–118

Fein JM, Flamm E (1979) Planned intracranial revascularization before proximal ligation for traumatic aneurysm. Neurosurgery 5(2):254–258

Fellus P, Lasjaunias P, Deffez JP (1979) Le contact bilabial: but à atteindre dans les traitements des retromandibulies. Actualités Odonto Stomatologiques 128: 733–746

Fenyes G, Kepes J (1956) Über das gemeinsame Vorkommen von Meningeomen und Geschwulsten anderen Typs im Gehirn. Zentralbl Neurochir 16:251–260

Ferlito A, Pesavento G, Recher G, Nicolai P, Narne S, Polidoro F (1984) Assessment and treatment of neurogenic and non-neurogenic tumors of the parapharyngeal space. Head Neck Surg 7:32–43

Fierstein SB, DeFeo D, Nutkiewicz A (1978) Complete obliteration of a carotid cavernous fistula with sparing of the carotid blood flow using a detachable balloon. Surg Neurol 9:277–280

Fincher EF (1951) Arteriovenous fistula between the middle meningeal artery and the greater petrosal sinus. Case report. Ann Surg 133:886–888

Finley JL, Barsky SH, Geer DE (1981) Healing of port-wine stains after argon laser therapy. Arch Dermatol 117:486

Finnerud CW (1960) Radiodermatis and cancer. Arch Dermatol 82:544

Finney LA, David NJ (1964) Aneurysm of extracranial internal carotid artery; report of case and discussion. Neurology (Minneap.) 14:376–379

Fisch U (1982) Infratemporal fossa approach for glomus tumors of the temporal bone. Ann Otol Rhin Laryng 91:474–479

Fisch U, Fagan P, Valavanis A (1984) The infratemporal fossa approach for the lateral skull base. Otolaryngol Clin North Am 17:513–552

Fisher ER, Hazard JP (1952) Non chromaffin paraganglioma of the orbit. Cancer 5:521–524

Fitzpatrick PJ, Rider WD (1973) The radiotherapy of nasopharyngeal angiofibroma. Radiology 109:171–178

Flechter JD, Dedd H, Newton TH, et al. (1975) Preoperative embolization of juvenile angiofibroma of the nasopharynx. Ann Otol Rhinol Laryngol 84:740–746

Fleisher AS, Kricheff II, Ransohoff J (1972) Postmortem findings following the embolization of an arteriovenous malformation. Case Report J Neurosurg 37:606–609

Flood LM, Kemink JL (1984) Surgery in lesions of the petrous apex. Otolaryngol Clin North Am 17:565–575

Folkman J (1975) Tumor angiogenesis: a possible control point in tumor growth. Ann Int Med 82:96–100

Foote GA, et al. (1974) Pulmonary complications of the flow directed balloon tipped catheter. New Engl J Med 290(17):927–931

Foster JH, Carter JW, Graham CP, et al. (1970) Arterial injuries secondary to the use of the Fogarty catheters. Annals of Surgery 171:6

Fourestier J, Ribault JY, Maria J et al. (1985) Les béances chez l'enfant, contribution à leur étude. Rev Stomatol Chir Maxillofac 86:147–152

Frederiks E (1973) Vascular pattern in embryos with clefts of primary and secondary palate. In: Advances in Anat Embryol Cell Biol. Springer, Berlin Heidelberg New York 46(6)

Freeny PC, Mennemeyer R, Kidd CR, et al. (1979) Long-term radiographic-pathologic follow-up of patients treated with visceral transcatheter occlusion using isobutyl-2-cyanoacrylate (bucrylate). Radiology 131:51–60

Freitas MAL, Cyro ABF, Lima R, et al. (1983) Traumatic ophthalmic fistula simulating carotid-cavernous fistula. Neurosurgery 12(1):102–104

Friedmann I, Osborn DA (1976) Systemic Pathology. Churchill Livingstone, Edinburgh, 2nd ed., Vol 1, 228–230

Fu YS, Perzin KH (1974) Non epithelial tumors of the nasal cavity, paranasal sinuses, and nasopharynx: a clinicopathologic study I. general features and vascular tumors. Cancer 33:1275–1287

Fujiwara S, Hachisuga S, Numaguchi Y (1980) Intracranial hypoglossal neurinoma: report of a case. Neuroradiology 20:87–90

Fukui M, Kitamura K, Ohgami S, Takaki T, et al. (1977) Radiosensitivity of meningioma-analysis of five cases of highly vascular meningioma treated by preoperative irradiation. Acta Neurochir (Wien) 36:47–60

Fuller AM, Brown HA, Harrison EG, Siekert RG (1967) Chemodectomas of the glomus jugulare tumors. Laryngoscope 77:218–238

Gaillard J, Haguenauer JP, Romanet P, Dubreuil C, Dumolard F (1978) Evolution insolite de deux chémotectomes tympano-jugulaires. J Oto-Rhino-Laryng 27:553–556

Ganti SR, Silver AJ, Hilal SK, Mawad ME, Sane P (1982) Computed tomography of cerebellar hemangioblastomas. J Comput Ass Tomogr 6:912–919

Garcia JC, Roach ES, McLean WT (1981) Recurrent thrombotic deterioration in the Sturge Weber syndrome. Child's brain 8:427–433

Gaston A, Chiras J, Leger JM, Bourbotte PH, Merland JJ (1984) Dural AV fistulas with direct drainage into the cerebral veins. J Neuroradiol 11:161–178

Geachan NE, Lambert J, Micheau C, Richard JM (1983) Synovialome malin du larynx. Ann Oto-Laryng 100:61–65

Gelber BR, Sundt TM Jr. (1980) Treatment of intracavernous and giant carotid aneurysms by combined internal carotid ligation and extra to intracerebral bypass. J Neurosurg 52:1–10

Geoffray A, Lee YY, Jings BS, Wallace S (1984) Extracranial meningiomas of the head and neck. AJNR 5:599–604

Gerlock AJ (1979) Embolisation of external carotid artery in the treatment of carotid cavernous sinus fistulae. Clin Radiol 30:111–116

Geuna E, Panzarasa G, Voci A, Arrigoni M (1985) Les hémangiopéricytomes du rocher, considérations à propos de 5 cas opérés. Neurochirurgie 31:51–59

Gianotta S, McGillicuddy JE, Kindt GW (1979) Gradual carotid artery occlusion in the treatment of inaccessible internal carotid artery aneurysm. Neurosurgery 5:417–421

Girgis IH, Fahmy SA (1973) Nasopharyngeal fibroma; its histopathological nature. J Laryngol 87:1107

Glasscock ME, Smith PG, Schwaber MK, Nissen AJ (1984) Clinical aspects of osseous hemangiomas of the skull base. Laryngoscope 94:869–873

Glenner GC, Grimley PM (1974) Tumors of the extra-adrenal paranglion system (including chemoreceptors). Atlas of Tumor Pathology, Second series, fascicle 9, Armed Forces Institute of pathology, Washington DC

Gold RE, Grace DM (1975) Gelfoam embolization of the left gastric artery for bleeding ulcers. Experimental considerations. Radiology 116:575–580

Golden AR (1976) Control of duodenal hemorrhage with cyanoacrylate. Br J Radiol 49:583

Goldenberg RA (1984) Surgeon's view of the skull base from the lateral approach. Laryngoscope 94, No. 12 suppl.

Golding-Wood PH (1970) Vidian neurectomy and other transantral surgery. Laryngoscope 80:1179–1189

Gomori JM, Dermer R, Shifrin E (1983) Aneurysm of the lingual artery. Neuroradiology 25:111–112

Goncalves CG, Briant TDR (1978) Radiologic findings in nasopharyngeal angiofibromas. J Can Assoc Radiol 29:209–215

Goodman SJ, Hasso A, Kirkpatrick D (1975) Treatment of vertebral jugular fistulas by balloon occlusion. Case report. J Neurosurg 43:362–367

Goody W, Schechter MM (1960) Spontaneous arteriovenous fistula of the vertebral artery. Br J Radiol 22:709–711

Gordeeff A, Mercier J, Bedhet N, Aillet G, Landais H, Delaire J (1986) Le kyste hématique du masseter: à propos de 2 observations. Rev Stomatol Chir Maxillofac. In Press.

Graf CJ (1965) Spontaneous carotid cavernous fistula: Ehlers Danlos syndrome and related conditions. Arch Neurol 13:262–272

Green JF, Fitzwater JE, Burgess J (1974) Arterial lesions associated with neurofibromatosis. Am J Pathol 62:481–487

Grisoli F, Vincentelli F, Fuchs S, Baldinin M, Raybaud C, Leclerc TA, Vigouroux RP (1984) Surgical treatment of tentorial arteriovenous malformations draining into the subarachnoid space. J Neurosurg 60:1059–1066

Gronski HW, Creely JJ Jr. (1975) Carotid-cavernous fistula: a complication of maxillofacial trauma. South Med J 68:1096–1102

Gross C, Vlahovitch B, Labauge R, et al. (1970) Les anevrysmes extracraniens de la carotide interne. Neurochirurgie 16:367–381

Guerrier Y, Guerrier B (1976) Anatomie topographique et chirurgicale du rocher. Acta Oto-Laryng Belg 30:22–50

Guillaume J, Roulleau J (1977) Experimental embolization with inflatable and releasable balloons in dogs. Neuroradiology 14:85–88

Gursoy G, Tolun R, Bahar S (1979) Aneurysmal dilatation of torcular. Neuroradiology 18:285–288

Haar F, Patterson RH Jr (1972) Surgery for metastatic intracranial neoplasm. Cancer 30:1241–1245

Haik BG, Jakobiec FA, Ellsworth RM, et al. (1979) Capillary hemangioma of the lids and orbit: an analysis of the clinical features and therapeutic results in 101 cases. Ophthalmology 86:760

Halasz NA, Kennady JC (1964) Excision of arteriosclerotic aneurysm of cervical internal carotid artery. J. Neurosurg 21:352–357

Halsted WS, Evans HM (1907) The parathyroid glands. Their blood supply and their preservation in operation upon the thyroid gland. Ann Surg 16:489–506

Hamby WB (1966) Carotid cavernous fistulas. Charles C. Thomas Springfield, III

Hamby WB, Gardner WJ (1933) Treatment of pulsating exophthalmos with report of two cases. Arch Surg 7:676–685

Handousa A, Farid H, Elwi AM (1954) Nasopharyngeal fibroma, clinico-pathological study of 70 cases. J Laryngol and Otol 68:647–666

Haratake J, Ishii N, Horie A, Yoshida A, Lin M (1984) Meningioma of the parapharyngeal space: unique extension of intracranial tumor. Laryngoscope 94:1372–1375

Harkins JC, Reed RJ (1969) Tumors of the peripheral nervous system. In: Atlas of tumor pathology, fasc 3. Washington D. C. Armed Forces Institute of Pathology

Harrison DFN (1954) Two cases of bleeding from ear from carotid aneurysm. Guy's Hosp. Rep. 103:207–212

Harrison DFN (1976) Juvenile postnasal angiofibroma. An evaluation. Clin Otolaryngol 1:187–193

Harrison DFN (1982) Use of estrogen in treatment of familial hemorrhagic telangiectasia. Laryngoscope 92:314–320

Harrison K (1974) Glomus jugulare tumors: their clinical behavior and management. Proc Roy Soc Med 67: 264–267

Harrison THM, Odom GL, Kunkle EC (1963) Internal carotid artery aneurysm arising in carotid canal. Arch Neurol Chicago 8:328–331

Hayes GJ (1963) External carotid cavernous sinus fistulas. J Neurosurg 20:692–700

Hayward E, Whitewell H, Paul KS, Barnes DM (1983) Steroid receptors in human meningioma (congress abstract) J Steroid Biochem 19 (Suppl):164

Healey JE, Gallager HS, Moore EG, et al. (1965) Experience with plastic adhesive in the nonsuture repair of body tumors. Am J Surg 109:416–423

Hekster REM, Lujendijk W, Matricali B (1973) Transfemoral catheter embolization: a method of treatment of glomus jugulare tumors. Neuroradiology 5:208–214

Helle TL, Conley FK (1980) Hemorrhage associated with meningioma: A case report and review of the literature. J Neurol Neurosurg Psychiat 43:725–729

Henderson JW, Campbell RJ (1977) Primary intraorbital meningioma with intraocular extension. May Clin Proc 52:504–508

Henderson JW, Schneider RC (1959) The ocular findings in carotid-cavernous fistula in a series of 17 cases. Am J of Ophthal 48(5):585–597

Henrikson P, Nilsson IM, Bergentz SE, Ljungqvist U, Rosengren B (1971) Giant hemangioma with a disorder of coagulation. Case report. Acta Pediat Scand 60:227–234

Heros RC, Nelson P, Ojemann RG, et al. (1983) Large and giant paraclinoid aneurysms. Surgical techniques, complications and results. Neurosurgery 12(2):153–163

Herrera M, Rysavy J, Kotula F (1982) Ivalon shaving: Technical considerations of a new embolic agent. Radiology 144:638–640

Hertzanu Y, Mendelsohn DB, Kassner G, Hockman M (1982) Haemangiopericytoma of the larynx. Brit J Radiol 55:870–873

Hidano A, Nakajima S (1972) Earliest features of the strawberry mark in the new born. Brit J Dermatol 87:138

Hidano A, Ogihara Y (1977) Cryotherapy with solid dioxyde in the treatment of naevus flammeus. J Dermatol Surg Oncol 3:213

Hieckman MS, Shenk G, Neems RL, Tinor BS (1979) Transfemoral cerebral arteriography: A comparison of complication rates. Radiology 132:93–97

Hieshima GB (1985) Therapeutic embolization of vascular injuries. In: Tsai FY (ed) Neuroradiology of Head Trauma. Baltimore Univ Park Press

Hieshima GB, Cahan LD, Berlin MS, Pribram H (1977) Calvarial, orbital and dural vascular anomalies in hereditary hemorrhagic telangiectasia. Surg Neurol 18:263–267

Hilal S, Michelsen WJ, Driller J (1969) Pod catheter: a means for small vessel exploration. J Appl Phys 40:1046

Hilal SK, Michelsen WJ (1975) Therapeutic percutaneous embolization for extraaxial base lesions of the head, neck and spine. J Neurosurg 43:275–281

Hill GJ, Khan E, Kochen JA (1984) Hemangioendiothelioma with intravascular coagulation and ischemic colitis. Cancer 54:2300–2304

Hiranandani LH, Melgeri RD, Juveker RV (1967) Angiofibroma of the ethmoidal sinus in female. J Laryngol Otol 81:935–939

Hitanant S, Sriumpai S, Na-Songla S, Pichyangkula C, Sindhavananda K, Viranuvatti V (1984) Paraganglioma of the common hepatic duct. Am J Gastr 79:485–488

Hite SJ, Grooves RA, Sharkey PC (1966) Superficial temporal artery aneurysms. Neurology 16:1044–1046

Hogemann KE, Gustafson G, Bjorlin G (1961) Ivalon surgical sponge used as temporary cover of experimental skin defects in rats. A preliminary report. Acta Chir. Scand. 121:83–89

Holman CM, Miller WE (1965) Juvenile nasopharyngeal angiofibroma. Am J Roentgenol 94:292–298

Hoover LA, Hanafee WN (1963) Differential diagnosis of nasopharyngeal tumors by computed tomography scanning. Arch Otolaryngol 109:43–47

Hora JF, Brown AK (1962) Paranasal juvenile angiofibroma. Arch Ontolaryngol 76:457–459

Hormia M, Koskinen O (1969) Metastasizing nasopharyngeal angiofibroma. Arch Oto Laryng 89:107–110

Horten BD, Ulrich H, Rubingstein LJ, et al. (1977) The angioblastic meningioma: A reappraisal of a nosological problem. J Neurol Sci 31:387–410

Horton JA, Marano GD, Kerber CW, et al. (1983) Polyvinyl alcohol foam – Gelfoam for therapeutic embolization. A synergetic mixture. AJNR 4:143

Hosobuchi Y (1975) Electrothrombosis of carotid-cavernous fistula. J Neurosurg 42:76–85

House WP, Glassock ME (1968) Glomus tympanicum tumors. Arch Oto Laryngol 87: 550–554

Houser OW, Baker HL (1968) Fibromuscular dysplasia and other uncommon disease of the cervical carotid artery: Angiographic aspects. Amer J Roentgenol 104:201–212

Houser OW, Baker HL, Rhoton AL, Okazaki H (1972) Intracranial dural arteriovenous malformations. Radiology 1105:55–64

Huber P (1976) A technical contribution to the exact angiographic localization of carotid cavernous fistulas. Neuroradiology 10:239–241

Hueper WC (1959) Carcinogetic studies on water-soluble and insoluble macromolecules. Arch Patol 67:589–617

Huntington GS, McClure CFW (1907) The development of the main lymph channels of the cat in their relations to the venous system. Anat Rec 1:36

Inceman S, Tangun Y (1969) Chronic defibrination syndrome due to a giant hemangioma associated with microangiographic hemolytic anemia. Am J Med 46:997–1002

Isamat F, Salleras V, Miranda AM (1970) Artificial embolization of carotid-cavernous fistula with post-operative patency of internal carotid artery. J Neurol Neurosurg Psychiat 33:674–678

Ishikawa M, Handa H, Taki W, Yoneda S (1982) Management of spontaneous carotid-cavernous fistulae. Surg Neurol 18:131–139

Ishimori S, Hattori M, Shibata Y (1967) Treatment of carotid cavernous fistulas by gelfoam embolization. J Neurosurg 27:315–319

Ito J, Imamura H, Kobayashi K, Tsuchida T, Sato S (1983) Dural arteriovenous malformations of the base of the anterior cranial fossa. Neuroradiology 24:149–154

Itzchak Y, Katznelson D, Boichis, et al. (1974) Angiographic features of arterial lesions in neurofibromatosis. AJR 122:643–647

Ivey DM, Delfino JL, Sclaroff A, Pritcherd LY (1980) Intramuscular hemangioma. Report of a case. Oral Surg Oral Med Oral Patho 50:295–300

Iwabuchi T, Sobota E, Suzuki M, Suzuki S, Yamashita M (1983) Dural sinus pressure as related to neurosurgical positions. Neurosurgery 12:203–207

Jafek BW (1983) Ultrastructure of human nasal mucosa. Laryngoscope 93:1576–1599

Jaieson KG (1965) Vertebral arteriovenous fistula caused by angiographic needle: report of one case. J Neurosurg 23:620–621

Jefferson G (1938) Sacular aneurysms of the internal carotid artery in the cavernous sinus. Br J Surg 26:267–302

Jellinger K, Slowik F (1975) Histologic subtypes and prognostic problems in meningiomas. J Neurol 208:279–298

Jiminez FP, Goree JA (1969) Traumatic arteriovenous fistula of the superficial temporal artery. Radiology 106:279–281

Johns ME, McLeod RM, Cantrell RW (1980) Estrogen receptors in nasopharyngeal angiofibromas. Laryngoscope 90:630–634

Johnston I (1979) Direct surgical treatment of bilateral intracavernous internal carotid artery aneurysms. Case Report. J Neurosurg 51:98–102

Kandel EI, Filatov YM (1966) Clinical picture and surgical treatment of meningiomas of the lateral ventricle. In Proceedings of the Third International Congress of Neurological Surgery. A C Devet (ed) Copenhagen, 1965, 719–723, Excerpta Medica, Amsterdam

Kaplan EN (1983) Vascular malformations of the extremities. In: Williams HB (ed), Symposium on Vascular Malformations and Melanotic Lesions, St. Louis, CV Mosby, 144–161

Karp LA, Zimmerman LE, Borit A, Spencer W (1974) Primary intraorbital meningiomas. Arch Ophthalmol 91:24–28

Kasabach HH, Merritt KK (1940) Capillary hemangioma with extensive purpura: report of a case. Am J Dis Child 59:1063–1080

Kataoka K, Taneda M (1984) Angiographic disappearance of multiple dural arteriovenous malformations. J Neurosurg 60:1275–1278

Kato T, Nemoto R (1978) Microencapsulation of mitomycion C for intra-arterial infusion chemotherapy. Proc Jpn Adad 54:413–417

Kato T, Nemoto R, Mori H, et al. (1980) Sustained released properties of microencapsulated Mitomycin C with ethyl cellulose infused into the renal artery of the dog kidney. Cancer 46:14–21

Kato T, Nemoto R, Mori H, et al. (1981) Transcatheter arterial chemoembolization of renal cell carcinoma with microencapsulated Mitomycin C. Urology 125:19–24

Kauffman GW, Rassweiler J, Richter G, Hauenstein KH, Rohrbach R, Friedburg H (1981) Capillary embolization with ethibloc: new embolization concept tested in dog kidneys. AJR 137:1163–1168

Kaufmann SL, Strandbert JD, Barth KH, et al. (1979) Therapeutic embolization with detachable silastic balloon: long term effects in swine. Invest. Radiol 14:156–161

Kendall B (1983) Results of treatment of arteriovenous fistulae with the Debrun technique. AJNR 4:405–408

Kepes, JJ (1982) Meningiomas. Biology, Pathology, and Differential Diagnosis. Masson, Chicago

Keplach GL, Wray SH, Roberson GH, Dallow RL (1978) Bilateral dural arteriovenous malformations simulating dysthyroid ophthalmopathy. Ann Ophthalmol 10:1519–1523

Kerber CW (1976) Balloon catheter with a calibrated leak, Radiology 120:547–550

Kerber CW (1976) A new system of catheter occlusive therapy. Invest Radiol 11:370

Kerber CW (1980) Flow controlled therapeutic embolization: A physiologic and safe technique. Am J Roentgenol 134:557–561

Kerber CW, Manke W (1983) Trigeminal artery to cavernous sinus fistula treated by balloon occlusion. Case report. J Neurosurg 58:611–613

Kerber CW, Bank WO, Horton JA (1978) Polyvinyl alcohol foam: prepacking emboli for therapeutic embolization. AJR 130:1193–1194

Kerber CW, Bank WO, Cromwell LD (1979) Calibrated leak balloon microcatheter: a new device for arterial exploration and occlusive therapy. AJR 132:202–207

Kessler LA, Wholey MH (1970) Internal carotid occlusion for treatment of intracranial aneurysms. A new percutaneous technique. Radiology 95:581–583

Khalifa MC, Bassyouni A (1981) "Nasal schwannoma" J Laryngol Otol 95:503–507

Kilian H (1951) Aneurysmen des branchiocephalen Stromgelueetes und weitere Erfahrungen mit der Mediatinotomia Sternoclavicularis. Arch Klin Chir 269:200–214

Klatzo L (1967) Neuropathological aspects of brain edema. J Neuropathol Exp Neurol 26:1–14

Knudsen RP, Alden ER (1979) Symptomatic arteriovenous malformation in infants less than 6 month of age. Pediatrics 64:238

Koch HJ, Escher GC, Lewis JS (1952) Hormonal management of hereditary hemorrhage telangiectasia. JAMA 149:1376–1380

Koegel L, Levine HL, Waldman SR (1982) Paraganglioma of the sphenoid sinus appearing as labile hypertension. Otolaryngol Head Neck Surg 90:704–707

Komisar A, Silver C, Kalnicki S (1985) Osteoradionecrosis of the maxilla and skull base. Laryngoscope 95:24–28

Koo AH, Newton TH (1972) Pseudoxanthoma elasticum associated with carotid rete mirabile. Am J Roentgenol Radium Ther Nucl Med 116:16–22

Korsgaard O, Lindholm J, Rasmussen P (1976) Endocrine function in patients with suprasellar and hypothalamic tumors. Acta Endocrinol 83:1–8

Kosnick EJ, Hunt WE, Miller CA (1974) Dural arteriovenous malformations. J Neurosurg 40:322–329

Kramer W (1969) Hyperplasie fibromusculaire et anevrisme extracranien de la carotide interne avec syndrome parapharyngien typique. Rev Neurol (Paris) 120:239–244

Krayenbuhl H (1967) Treatment of carotid cavernous fistula consisting of one stage operation by muscle embolization of the fistulous carotid segment in Donaghy RMP, Yasargil MD (eds.): Microvascular Surgery. Thieme, Stuttgart 151–167

Kricheff II, Berenstein A (1979) Simplified solid particle embolization with a new introducer. Radiology 131:794–795

Kuhner A, Krastel A, Stolle W (1976) Arteriovenous malformations of the transverse dural sinus. J Neurosurg 45:12–19

Kupersmith MJ, Berenstein A, Choi IS, et al. (1984) Percutaneous transvascular treatment of giant carotid aneurysms: neurophthalmic findings. Neurology 34(3):328–335

Kupersmith M, Berenstein A, Flamm E, et al. (1986) Neuroophthalmologic abnormalities and intravascular therapy of traumatic carotid cavernous fistulas. Ophthalmology 93:906–912

Laccourreye H, Beutter P, Brasnu D, Lacau-Saint-Guily J, Candauz P, Laval-Jeantet M, Buy JN (1983) Interêt de la tomodensitométrie dans les tumeurs du pharyngo-larynx. Ann Oto-Laryng 100:341–345

Lack EE, Cubilla AL, Woodruff JM, Farr HW (1977) Paragangliomas of the head and neck region. A clinical study of 69 patients. Cancer 39:397–409

Lacour P, Doyon D, Manelfe C, Picard L, Salisachs P, Schwaab G (1975) Treatment of chemodectomas by arterial embolization (glomus tumors). J Neuroradiol 2:275–287

Laine E, Galibert P, Lopez C, Delahouse J, Delandtsheer JM, Christiaens JL (1963) Anévrysmes arterioveineux intra-duraux (developpés dans l'epaisseur de la duremère) de la fosse postérieure. Neurochirurgie 9:147–158

Laitiner L, Servo A (1978) Embolization of cerebral vessels with inflatable and detachable balloon. J Neurosurg 48:307–308

Lamas E, Lobato RD, Esparza J, Escudero L (1977) Dural posterior fossa AVM producing raised sagittal sinus pressure. J Neurosurg 46:804–809

Landolt AM, Millikan CH (1970) Pathogenesis of cerebral infarction secondary to mechanical carotid artery occlusion. Stroke 1:52–62

Lansky LL, Maxwell JA (1975) Mycotic aneurysms of the internal carotid artery in an unusual intracranial location. Dev Med Child Neurol 17:79–88

Laplane D, Carydakis C, Baulac M, Elhadi D, Chiras J (1986) Sténoses des artères intracraniennes 44 ans après radiothérapie craniofaciale. Rev Neurol 142:65–67

Lapresle J, Lasjaunias P, Verret JM (1979) Anevrisme geant de la carotide intracaverneuse compliqué d'hemorrhagie meningée. Nouv Presse Med 8:3037–3040

Lasjaunias P (1980) Nasopharyngeal angiofibromas. Hazards of embolization. Radiology 136:119–123

Lasjaunias P, Doyon D (1978) The ascending pharyngeal artery and the blood supply of the lower cranial nerves. J Neuroradiol 5:287–301

Lasjaunias P, Doyon D (1980) Malformations vasculaires de la cavité buccale; evaluation diagnostique et thérapeutique par l'angiographie, revue de 25 cas. J Neuroradiol 7:243–270

Lasjaunias P, Doyon D (1981) Angiographie diagnostique et thérapeutique en neuropédiatrie. Revue de 31 cas de lésions maxillo-faciales et cervicales entre 1977 et 1981. Ann Oto Laryng 98:625–628

Lasjaunias P, Moret J (1978) Normal and non pathological variations in the angiographic aspects of the arteries of the middle ear. Neuroradiology 15:213–219

Lasjaunias P, Picard L, Manelfe C, Moret J, Doyon D (1980) Angiofibrome nasopharyngien; revue de 53 cas avec embolisation. Place de l'angiographie préthérapeutique, hypothèses physio-pathogéniques. J Neuroradiol 7:73–95

Lasjaunias P, Menu Y, Bonnel D, Doyon D (1981) Paragangliomes non chromaffines de la tête et du cou. J Neuroradiol 8:239–281

Lasjaunias P, Appel B, Carriere T (1983) Maladie de Rendu Osler Weber, evaluation diagnostique et thérapeutique par l'angiographie. Ann Oto Laryng 100:203–215

Lasjaunias P, Halimi PH, Lopez-Ibor L, Sichez JP, Hurth M, De Tribolet N (1984) Traitement endovasculaire des malformations vasculaires durales (MVD) pures "spontanées". Revue de 23 cas explorés et traités entre mai 1980 et octobre 1983. Neurochirurgie 30:207–223

Lasjaunias P, Deffez JP, Fellus P, Huard JL, Franchi-Deffez I (1985) Les malformations vasculaires linguales, leurs conséquences sur la croissance de l'étage inférieur. Rev Stomatol Chir Maxillofac 86:99–102

Lasjaunias P, Ming C, Terbrugge K, Tolia A, Hurth M, Bernstein M (1986) Neurological manifestations of intracranial dural arteriovenous malformations. J Neurosurg 64:724–730

Latchaw R, Gold LH (1979) Polyvinyl foam embolization of vascular neoplastic lesions of the head and neck and spine. Radiology 131:669–679

Lehmann RAW, Hayes GJ (1966) Toxicity of alkyl 2-cyanoacrylates. I. Peripheral nerve. Arch Surg 93:441–446

Lehmann RAW, Hayes GJ (1967) The toxicity of alkyl 2-cyanoacrylate tissue adhesive: brain and blood vessels. Surgery 61:915–922

Leikensohn JR, Benton C, Cotton R (1976) Subglottic hemangioma. J Otolaryngol 58:487

Leikensohn JR, Epstein LI, Vasconez LO (1981) Superselective embolization and surgery of noninvoluting hemangiomas and A. V. malformations. Plast Reconstr Surg, 143–152

Lepoire J, Montaut J, Bouchet M, Laxenaire M (1963) Anevrysmes arterioveineux intra-frontaux vascularisés par l'artère ethmoidale antérieure à propos de trois observation. Neurochirurgie 9:159–166

Lester J (1966) Arteriovenous fistula after percutaneous vertebral angiography. Acta Radiol (Diagn) 5:337–340

Lewis RJ, Ketcham AS (1973) Maffucci's syndrome: functional and neoplastic significance. J Bone Joint Surg 55:1456

Lindenauer SM (1965) The Klippel Trenaunay syndrome: varicosity hypertrophy and hemangioma with no arteriovenous fistula. Ann Surg 162:303

Lister WA (1938) The natural history of strawberry naevi. Lancet 1:1429

Llena JF, Wisoff HS, Hirano A (1982) Gangliocytic paraganglioma in cauda equina region, with biochemical and neuropathological studies. J Neurosurg 56:280–282

Lloyd GA (1982) Primary orbital meningioma: a review of 41 patients investigated radiologically. Clin Radiol 33:181–187

Lloyd GAS, Phelps PD (1982) The investigation of petro-mastoid tumors by high resolution CT. Brit J Radiol 55:483–491

Loch WE (1950) Tumors in the ear. In diagnosis and treatment of Tumors of the Head and Neck (Not Including the Central Nervous System). Edited by Ward GE and Hendrick JW. Williams & Wilkins, Baltimore, 578–589

Lopez DA, Silvers DN, Hellwig EB (1974) Cutaneous meningiomas – A clinicopathologic study. Cancer 34:728–744

Lord JW, Stone PW, Cloutheir WA, et al. (1958) Major blood vessel injury during elective surgery. Arch Surg 77:282–288

Loskutoff DJ, Edgington TS (1977) Synthesis of a fibrinolytic activator and inhibitor by endothelial cells. Proc Natl Acad Sci USA 74:3903–3907

Louvel A, Abelanet R (1979) Anatomie pathologique des polunéoplasies endo-craniennes. Ann Med Interne 12:583–589

Lucas RB (1976) Pathology of tumors of the oral tissues. Churchill Livingstone Edinburgh, London and New York

Luessenhop AJ, Spence WT (1960) Clinical Notes: Artificial embolization of cerebral arteries. JAMA 172:1153–1155

Luessenhop AJ, Velasquez AC (1964) Observation on the tolerance of the intracranial arteries to catheterization. J Neurosurg 21:85–91

MacConnell EM (1953) The arterial blood supply of the human hypophysis cerebri. Anat Rec 115:175–203

Maceri DR, Makielski KH, Arbor A (1984) Intraoral ligation of the maxillary artery for posterior epistaxis. Laryngoscope 94:737–741

Maddison FE (1970) Arteriographic evaluation of carotid artery surgery. AJR 109:121–126

Madoule PH, Trampont PH, Doyon D, et al. (1981) Experimentation chez le chien de micro-billes utisasbles en angiographic therapeutique. J Radiol 62:457–462

Madoule PH, Trampont PH, Roche A (1984) Chimoembolization: principles and perspectives. J Microencapsulation 1:21–25

Mahaley MS Jr., Brooks WH, Roszman TL, et al. (1977) Immunobiology of primary intracranial tumors. Part I: Studies of the cellular and humoral general immune competence of brain tumor patients. J Neurosurg 46:467–476

Mahe E, Poncet P, Basset JM, Le Doussal V (1983) Tumeurs bénignes rares des fosses nasales et des sinus de la face (schwannomes bénins, fibromyxome). Ann Otolaryng 100:347–351

Malan E, Azzolini A (1968) Congenital arteriovenous malformations of the face and scalp. J Cardiovasc Surg 2:109–140

Malik GM, Pearce JE, Ausman JL, Mehta B (1984) Dural arteriovenous malformations and intracranial hemorrhage. Neurosurgery 15:332–339

Manelfe C, Berenstein A (1980) Treatment of carotid cavernous fistulas by venous approach. J Neuroradiology 7:13–19

Manelfe C, Roulleau J, Julian A, Giudicelli G (1972) Glomus tympanicum tumors: early diagnosis by arteriography. Neuroradiology 4:226–232

Manelfe C, Clarisse J, Fredy D, et al. (1974) Dysplasies fibromusculaires des artères cervico-cephalique. J Neuroradiol 1:149–231

Manelfe C, Espagno B, Guiraud M, et al. (1975) Therapeutic embolization of cranio-cerebral tumors. J Neuroradiol 2:257–274

Marc JA, Takei Y, Schechter MM et al. (1975) Intracranial hemangiopericytomas: angiography, pathology and differential diagnosis. AJR 125:823–832

Margolis MT, Stein RL, Newton TH (1972) Extracranial aneurysms of the internal carotid artery. Neuroradiology 4:78–89

Margolis MT, Freeny PC, Kendrick MM (1979) Cyanoacrylate occlusion of a spinal cord arteriovenous malformation. Case report. Neurosurgery 51:107–110

Markham JW (1961) Arteriovenous fistula of the middle meningeal artery and the greater petrosal sinus. J Neuro Surg 18:857–849

Markham JW (1969) Spontaneous arteriovenous fistula of the vertebral artery and veins. Case report. J Neurosurg 31:220–223

Marks PV, Brookes GB (1983) Malignant paraganglioma of the larynx. J Laryng and Otol 97:1183–1188

Martin H, Martin C (1984) Les injections de colle de fibrine dans les epistaxis graves et la maladie de Rendu-Osler. Ann Oto Laryng 101:561–563

Martin H, Ehrlich HE, Abels JC (1984) Juvenile nasopharyngeal angiofibroma. Ann Surg 127:513–536

Massoud GE, Awwad HK (1960) Nasopharyngeal fibroma: its malignant potentialities and radiation therapy. Clin Radiol 11:156–161

Matsuda A, Matsuda I, Sato M, Handa J (1982) Superior sagittal sinus thrombosis followed by subdural hematoma. Surg Neurol 18:206–211

Matsumoto T, Nemhauser GM, Soloway HB et al. (1969) Cyanoacrylate tissue adhesives: an experimental and clinical evaluation. Milit med 134:247–252

Maurice M, Milad M (1981) Pathogenesis of juvenile nasopharyngeal fibroma (a new concept). J Laryng Otol 95:1121–1126

Maxwell JA, Goldware SI (1973) Use of tissue adhesive in the surgical treatment of cerebrospinal fluid leaks. Experience with isobutyl 2-cyanoacrylate in 12 cases. J Neurosurg 39:332–336

Mazzei TS, Mazzei CM, Sonener A (1976) Hypocalcemia y tetania en el meningioma. Desaparicion despues de su extirpacion. Sindrome paraneoplasico. Rev Clin (Espanol) 141:183–186

McCormick WF, Kelly PJ, Sarwar M (1980) Fatal paradoxical muscle embolization in traumatic carotid cavernous fistula repair. J Neurosurg 52:321–329

McDowell HA (1971) Postarteriographic arteriovenous fistula of the cervical vertebral artery. South Med J 64:119–120

Melon C (1964) Physiopathologie generale de la muqueuse nasale. Acta Oto Rhino Laryng Belgica 18:219–279

Melot GH, Jeanmart L, Brihaye J, et al. (1966) Atypies arterielles cervicales infantiles. J Belge Radiol 49:229–233

Merland JJ, Riche MC, Monteil JP (1980) Classification actuelle des malformations vasculaires. Ann Chir Plast 25:105

Merlis AL, Schaiberger CL, Adler R (1982) External carotid-cavernous sinus fistula simulating unilateral Graves' ophthalmopathy. J Comput Ass Tomogr 6:1006–1009

Mettinger KL (1982 b) Fibromuscular dysplasia and the Brain. II. Current concept of the disease. Stroke 13(1)53–56

Mettinger KL, Ericson K (1982 a) Fibromuscular dysplasia and the Brain. Observations on angiographic, clinical and genetic characteristics. Stroke 13(1):46–52

Michelsen JJ, New PFJ (1969) Brain tumor and pregnancy. J Neurol Neurosurg Psychiatry 32:305–307

Miller JD, Jawad K, Jennett B (1977) Safety of carotid ligation and its role in the management of intracranial aneurysms. J Neurol Neurosurg Psychiat 40:64–72

Miller JDR, Grace MG, Russell DB, Zacks DJ (1977) Complications of cerebral angiography and pneumography. Radiology 124:741–744

Miller RE, Hieshima GB, Giannotta SL, et al. (1984) Acute traumatic vertebral arteriovenous fistula: Balloon occlusion with the use of a contralateral approach. Neurosurgery 14(2):225–229

Miller SH, Smith RL, Schochat SJ (1976) Compression treatment of hemangiomas. Plast Reconstr Surg 58:573

Million RR, Dickens WJ, Cassidi PG (1982) Chemodectomas arising in temporal bone structures. Laryngoscope 92:188–191

Mineua DE, Miller FJ, Lee RG, Nakashima EN, Nelson JA (1982) Experimental transcatheter splenectomy using absolute ethanol. Radiology 142:355–359

Mira JG, Chu FCH, Forther JG (1977) The role of radiotherapy in the management of malignant hemangiopericytoma. Cancer 39:1254–1259

Mirrizi PC (1935) Tumeur du corpuscule carotidien. Presse Med 43:1804–1907

Mische RE, Balkany TJ (1980) Skull base approach to glomus jugulare. Laryngoscope 90:189–191

Miyasaka K, Takei H, Nomura M, Sugimoto S, Aida T, Abe H, Tsuru M (1980) Computerized tomography findings in dural arteriovenous malformations. J Neurosurg 53:698–702

Modan B, Baidatz D, Mart H, et al. (1974) Radiation induced head and neck trauma. Lancet 1:277–279

Modesti LM, Binet EF, Collins GH (1976) Meningiomas causing spontaneous intracranial hematomas. J Neurosurg 45:437–441

Moody DM, Ghatak NR, Kelly DL (1976) Extensive calcification in a tumor of the glomus jugulare. Neuroradiology 12:131–135

Moore MT (1954) The fate of clinically unrecognized intracranial meningiomas. Neurology (Minneapolis) 4:837–856

Moret J, Lasjaunias P (1986 a) Abnormal vessel in the middle ear. In the ear (Vignaud J, Jardin C, Rosen L), Masson, Paris 136–145

Moret J, Lasjaunias P (1986 b) Vascular architecture of tympano-jugular glomus tumor. In the ear (Vignaud J, Jardin C, Rosen L), Masson, Paris 289–303

Moret J, Roulleau J, Poncet E, Vignaud J (1977) Interêt de l'artériographie thérapeutique dans le traitement des glomus tympano-jugulaires. Ann Oto Laryngol 94:491–498

Moret J, Lasjaunias P, Doyon D (1979) Occipital approach for treatment of arteriovenous malformations of the vertebral artery by balloon occlusion. Neuroradiology 17:269–273

Morley TP, Barr HWK (1969) Giant intracranial aneurysms. Diagnosis, course and management. Clin Neurosurg 16:73–94

Morris G (1969) Delayed perforation of the internal carotid artery by an ingested foreign body. Br J Surg 56:711–712

Mortimer H, Wright RP, Collip JB (1936) The effect of oestrogenic hormones on the nasal mucosa; their role in the nasosexual relation; and their significance in clinical rhinology. J Canad Med Assoc 35:615

Mujica RH, Rosenblat AM, Luessenhop AJ (1981) Subarachnoid hemorrhage secondary to an aneurysm of the ascending pharyngeal artery case report. J Neurosurg 54:818–820

Mullan S (1974) Experiences with surgical thrombosis of intracranial berry aneurysms and carotid cavernous fistulas. J Neurosurg 41:657–670

Mullan S (1979) Treatment of carotid-cavernous fistulas by cavernous sinus occlusion. J Neurosurg 50:131–144

Muller H (1971) Fibrome nasopharyngien. Ann Oto Laryngol 88:455

Mulliken JB, Glowacki J (1982) Hemangiomas and vascular malformations in infants and children: a classification based on endothelial characteristics. Plast Reconstr Surg 69:412–420

Mulliken JB, Murray JE, Castaneda AR (1978) Management of vascular malformation of the face using total circulatory arrest. Surg Gynecol Obstr 146:168

Mulliken JB, Zetter BR, Folkman J (1982) In vitro characteristics of endothelium from hemangiomas and vascular malformations. Surgery 92:348–353

Nagamine Y, Komatsu S, Suzuki J (1983) New embolization method using estrogen: effect of estrogen on microcirculation. Surg Neurol 20:269–275

Nasashima C, Iwasaki T, Kawanuma, et al. (1977) Traumatic arteriovenous fistula of the vertebral artery with spinal cord symptoms. Case report. Neurosurgery 46:681–687

Neel HB, Whicker JH, Devine KD, Weiland LH (1973) Juvenile angiofibromas: review of 120 cases. Am J Surg 126:547–556

Negoro M, Kageyama N, Ishiguchi T (1983) Cerebrovascular occlusion by catheterization and embolization: clinical experience. AJNR 4:362–365

Neidhart JA, Roach RW (1982) Successful treatment of skeletal hemangioma and Kasabach Merritt syndrome with aminocaproic acid; is fibrinolysis "defensive"? Am J Med 73:434–438

Nelson DA, Mahru MM (1963) Death following digital carotid artery occlusion. Arch Neurol 8:640–643

Nelson RA, Banitt EH, Robertson JK, et al. (1968) New fluoroalkyl cyanoacrylates as surgical adhesives. Fed Proc 27:707

New PJR, Momose KJ (1969) Traumatic dissection of the internal carotid artery at the atlanto-axial level secondary to nonpenetrating injury. Radiology 93:41–49

Newton TH, Cronqvist S (1969) Involvement of dural arteries in intracranial arteriovenous malformations. Radiology 93:1071–1078

Newton TH, Hoyt WF (1970) Dural arteriovenous shunts in the region of the cavernous sinus. Neuroradiology 1:71–78

Newton TH, Potts DG (1974) Radiology of the Skull and Brain. Vol 3. St. Louis CV Mosby

Newton TH, Weidner W, Greitz T (1968) Dural arteriovenous malformations in the posterior fossa. Radiology 90:27–32

Nishijima M, Kamiyama K, Oka N, Endo S, Takaku A (1984) Electrothrombosis of spontaneous carotid-cavernous fistula by copper needle insertion. Neurosurgery 14:400–405

Nishioka H (1966) Results of the treatment of intracranial aneurysms by occlusion of the carotid artery in the nerve. J Neurosurg 25:600–687

Norman D, Newton TH, et al. (1983) Carotid cavernous fistula closure with detachable silicone balloons. Radiology 149:149

Norman JA, Schmidt KW, Grow JB (1950) Congenital arteriovenous fistulas of the cervical vertebral vessels with heart failure in an infant. J Pediat 36:598–604

Noyek AM, Greyson ND, Steinhart MI, Kassel EE, Shulman HS, Rothberg R, Goldfinger M, Miskin M, Freeman JL (1983) Thyroid tumor imaging. Arch Otolaryng 109:205–224

Obley DL, Winzelberg GG, Qjarmolowski CR, Hydovitz JD, Danowski TS, Wholey MH (1984) Parathyroid adenomas studied by digital substraction angiography. Radiology 153:449–451

Obrador S, Soto M, Sileva J (1975) Clinical syndromes of arteriovenous malformations of the transverse sigmoid sinus. J Neurol Neurosurg Psy 38:436–451

Ogura JH (1978) Glomus jugulare and vagale. Ann Otol, Rhinol, Laryngol 87:622–629

Ohara I, Utsumi N, Ouchi H (1968) Resection of extracranial internal carotid artery aneurysms with arterial reconstruction. J Cardiovasc Surg (Torino) 9:365–373

Ohi M, Sakakura Y, Nozaki S, Mitsui H, Yatani R, Moriwaki K (1979) Subglottic hemangioma: a case report and review of the literature. Mie Medical Journal 2–3:107–113

Olcott CIV, Newton TH, Stoney RJ (1976) Intra-arterial embolization in the management of arteriovenous malformations. Surgery 79:3

Oller DW, Gee W, Kingsley JR (1976) Treatment of high extracranial internal carotid artery aneurysms. Ann Surg 42:311–315

Olutola PS, Eliam M, Molot M, Talalla A (1983) Spontaneous regression of a dural arteriovenous malformation. Neurosurgery 12:687–690

Oppenheimer BS, Oppenheimer ET, Danishefsky I, et al. (1980) Further studies of polymers as carcinogenic agents in animals. Cancer Res 15:333–340

Osborn A (1981) Craniofacial venous plexuses; angiographic study. AJR 136:139–143

Osborn DA (1959) So-called juvenile angiofibroma of nasopharynx. J Laryngol Otol 73:295–316

Osborn DA, Sokolovski A (1965) Juvenile angiofibroma in a female. Arch Otolaryng 82:629–632

Osborne AG, Anderson RE (1977) Angiographic spectrum of cervical and intracranial fibromuscular dysplasia. Stroke 8:617–626

Owen WG, Esmon CT (1981) Functional properties of an endothelial cell cofactor for thrombincatalyzed activation of protein C. J Biol Chem 256:5532–5535

Packer P (1960) Severe epistaxis due to a leaking extracranial aneurysm of the internal carotid artery. S Afr Med J 34:641–642

Page RC, Larson EJ, Siegmund E (1966) Chronic toxicity studies of methyl-2-cyanoacrylate in dogs and rats (In) Healey JE Jr, ed: Proceedings of the Symposium on Physiological Adhesives, University of Texas, Houston, Texas Feb 3–4, p. 11–23, (available from Ethicon Corp., Somerville NJ 08876)

Parisier SC, Sinclair GM (1967) Glomus tumor of the nasal cavity. Laryngoscope, 2013–2024

Parkinson D (1973) Carotid cavernous fistula: direct repair with preservation of the carotid artery. Technical note. J Neurosurg 38:99–106

Pasyk KA, Dingman RO, Argental LC et al. (1984) The management of hemangiomas of the eyelid and orbit. Head Neck Surg 6:851–857

Pearse AGE (1977) The diffuse neuroendocrine system and the apud concept: related "endocrine" peptides in brain, intestine, pituitary, placenta, and anuran cutaneous glands. Med Biol 55:115–125

Pecker J, Bonnal J, Javalet A (1965) Deux nouveaux cas d'anevrismes arterioveineux intraduraux de la fosse postérieure alimentés par la carotide externe. Neurochirurgie 11:327–332

Peeters FLM (1982) Angiographically demonstrated large vascular malformation in a patient with a normal angiogram 23 years before. A case report. Neuroradiology 23:113–114

Peeters FLM, Kroger R (1979) Dural and direct cavernous sinus fistulas. AJR 132:599–606

Perry MO, Thal ER, Shires GT (1961) Management of arterial injuries. Ann Surg 173:403–408

Persky MS, Berenstein A, Cohen NL (1984) Combined treatment of head and neck vascular masses with preoperative embolization. Laryngoscope 94:20–27

Pertuiset B, Morel-Maroger A, Philippon J, et al (1967) Les anevrysmes arterio-veineux traumatiques de l'artère meningée moyenne. La Presse Medicale 54:2775–2328

Pertuiset B, Sichez JP, Yacoubi A, Gardeur D, Melon E, Haddad K (1983) Quatrevingt-seize cas d'hémorragie cérébrale médicale spontanée. Expérience diagnostique et thérapeutique. Rev Neurol 139:359–366

Pesavento G, Ferlito A (1982) Hemangiopericytoma of the larynx. A clinico-pathological study with review of the literature. J Laryng and Otol 96:1065–1073

Peterman AF, Hayles AB, Dockerty MD (1969) Encephalotrigeminal angiomatosis (Sturge-Weber disease): clinical study of thirty-five cases. JAMA 167:21

Peters FLM, van de Werf AJM (1980) Detachable balloon technique in the treatment of direct carotid-cavernous fistulas. Surg Neurol 14:11–19

Pettet JR, Woolner LB, Judd ES (1937) Carotid body tumors of the carotid body. Review of 159 histologically verified cases. Report of case. West J Surg 45:42–46

Pevsner PH (1977) Micro-balloon catheter for superselective angiography and therapeutic occlusion. Am J Roentgenol 128:225–230

Pevsner PH, George ED, Doppman LJ (1982) Interventional radiology polymer update: Acrylic. Neurosurgery 10:314–316

Pia HW (1978) Classification of aneurysms of the internal carotid system. Acta Neurochir (Wien) 40:5–31

Picard JM, Andre R, Djindjian J (1974) Angiographie superséléctive et embolisation des localisations oto-rhinolaryngologiques de l'angiomatose de Rendu Osler. J Neuroradiol 1:351–363

Picard L, Arnould G, Dureux JB, Tridon P, Weber M, Thiriet M, Floquet J (1968) Malformations vasculaires cérébrales et angiomatose de Rendu Osler. Rev Neurol 11:230–235

Picard L, Lepoire J, Mantaut J, et al. (1974) Endarterial occlusion of carotid cavernous fistulas using a balloon tipped catheter. Neuroradiology 8:5–10

Picard L, Robert J, Andre JM, et al. (1976) Embolization with iodine 131 marked sponge. 1. Technique, indications and results. J Neuroradiol 3:53–74

Picard L, Rebstock J, Marchal AL, et al. (1980) Release of endovascular occlusion balloons using a thermoresistive technique. J Neuroradiol 7:231–242

Pinto R, Kircheff II, Butler A, et al. (1979) Correlation of computed tomographic angiographic and neuropathological changes in giant cerebral aneurysms. Radiology 132:85–92

Pitanguy I, Caldeira AML, Calixto CA et al. (1984) Clinical evaluation and surgical treatment of hemangiomata. Head Neck Surg 7:47–59

Poisson M, Magdelenat H, Foncini JF et al. (1980) Recepteurs d'estrogènes et de progestérone dans les meningiomes. Etude de 22 cas. Rev Neurol (Paris) 136:193–203

Pool JL, Potts DG (1965) Aneurysms and arteriovenous anomalies of the brain: diagnosis and treatment. Harper & Row, New York

Popescu V (1985) Intratumoral ligation in the management of orofacial cavernous hemangiomas. J Maxillofac Surg 13:99–107

Prabhakar S, Sawhney IM, Chopra JS, Kak VK, Banerjee AK (1984) Hemibase syndrome: an unusual presentation of intracranial paraganglioma. Surg Neurol 22:39–42

Probst FP (1980) Vascular morphology and angiographic flow patterns in Sturge Weber angiomatosis: facts, thoughts and suggestions. Neuroradiology 20:73–78

Prolo DJ, Hanbery JW (1971) Intraluminal occlusion of a carotid cavernous fistula with a balloon catheter. Technical Note. J Neurosurg 35:237–242

Prolo DJ, Burres KP, Hanberg JW (1977) Balloon occlusion of carotid cavernous fistula: Introduction of a new catheter. Surg Neurol 7:209–214

Pudenz RH, Odom FL (1942) Meningocerebral adhesions. An experimental study of human amniotic membrane, amnioplastin, beef allantoic membrane, cargile membrane, tantalum foil, and polyvinyl alcohol foam. Surgery 12:318–344

Quattlebaum JK, Jr., Upson ET, Neville RL (1959) Stroke associated with elongation and kinking of internal carotid artery: report of three cases treated by segmental resection of carotid artery. Ann Surg 150:824–832

Quisling RG, Mickley JP et al. (1984) Histopathologic analysis of intra-arterial polyvinyl alcohol microemboli in rats cerebral cortex. AJNR 5:101–104

Rabson AS, Elliot JL (1957) Carotid body tumors with regional lymph node involvement with report of a case. Surgery 42:381–385

Raphael HA, Bernatz PE, Spittell JA Jr., et al. (1963) Cervical carotid aneurysms: treatment by excision and restoration of arterial continuity. Amer J Surg 105:771–778

Rappaport I, Rappaport J (1977) Congenital arteriovenous fistula of the maxillofacial region. Am J Surg 134:38

Reese AB (1976) Tumors of the eye, 3rd ed. Harper & Row. Hagerstown, pp 148–153

Reich NE, Adler LM, Duchesneau PM, Schumacher PO, Hall PM (1975) Norepinephrine and epinephrine secreting paraganglioma of the jugular glomus. Neuroradiology 8:263–265

Reid TL, Cornell B, Murtagh R et al. (1985) Port wine nevus associated with ipsilateral saccular aneurysms: treatment by intraarterial balloon trapping. Surg Neurol 23:541–544

Reivich M, Holling HE, Robert B, Toole JF (1961) Reversal of blood flow through the vertebral artery and its effect on cerebral circulation. N Engl J Med 265:878–885

Reizine D, Merland JJ, Birkur P, Leban M, Riche MC (1985) Treatment of spontaneous intraparotid direct arteriovenous fistulae using a detachable balloon technique. J Neuroradiol 12:35–43

Rensburg JCJ, van (1964) Aneurysm of the internal carotid artery presenting as a peritonsillar abscess. S Afr Med J 38:567–569

Rich NM, Baugh JH, Hughes CW (1970) Acute arterial injuries in Vietnam: 1000 cases. J Trauma 10:35–369

Riche MC, Hadjean E, Tran-Ba-Huy T, Merland JJ (1983) The treatment of capillary venous malformations using a new fibrosing agent. Plast Reconstr Surg 71:607–612

Rob RC (1954) Arterial aneurysms. Ann Roy Coll Surg Eng 14:35–49

Robbins SL, Cotran RS (1979) Pathologic Basis of Disease. 2nd ed. Saunders Philadelphia, p. 165

Roberson GH, Price AC, Davis JM, Gulati A (1979) Therapeutic embolization of juvenile angiofibroma. AJR 133:657–663

Robertson JH, Clark WG, Acker JD (1982) Bilateral occipital epidural hematomas. Surg Neurol 17:468–472

Robinson JL, Sedzimir CB (1970) External carotid transverse sinus fistula. Case report. J Neurosurg 33:718–720

Rodriquez-Erdmann F, Button L, Murray JE (1971) Kasabach-Merritt syndrome: coagulo-analytical observations. Am J Med Sci 261:9–15

Roman G, Fischer M, Perl D, Poser C (1978) Neurological manifestations of hereditary hemorrhagic telangiectasia (Rendu Osler Weber disease); report of 2 cases and review of the literature. Ann Neurol 4:130–144

Romodanov AP, Shcheglov VL (1982) Intravascular occlusion of saccular aneurysms of the cerebral arteries by means of a detachable balloon catheter. In: Krayenbühl H (ed) Advances and Technical Standards in Neurosurgery. Vol 9, Springer, Wien

Rosenwasser H (1958) Metastasis from glomus jugulare tumors. Arch Otolaryng 67:197–203

Rosenwasser H (1968) Monograph on glomus jugulare tumors. Arch Otolaryng 88:29–66

Rosenwasser H (1974) Glomus jugulare tumors. Proc Roy Soc Med 67:259–264

Roski RA, Owen M, White RJ, et al. (1982) Middle meningeal artery trauma. Surg Neurol 17(3):200–203

Rubi F (1945) Neurofibromatose et lesions vasculaires. Schweiz Med Wochenschr 75:463–465

Rubinstein LJ (1972) Atlas of Tumor Pathology. Tumors of the Central Nervous System. Armed Forces Institute of Pathology, Washington, D. C.

Russell DS, Rubinstein LJ (1977) Pathology of Tumors of the Nervous System. 4th ed. Williams & Wilkins, Baltimore, p. 89

Sabin FR (1901) On the origin of the lymphatic system from the veins and the development of the lymph and thoracic duct in the pig. Am J Anat 1:367

Sachs E (1977) Diagnosis and treatment of brain tumors and care of the neurosurgical patient. J Neuroradiol 4:385–398

Salama N, Stafford N (1982) Meningiomas presenting in the middle ear. Laryngoscope 92:92–97

Saldana MJ, Salem LE, Travezan R (1973) High altitude hypoxia and chemodectomas. Human Pathol 4:251–263

Salvolini U, Cabanis E, Iba-Zizen MT, Hemmy D (1984) Apport diagnostique de la reconstruction tri-dimentisionnelle en scanner. RX: coupes et surfaces de l'anatomie céphalique. Ann Chir Plast Esthé 29:339–357

Samy LL, Hashem M (1962) Nonchromaffin paraganglioma of the ear with a report of six cases with abnormal features. J Laryngol Otol 76:499–534

Sano K, Jimbo M, Saito I (1975) Artificial embolization of inoperable angiomas with polymerizing substance. In: Pia HW, Glaeve, et al. (eds) Cerebral angiomas: Advances in Diagnosis and Therapy. Springer, Berlin Heidelberg New York, pp. 222–229

Sano K, Wakai S, Ochiai C, Takakura K (1981) Characteristics of intracranial meningiomas in Childhood. Child's Brain 8:98–106

Sanoudos GMN, Ramp, Imparato I (1973) Internal carotid aneurysms. Am Surg 39:118

Satoh T, Sakurai M, Yamamoto Y, Asari S (1983) Spontaneous closure of a traumatic middle meningeal arteriovenous fistula. Neuroradiology 25:105–109

Sattler CH (1920) Beitrag zur Kenntnis des pulsierenden Exophthalmus. Augenh 43:534–552

Saylor WR, Saylor DC (1974) Vascular lesions of neurofibromatosis. Angiology 25:510–519

Scarcella JV, Dykes ER, Anderson R (1975) Hemangiomas of the parotid gland. Plast Reconstr Surg 56:642

Schechter DC (1979) Cervical carotid arteries. NY State J Med 79:892–901

Schiff M (1959) Juvenile nasopharyngeal angiofibroma: a theory of pathogenesis. Laryngoscope 69:981–1016

Schnegg JF, Gomes F, LeMarchand-Beraud T, Tribolet N (1981) presence of sex steroid hormone receptors in meningioma tissue. Surg Neurol 15:418

Schoenberg BS, Christine BW, Whisnant JP (1975) Nervous system neoplasms and primary malignancies of other sites. Neurology (Minneapolis) 25:705–712

Schuller DE, Lucas JG (1982) Nasopharyngeal paraganglioma, report of a case and review of literature. Arch Otolaryngol 108:667–670

Schwartz ML, Israel HL (1983) Severe anemia as a manifestation of metastatic jugular paraganglioma. Arch Otolaryngol 109:269–272

Scialfa G, Valsecchi F, Tonon C (1979) Treatment of external carotid arteriovenous fistula with detachable balloon. Neuroradiology 17:265–267

Scialfa G, Valsecchi F, Scotti G (1983) Treatment of vascular lesions with balloon catheters. AJNR 4:395–398

Scott JA, Berenstein A, Blumenthal D (1987) The use of the activated coagulation time during interventional procedures. Radiology

Sedzimir BC, Occleshaw JV (1967) Treatment of carotid-cavernous fistula by muscle embolization and Jaeger's maneuver. J Neurosurg 27:309–314

Seljeskog EL, Rogers HM, French LA (1968) Arteriovenous malformation involving the inferior sagittal sinus in an infant. J Neurosurg 29:623–624

Serbinenko FA (1971 a) Catheterization and occlusion of major vessels of the brain In, Perviy vseosouzniy s'ezd neuoshirurgov, Tom 1, Moscova 114–119

Serbinenko FA (1971 b) Surgical treatment of arteriosinus fistulae, formed by arteries of dura mater and sinus cavernous. In Perviy vsisouzniy s'ezd neurochirurgov Tom. 1 Moscva 119–123

Serbinenko FA (1971 c) Balloon occlusion of cavernous portion of the carotid artery as a method of treatment carotid cavernous fistulae. Zh Copr Neirokhr 6:3–9

Serbinenko FA (1972) Reconstruction of cavernous part of carotid artery in case of carotid cavernous fistula. Vopr Neirokhir 36:309

Serbinenko FA (1974) Balloon catheterization and occlusion of major cerebral vessels. J Neurosurg 41:125–145

Serbinenko FA (1979) Six Hundred endovascular neurosurgical procedures in vascular pathology A ten year experience. Acta Neurochir (Suppl. 28):310–311

Serbinenko FA, Promyslow MS, Bagigov GA et al. (1973) Catheterization method of preoperative staining of intracerebral tumors. Vopr Neiokhir 37:3–7

Sharbrough FW, Messick MJ Jr., Sundt TM Jr. (1973) Correlation of continous electroencephalograms with cerebral blood flow measurements during carotid endartarectomy. Stroke 4:674–683

Sharma PD, Johnson AP, Whitton AC (1984) Radiotherapy for jugulo-tympanic paragangliomas (glomus jugulare tumors) J Laryng Otol 98:621–629

Shea PC jr., Glass LF, Reid WA, Harland A (1955) Anastomosis of common and internal carotid arteries following excision of mycotic aneurysm. Surgery 37:829–832

Shim WKT (1969) Hemangiomas of infancy complicated by thrombo-cytopenia. Am J Surg 116:896–906

Shumacker HB, Jr., Campbell RL, Hineberger RG (1966) Operative treatment of vertebral arteriovenous fistulas. J Trauma 6:3–19

Siekert RG (1956) Neurologic manifestations of tumors of the glomus jugulare. Arch Neurol Psychiatry 76:1–13

Skultety FM (1968) Meningioma simulating ruptured aneurysm. Case report. J Neurosurg 28:380–382

Smit LME, Barth PG, Stam FE et al. (1981) Congenital multiple angiomatosis with brain involvement. Child's Brain 8:461–467

Snyder M, Renaudin J (1977) Intracranial hemorrhage associated with anticoagulation therapy. Surg Neurol 7:31–34

Soffer D, Pittaluga S, Feiner M, et al. (1983) Intracranial meningiomas following low-dose irradiation to the head. J Neurosurg 59:1048–1053

Solis OJ, Davis KR, Ellis GT (1977) Dural arterio-venous malformation associated with subdural and intracerebral hematoma: a CT scan and angiographic correlation. J Comput Ass Tomogr 1:145–150

Soloman H, Goldman L, Henderson B (1968) Histopathology of the laser treatment of port-wine lesions. J Invest Dermatol 50:141

Som PM, Cohen BA, Scher M, Choi IS, Bryan NR (1982) The angiomatous polyp and the angiofibroma: two different lesions. Radiology 144:329–334

Som PM, Reede DL, Bergeron RT, Parisier SC, Shugar JAMN, Cohen NL (1983) Computed tomography of glomus tympanicum tumors. J Comput Ass Tomogr 7:14–17

Spector FJ, Maisel RH, Ogura JH (1973) Glomus tumors in the middle ear. I. An analysis of 46 patients. Laryngoscope 83:1652–1672

Spector GJ, Sobol S, Thawley SE, Maisel RH, Ogura JH (1979) Panel discussion: glomus jugulare tumors of the temporal bone. Patterns invasion of the temporal bone. Laryngoscope 98:1628–1639

Spector GJ, Drucks NS, Gado M (1976) Neurologic manifestation of glomus tumor in the head and neck. Arch Neurol 8:239–281

Standefer J, Holt GR, Brown WE, Gates GA (1983) Combined intracranial and extracranial excision of nasopharyngeal angiofibroma. Laryngoscope 93:772–779

Stappleford RG, Gruenberg JC, Wolford DG, Kerchner JB (1981) Vertebral artery injury. Case report and review of operative approaches. Henry Ford Hosp Med 29:148–152

Stecker RH, Lake CF (1965) Hereditary telangiectasia: review of 102 cases and presentation of an innovation of septodermoplasty. Arch Otolaryngol 82:522–526

Stevens JM, Ruiz JS, Kendall BE (1983) Observation on peritumoral oedema in meningioma. Part I: Distribution, spread and resolution of vasogenic oedema seen on computed tomography. Neuroradiology 25:71–80

Stiller D, Ketenkamp D, Kuttner K (1976) Cellular differentiation and structural characteristics in nasopharyngeal angiofibromas: an electron-microscopic study. Virchows Arch (Pathol Anat) 371:273

Stock JL, Krudy AG, Doppman JL, et al. (1981) Parathyroid imaging after intraarterial injections of (75 SE) selenomethionine. J Clin Endocr Met 52:835–839

Straub PW, Kessler S, Schreiber A, Frick PG (1972) Chronic intra-vascular coagulation in the Kasabach-Merritt syndrome: preferential accumulation of fibrinogen. I 131 in a giant hemangioma. Arch Intern Med 129:475–478

Strauss M (1983) Long-term complications or radiotherapy confronting the head and neck surgeon. Laryngoscope 93:310–313

Strauss M, Nicholas GG, Abt AB, Harrison TS, Seaton JF (1983) Malignant catecholamine-secreting carotid body paraganglioma. Otolaryng Head Neck Surg 91:315–321

Strenger L (1966) neurological deficits following therapeutic collapse of intracavernous carotid aneurysm. J Neurosurg 25:215–218

Sugar HP (1979) Neovascular glaucoma after carotid cavernous fistula formation. Ann Ophthalmol 1667–1668

Sundt TM, Piepgras DG (1983) The surgical approach to arteriovenous malformations of the lateral and sigmoid dural sinuses. J Neurosurg 59:32–39

Suwanwela C, Suwanwela N, Charuchinda S, et al. (1972) Intracranial mycotic aneurysms of extravascular origin. J Neurosurg 36:552–559

Suzuki J, Komatsu S (1981) New embolization method using estrogen for dural arteriovenous malformation and meningioma. Surg Neurol 16:438–442

Svoboda DJ, Kirschner F (1966) Ultrastructure of nasopharyngeal angiofibroma. Cancer 19:1949

Swan HJC, Banz E, et al. (1970) Catheterization of the heart in man with use of a flow direct balloon tipped catheter. New Eng J Med 283:447–451

Tadavarthy SM, Knight L, Ovitt TW, et al. (1974) Therapeutic transcatheter arterial embolization. Radiology 113:13–16

Takahashi M, Killeffer F, Wilson G (1969) Iatrogenic carotid cavernous fistulas: case report. J Neurosurg 30:498–500

Taki W, Handa H, Yamagata S, et al (1970) A combined technique for treating certain aneurysms of the anterior communicating artery. J Neurosurg 33:41–47

Taki W, Handa Y, Yamagata S, et al. (1979) Embolization and superselective angiography by means of balloon catheters. Surg Neurol 12(1):7–14

Taki W, Handa H, Yamagata S, et al. (1979) Balloon embolization of a giant aneurysm using a newly developed catheter. Surg Neurol 12(5):363–365

Taki W, Handa H, Yamagata S, et al. (1980) Radiopaque solidifying liquids for releasable balloon technique: A technical note. Surg Neurol 13(2):140–142

Taki W, Handa H, Yamagata S, et al. (1980) The released balloon technique with activated high frequency electrical current. Surg Neurol 13:405–408

Taki W, Handa H, Yonekawa Y, et al. (1981) Detachable balloon catheter systems for embolization of cerebrovascular lesions. Neurologia Medicochir 21(7):709–719

Taki W, Handa H, Miyake H, et al. (1985) New detachable balloon Technique for Traumatic carotid cavernous sinus fistulae. AJNR 6:961–964

Tapia Acuna R (1965) The nasopharyngeal fibroma and its treatment. Arch Otolaryng 64:451–455

Taptas JN (1961) Intracranial meningioma in a four month old infant simulating subdural hematoma. J Neurosurg 18:120–121

Taxy JB (1977) Juvenile nasopharyngeal angiofibroma: an ultrastructural study. Cancer 39:1044

Teal JS, Bergeron RT, Rumbaugh CL, et al. (1972) Aneurysms of the cervical portion of the internal carotid artery associated with neck trauma. Radiology 105:353–358

Terada T, Kikuchi H, Karasawa J, Nagata I (1984) Intracerebral arteriovenous malformations fed by the anterior ethmoidal artery: case report. Neurosurgery 14:578–582

Tessier P (1976) Anatomical classification of facial, cranio facial and laterofacial clefts. J Maxillofac Surg 4:69–92

Theron J, Lasjaunias P (1976) Participation of the external and internal carotid arteries in the blood supply of acoustic neurinomas. Radiology 118:83–88

Thibaut A (1963) Angiographic carotidienne sélective dans le diagnostique et le traitement des angiofibromes nasopharyngiens. Acta Radiol Diagn 1:468–480

Thomas HG, Dolman CL, Berry K (1981) Malignant meningioma: clinical and pathological features. J Neurosurg 55:929–934

Thomson HG, Ward CM, Crawford JS, Stigmar G (1979) Hemangiomas of the eyelid: visual complications and prophylactic concepts. Plast Reconstr Surg 63:641–647

Tindall G, Kapp J, Odom G (1966) The use of tantalum dust as an adjunct in the postoperative management of subdural hematomas. J Neurosurg

Tönnis W (1936) Aneurysma arteriovenosum. In: Bergstrand H, Olivecrona H, Tönnis E (eds): Gefäßmißbildungen und Gefäßgeschwülste des Gehirns. Thieme, Leipzig, S. 88–134

Tomita T, McLone DG, Naidich TP (1981) Mycotic aneurysm of the intracavernous portion of the carotid artery in childhood. Case report. J neurosurg 54:681–684

Toppozada H, Michaels L, Toppozada M, El-Ghazzawi E, Talaat A, Elwany S (1981) The human nasal mucosa in the menstrual cycle. J Laryng Otol 95:1237–1247

Toppozada H, Michaels L, Toppozada M, El-Ghazzawi E, Talaat A, Elwany S (1982) The human respiratory nasal mucosa in pregnancy. An electron microscopic and histochemical study. J Laryng Otol 96:613–626

Toya S, Shiobara R, Izumi J, Shinomiya Y, Shiga H, Kimura C (1981) Spontaneous carotid-cavernous fistula during pregnancy or in the postpartum stage. J Neurosurg 54:252–256

Treil J, Morel C, Bonafe A, Manelfe C (1977) Traumatic rupture of the middle meningeal artery. Angiographic appearance. A review of 30 cases. J Neuroradiol 4:399–414

Tsai FY, Hieshima GB, Mehringer CM, Grinnell V, Pribram HW (1983) Delayed effects in the treatment of carotid-cavernous fistulas. AJNR 4:357–361

Turner DM, Vangiler JC, Mojtahedi S, Pierson EW (1983) Spontaneous intracerebral hematoma in carotid-cavernous fistula. Report of three cases. J Neurosurg 59:680–686

Turpin G, Jambart S (1970) Physiologie, physiopathologie et classification des polyadénomatoses endocrines. Ann Méd Interne 130:591–599

Ulrich DP, Sugar O (1960) Familial cerebral aneurysms including one extracranial internal carotid artery aneurysms. Neurology 10:228–294

Valavanis A, Fisch U (1983) The contribution of computed tomography in the management of glomus tumors of the temporal bone. Rev Laryng 104:411–415

Valavanis A, Schubiger O, Hayek J, Pouliadis G (1981) CT of meningiomas of the posterior surface of the petrous bone. Neuroradiology 22:111–121

Valavanis A, Schubiger O, Oguz M (1983) High resolutions CT investigation of non chromaffin paragangliomas of the temporal bone. AJNR 4:516–519

Valdazo A, Theron J, Houtteville JP, Lechevalier B (1978) Exérèse d'une volumineuse tumeur du glomus jugulaire après embolisation pré-opératoire. Oto-Neuro-Opth 50:413–420

Van de Werf AJ (1964) Sur un cas d'anévrisme arterioveineux intradural bilateral de la fosse postérieure chez un enfant. Neurochirurgie 10:140–144

Vase P, Lorentzen M (1983) Histological findings following estrogen treatment of hereditary hemorrhagic telangiectasia; a controlled double blind investigation. J Laryng Otol 97:427–429

Verbiest H (1951) L'anévrisme arterioveineux intradural. Rev neurol 85:189–199

Vinters HV (1985) The hystotoxicity of cyanoactrylate. Neuroradiology 27:279–291

Vinters HV, Debrun G, Kaufmann JCE et al. (1981) Pathology of arteriovenous malformations embolized with isobutyl-2-cyanoacrylate. J Neurosurg 55:819–825

Viñuela F, Debrun G, Fox AJ, Kan S (1983) Detachable calibrated-leak balloon for superselective angiography and embolization of dural arteriovenous malformations. J Neurosurg 58:817–823

Viñuela F, Fox AJ, Kan S, Drake CG (1983) Balloon occlusion of a spontaneous fistula of the posterior cerebellar artery. J Neurosurg 58:287–290

Viñuela F, Fox AJ, Debrun G, Peerless SJ, Drake CG (1984) Spontaneous carotid-cavernous fistulas: clinical, radiological, and therapeutic considerations. Experience with 20 cases. J Neurosurg 60:976–984

Vorra FH, et al. (1974) Massive thrombosis with the use of a Swan-Ganz catheter. Chest 65(6):682–684

Waga S, Handa J, Teraura T, Handa H (1974) Traumatic vertebral arteriovenous fistula. Surg Neurol 2:279–281

Wagas S, Fugimoto K, Morikawa D, Morooka Y, Okada M (1978) Dural arteriovenous malformation of the anterior fossa. Surg Neurol 8:356–359

Waldman SR, Levine HL, Astor F, Wood BJ, Weinstein M, Tucker HM (1981) Surgical experience with nasopharyngeal angiofibroma. Arch Ontolaryngol 107:677–682

Walike JW, Bailey BJ (1971) Head and neck hemangiopericytoma. Arch Otolaryngol 93:345–353

Walike JW, MacKay B (1970) Nasopharyngeal angiofibroma: light and electron microscopic changes after stilbesterol therapy. Laryngoscope 80:1109

Walsh JW, Winston KR, Smith T (1977) Meningioma with subdural hematoma. Surg Neurol 8:293–295

Ward PH, Thompson R, Calcaterra T, Kadin MR (1974) Juvenile angiofibroma: a more rational therapeutic approach based upon clinical and experimental evidence. Laryngoscope 84:2181–2194

Warrell RP, Sanford JK (1985) Treatment of severe coagulopathy in the Kasabach-Merritt syndrome with aminocaproic acid and cryoprecipitate. New Engl J Med 313:309–312

Watanabe A, Takahara Y, Ibuchi Y, Mizukami K (1984) Two cases of dural arteriovenous malformation occuring after intracranial surgery. Neuroradiology 26:375–380

Watkins E Jr, Hering AG, Lerna R, et al. (1960) The use of intravascular balloon catheters for isolation of the pelvic vascular bed during pump oxygenator perfusion of cancer chemotherapeutic agents. Surg Gynecol Obstet 111:464

Welti H, Jung A (1933) La chirurgie des parathyroides. Anatomie chirurgicale des parathyroides. J Chir 42:501–504

Wemple JB, Smith GW (1966) Extracranial carotid aneurysm: report of four cases. J Neurosurg 24:667–671

Wepsic JG, Pruett RC, Tarlov W (1972) Carotid-cavernous fistula due to extradural subtemporal retrogasserian rhizotomy. Case Report. J Neurosurg 37:498–500

Weyand RD, MacCarthy CS, Wilson RB (1951) The effect or pregnancy on intracranial meningiomas occurring around the optic chiasm. Clin North Am 31:1225–1233

Whelan MA, Reede DL, Meisler W, Bergeron RT (1984) CT of the base of the skull. Radiologic Clinics of North America 22:177–217

Whicker JH, Devine KD, McCarty CS (1973) Diagnostic and therapeutic problems in extracranial meningiomas. Am J Surg 126:452–457

White RI, Strandbert JV, Gross GS, et al. (1977) Therapeutic embolization with longterm occluding agents and their affects on embolized tissues. Radiology 125:677–687

White RI, Kaufman SL, Barth KH, et al. (1979 a) Embolotherapy with detachable silicone balloons. Technique and clinical results. Radiology 13:619–627

White RI, Kaufman SL, Barth KH, et al. (1979 b) Therapeutic embolization with detachable silicone balloons. Early clinical experience. JAMA 241(12):1257–1260

White RI, Barth KH, Kaufman SL, et al. (1980) Therapeutic embolization with detachable balloon. Cardiovasc. Intervent Radiol 3:229–241

Wholey MH, Kessler L, Boehnke MA (1972) Percutaneous balloon catheter technique for the treatment of intracranial aneurysms. Acta Radiol Diagn 18:286

Williams HB (1975) Hemangiomas of the parotid gland in children. Plast Reconstr Surg 56:29

Williams HB (1979) Facial bone changes with vascular tumors in children. Plast Reconstr Surg 63:309

Williams JJB Edit (1983) Symposium on vascular malformation and melanotic lesions. St. Louis CV, Mosby

Willis AG, Birrell JH (1955) The structure of a carotid body tumor. Acta Anat (Basel) 25:220–265

Wilson AJ, Ratliff JL, Lagios MD, et al. (1979) Mediastinal meningioma. Am J Surg Pathol 3:557–562

Wilson GH, Hanafee WN (1969) Angiographic findings in 16 patients with juvenile nasopharyngeal angiofibroma. Radiology 92:279–284

Wilson JR, Jordon PH Jr. (1961) Excision of an internal carotid aneurysm: restitution of continuity by substitution of external for internal carotid artery. Ann Surg 154:45–47

Wilson WW (1959) X-ray treatment of hemangiomas: a review of 500 cases on 15 years experience. South Med J 52:1355

Wing V, Scheible W (1983) Sonography of jugular vein thrombosis. AJR 140:333–336

Winslow N (1926) Extracranial aneurysms of internal carotid artery history and analysis of cases registered to Aug. 1, 1925. Arch Surg 13:689–729

Winslow N, Edwards M (1934) Aneurysm of temporal artery: report of case. Bull School Med Univ., Maryland 19:57–72

Wisnicki JL (1984) Hemangiomas and vascular malformations. Ann Plastic Surg 12:41–59

Wolf EJ, Hubler WR (1975) Tumor angiogenic factor and human skin tumors. Arch Dermatol 111:321

Wolverson MK, Sundaram M, Eddelston B, Prendergast J (1981) Diagnosis of parathyroid adenoma by computed tomography. J Comput Ass Tomogr 5:818–826

Wood EH, Correll JW (1969) Atheromatous ulceration in major neck vessels as a cause of cerebral embolism. Acta Radiol (Diagn.) 9:520–536

Wood MW, White RJ, Kernohan JW (1957) One hundred intracranial meningiomas found incidentally at necropsy. J Neuropathol Exp Neurol 16:337–340

Woodard SC, Hermann JB, Cameron JL, et al. (1965) Histotoxicity of cyanoacrylate tissue adhesive in the rat. Ann Surg 162:113–122

Woolard HH (1922) The development of the principal arterial stems in the forelimb of the pig. Contrib Embryol 14:139

Work WP, Hybels RL (1974) A study of tumors of the parapharyngeal space. Laryngoscope 84:1748–1755

Wortzman G (1963) Traumatic pseudoaneurysms of the superficial temporal artery. Radiology 80:444–446

Wosnessenski WP (1923) Geschwulst der Carotisdrüse. Medizinskaja Myssl 2:732–739

Wu B (1981) Orbital chemodectoma, clinical and pathological analysis of 2 cases. Chin Med J 94:419–422

Wychulis AR, Beahrs OH, Bernatz PE (1964) Aneurysms of internal carotid artery treated by excision and anastomosis to external carotid artery. Arch Surg (Chicago) 88:803–806

Wyke BD (1949) Primary hemangioma of the skull, a rare cranial tumor: review of the literature and report of case with special reference to roentgenographic appearance. Am J Roentgenol Radium Ther Nucl Med 61:302

Yamada S, Kindt GW, Youman JR (1967) Carotid artery occlusion due to nonpenetrating injury. J Trauma 7:333–342

Yamakawa Y, Kinoshita K, Fukui M, et al. (1980) Radiosensitive meningioma. Surg Neurol 13:471–475

Yasargil MG (1984) Microneurosurgery, Vol 2. Thieme, Stuttgart New York

Young N (1941) Bleeding from ear as sign of leakage aneurysm of extracranial portion of internal carotid artery. J Laryng 56:35–64

Zachrisson BF (1976) Thyroid arteriography. Acta Radiol, Suppl 350:122

Zak FG, Lawson W (1982) The paraganglionic chemoreceptor system. Physiology, pathology and clinical medicine. Springer Verlag Edit, New York

Zakka KA, Summerer RW, Yee RD, et al. (1979) Optociliary veins in a primary optic nerve sheath meningioma. Am J. Ophthalmol 87:91–95

Zanetti PH, Sherman FE (1972) Experimental evaluation of a tissue adhesive as an agent for the treatment of aneurysms and arteriovenous anomalies. J Neurosurg 36:72–79

Zang KD, Singer H (1967) Chromosomal constitution of meningiomas. Nature 216:84–85

Zilkha A, Daiz AS (1980) Computed tomography in carotid cavernous fistula. Surg Neurol 14:325–329

Zollikofer C, Castaneda-Zuniga WR, Galliani G, et al. (1980) Therapeutic blockage of arteries using compressed Ivalon. Radiology 136:635–640

Zülch KJ (1980) Principles of the new World Health Organization (WHO) classification of brain tumors. Neuroradiology 19:59–66

Subject Index

Numbers preceded by an F refer to figure numbers

Printed in the United States
by Baker & Taylor Publisher Services